TECHNIQUES IN CLINICAL ENDODONTICS

HAROLD GERSTEIN, B.S., D.D.S.

Professor and Chairman
Department of Endodontics
Marquette University
School of Dentistry
Milwaukee, Wisconsin

1983

W.B. SAUNDERS COMPANY

Philadelphia   London   Toronto   Mexico City   Rio de Janeiro   Sydney   Tokyo

W. B. Saunders Company: West Washington Square
                           Philadelphia, PA   19105

                           1 St. Anne's Road
                           Eastbourne, East Sussex BN21 3UN, England

                           1 Goldthorne Avenue
                           Toronto, Ontario M8Z 5T9, Canada

                           Apartado 26370 — Cedro 512
                           Mexico 4, D.F., Mexico

                           Rua Coronel Cabrita, 8
                           Sao Cristovao Caixa Postal 21176
                           Rio de Janeiro, Brazil

                           9 Waltham Street
                           Artarmon, N.S.W. 2064, Australia

                           Ichibancho, Central Bldg., 22-1 Ichibancho
                           Chiyoda-Ku, Tokyo 102, Japan

Library of Congress Cataloging in Publication Data

Gerstein, Harold.
  Technics in clinical endodontics.

  1. Endodontics.   2. Root canal therapy.
I. Title.   [DNLM: 1. Endodontics–Methods. WU 230 G383t]
RK351.G47   617.6'342059   81-40896
ISBN 0-7216-4087-7   AACR2

Techniques in Clinical Endodontics   ISBN   0-7216-4087-7

Last digit is the print number: 9   8   7   6   5   4   3   2   1

DEDICATION

I dedicate this effort to Bernice, my loved wife and companion, for her willing cooperation and accordance with my professional decisions and those people who most influenced and guided my endodontic career efforts in a personal way: Dr. Edgar D. Coolidge, Dr. Irving Abramson, Dr. Victor H. Dietz, Dr. Harold H. Epstein, Dr. Harold A. Maxmen, Dr. Samuel S. Patterson, Dr. Bertram L. Wolfsohn, and many others too numerous to mention. I would like to pay special homage to two general practitioners who have made substantial contributions to endodontics and, in particular, to my professional life—Dr. Henry Kahn and the late Dr. Leo D. Pinsky.

CONTRIBUTORS

WALTER T. CUNNINGHAM, D.D.S., M.S.

Commander, U.S. Navy Dental Corps; Research Endodontist, Dental Sciences Branch, Naval Medical Research Institute, National Naval Medical Center, Bethesda, Maryland.

Endosonic Endodontics.

HAROLD GERSTEIN, B.S., D.D.S.

Professor and Chairman, Department of Endodontics, Marquette University School of Dentistry, Milwaukee, Wisconsin; Clinical Professor, Loyola University School of Dentistry, Maywood, Illinois; Visiting Lecturer, Northwestern University School of Dentistry, Chicago, Illinois.

Access Cavity Preparation; Modifications and Special Hints.

MELVIN GOLDMAN, D.D.S.

Clinical Professor of Endodontics, Director of Post-Graduate Endodontics, Tufts University School of Dental Medicine, Boston, Massachusetts.

New Directions—Introduction.

LEO GRUDIN, B.S., D.D.S.

Clinical Professor, Department of Endodontics, University of Southern California School of Dentistry, International Students Program, Los Angeles, California.

Softened Gutta Percha Technique.

MICHAEL A. HEUER, D.D.S., M.S.

Professor and Chairman, Department of Endodontics, Northwestern University School of Dentistry; Dental Staff, Northwestern Memorial Hospital, Chicago, Illinois.

Silver Point: The Rigid Core Technique.

JAY MARLIN, D.M.D.

Assistant Clinical Professor of Endodontics, Harvard University School of Dental Medicine, Associate Clinical Professor of Endodontics, Forsyth Dental Research Center, Boston, Massachusetts; Staff Appointments, Memorial Hospital, Worcester, Massachusetts; Burbank Hospital, Fitchburg, Massachusetts; Leominster Hospital, Leominster, Massachusetts.

Injection Molded Gutta Percha.

HOWARD MARTIN, D.M.D.

Professorial Lecturer in Endodontics, Georgetown University School of Dentistry, Washington, D.C.

Endosonic Endodontics.

CARL W. NEWTON, D.D.S., M.S.D.

Associate Professor and Acting Chairman, Department of Endodontics, Indiana University School of Dentistry; Consultant, Veterans Administration; Associate Member, St. Vincent Hospital, Section of Comprehensive Dentistry, Indianapolis, Indiana.

Lateral Condensation.

ROBERT J. OSWALD, D.D.S.

Associate Professor and Chairman of Endodontics, Department of Endodontics, School of Dentistry, University of Washington, Seattle, Washington.

Calcium Hydroxide Root Closure.

SAMUEL S PATTERSON, D.D.S., M.S.D.

Professor and Chairman, Department of Endodontics, Indiana University School of Dentistry; Dentist-in-Residence, Veterans Administration (Endo); Consultant, Veterans Administration, Active Staff, Section of Comprehensive Dentistry, St. Vincent Hospital, Indianapolis, Indiana.

Lateral Condensation.

RONALD J. PRUHS, D.D.S., M.S.

Associate Professor and Chairman, Department of Pedodontics, Marquette University School of Dentistry; Active Staff, Milwaukee Children's Hospital, Milwaukee, Wisconsin.

Pulp Therapy for Children and Adolescents.

HERBERT SCHILDER, B.A., D.D.S.

Assistant Dean, Continuing Education, Professor and Chairman, Department of Endodontics, Goldman School of Graduate Dentistry, Boston University; Dental Surgeon, Riesman Dental Clinic, Beth Israel Hospital, Boston, Massachusetts.

Warm Gutta Percha Vertical Condensation.

JAMES H. SHERARD Jr., D.D.S.

Private Practitioner in Endodontics, Atlanta, Georgia (formerly, Chairman of Department of Endodontics, Emory University School of Dentistry, Atlanta, Georgia).

Diffusion Update.

JOHN T. STREIFF, D.D.S., M.S.D.

Associate Adjunct Professor, Department of Endodontics, Marquette University School of Dentistry, Milwaukee, Wisconsin.

Access Cavity Preparation.

GARY N. TAYLOR, D.D.S., M.S.

Associate Professor and Director, Loyola University, School of Dentistry, Maywood, Illinois; Consultant, Veterans Administration, Hines, Illinois.

Restoration Selection.

HENRY J. VAN HASSEL, D.D.S., M.S.D., Ph.D.

Professor of Endodontics and Director, Graduate Endodontics, University of Maryland, Baltimore, Maryland.

Calcium Hydroxide Root Closure.

RAYMOND T. WEBBER, D.D.S., M.S.

Clinical Assistant Professor, Department of Oral Medicine, College of Dentistry, University of Florida, Gainesville, Florida.

Traumatic Injury and Calcium Hydroxide.

PREFACE

The impetus for the creation of this book was quite simple — virtually no day goes by without someone asking me what is the best way to prepare and fill a root canal given a special set of circumstances. There are many modalities used to accomplish the preparing and filling of root canals, and this book is designed to demonstrate the various techniques in common use. No one procedure will suffice for all the problems encountered in an endodontic practice. The philosophy of thorough debridement and root fill is recognized as basic to success, and various means to achieve this end have been developed.

We attempt here to bring together recognized authorities to describe the various endodontic approaches and to provide an explanation of the differences. We have all built upon studies and recommendations of many scientists and practitioners. We owe much to people like G. V. Black and later Edgar D. Coolidge, Kronfeld, and Kessel, as well as more modern leaders such as Burns, Cohen, Grossman, Healy, Ingle, Kaiser, Morse, Sommer, Weine, and others. The outstanding individuals who are coauthors of this book have been chosen for their special expertise and contributions to the profession.

This book is not intended to be a text in the classic sense. It does not address the basic science issues, diagnoses, or interdisciplinary relationships. If one desires that information, a standard school text is in order. Instead, this book starts when endodontic treatment is recognized as the treatment of choice. It describes techniques that are accepted by recognized teachers and taught in dental schools. Experimental procedures are not included.

One chapter is devoted to "newer concepts" born of advanced technology, all of which have been researched and studied and are predicated upon the proven basic ideas of controlled preparation and filling.

A great deal of attention has been paid to a description of access to the pulp chamber and canal — the foundation of sound treatment. This is followed by separate sections devoted to specific techniques. There is a growing awareness of the use of calcium hydroxide in endodontics, and an excellent chapter covers that subject as thoroughly as possible in describing all the clinical uses for the material.

Chapter 10 describes some modifications and special hints for clinical simplification, whereas the last chapter, devoted to restoration, is purposefully given special consideration, since treatment of the root is of no avail without returning it to useful purpose.

HAROLD GERSTEIN

ACKNOWLEDGMENTS

I'd like to thank the authors of each section for sharing their wealth of knowledge. These individuals have been recognized as leaders and teachers by their peers.

Each will recognize people of special importance to them at the beginning of the chapter.

I would like to thank Mr. Jeffery F. Seipel for his photographic help, Mr. John Jones for his art, and especially our secretary, Miss Dana Fuys, for her continual help and assistance.

CONTENTS

1

Access Cavity Preparation

JOHN T. STREIFF, D.D.S., M.S.D.
HAROLD GERSTEIN, B.S., D.D.S.

One of the most frequent errors occurring in endodontic therapy is the lack of an adequate access cavity. Since this occurs early in treatment, it has a considerable effect on the remainder of the procedure. An inadequate access cavity preparation greatly increases the difficulty of the remaining endodontic treatment. Conversely, adequate access will help to simplify the remaining procedures.

The purpose of this chapter is to provide objectives and techniques for the access cavity preparation of any tooth regardless of anatomic variations and to provide specific illustrations and examples of access cavity preparations in incisors, canines, bicuspids, and molars.

PRINCIPLES OF ACCESS CAVITY PREPARATION

There are only two objectives in access cavity preparation: first, to gain access to the apical foramen, not just the orifice of the root canal, and second, to completely debride the contents of the pulp chamber, including the pulp horns.

TECHNIQUES OF ACCESS CAVITY PREPARATION

The following list is an orderly progression of the steps necessary for access cavity preparation:

1. Visualize the internal anatomy.
2. Reduce posterior teeth from occlusion (see Exceptions, page 6).
3. Remove caries, unsupported enamel, and unsound restorations.
4. Locate the pulp chamber.
5. Remove the entire roof of the pulp chamber and flare the walls.
6. Locate the orifices of the root canals.
7. Complete the debridement of the chamber.

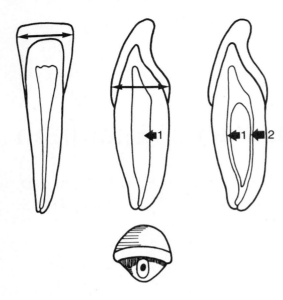

Figure 1–1 Mandibular incisor showing the narrow mesio-distal dimension, and wide buccal-lingual dimension with the two most common canal configurations. The incisal view shows the wide buccal-lingual access cavity preparation.

Visualizing the Internal Anatomy

Many access cavity preparations and subsequent instrumentation errors are made because the pulp is not viewed in three dimensions. There is a tendency to think of the pulpal anatomy only in terms of the mesio-distal view given by the radiographs. Instead, visualize the location and shape of the pulp chamber and root canals in three dimensions before starting your access cavity. To do this you are aided by the external anatomy of the tooth, radiographs, extrinsic factors, and age of the patient.

External Anatomy. The internal or pulpal anatomy (chamber and root canals) has approximately the same shape as the outside of the tooth or external anatomy. For example:

1. The mandibular incisors are very narrow mesio-distally, which is the view we are most accustomed to seeing, but are wide in a buccal-lingual

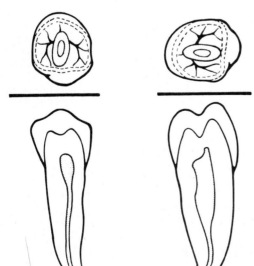

Figure 1–2 Mandibular bicuspid comparing the buccal-lingual dimensions with the mesio-distal dimensions and the oval access cavity preparation.

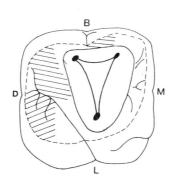
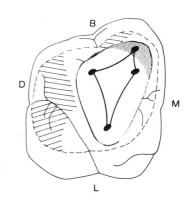

Figure 1–3 The two most common anatomic configurations of the crown of maxillary first molars and the shape of the access cavity preparation for each one. Note how the pulp chamber follows the shape of the external anatomy.

direction. Consequently, their pulpal anatomy will be narrow mesio-distally, but wide buccal-lingually, having one very wide canal, or frequently two canals (Fig. 1–1).[1, 2]

2. Bicuspids have a somewhat oval crown and either one oval root or two round roots (Fig. 1–2). The pulp chamber will be oval, requiring an oval access cavity preparation, and the root canals will have an anatomy similar to the roots.

3. If a molar has a bulbous cusp, as is frequently found on the mesio-buccal surface of maxillary first molars, the pulp chamber will usually extend into that bulbous portion (Fig. 1–3).

Preoperative Radiographs. Preoperative radiographs are essential to help show the shape and location of the chamber and root canals. Radiographs are only two dimensional and therefore preoperative films of all teeth, with the possible exception of maxillary anteriors, should be taken from more than one angle to get a better view of tooth curvature and otherwise superimposed structures (Fig. 1–4). One of these views should always be straight on and the other from a mesial or distal angle.

Figure 1–4 The straight-on radiographs are helpful, but occasionally, as in the figure on the left, the buccal and lingual roots are completely superimposed and one of the roots is not apparent. The figure on the right shows that if the radiograph is taken from a mesial or distal angle, the two roots are separated and both become apparent.

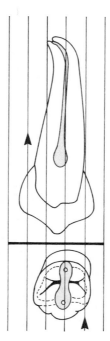
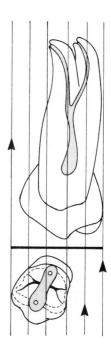

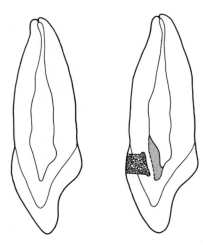

Figure 1–5 The illustration (*left*) is a buccal-lingual view of normal external and pulpal anatomy. The illustration (*right*) shows reparative dentin formation (light gray) pulpal to Class V caries and subsequent restoration.

It is difficult to take radiographs of bicuspids from a distal angle because they often are projected anterior to the x-ray film. However, for maxillary molars, taking a radiograph from a distal angle will provide the best view of the mesio-buccal root. Therefore, a convenient guide for routine preoperative radiographs is to take one radiograph straight on and take the angle radiograph from a mesial angle, except for maxillary molars, which should be taken from a distal angle. Remember, this is only a guide and should be altered to meet the needs of the individual tooth.

Extrinsic Factors. Extrinsic factors such as caries, restorations, attrition, abrasion, and trauma will stimulate the formation of reparative dentin, which in turn will alter the internal anatomy. Note how reparative dentin forms pulpally to a Class V restoration, reducing the size of the chamber (Fig. 1–5). The same type of reparative dentin formation will form pulpally as a response to any low-grade chronic irritant, such as erosion, abrasion, some caries, and some operative procedures, in an attempt to protect the remaining pulp from that irritant. This, in turn, alters the anatomy of the pulp chamber or even the root canals if the irritant is on or near the root

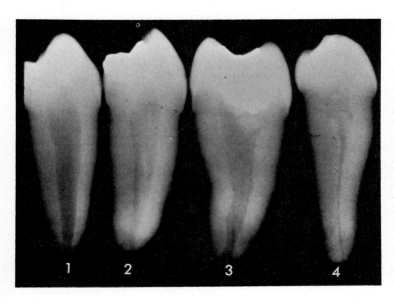

Figure 1–6 The four bicuspids illustrated left to right: first, a normal pulpal anatomy; second, a recent irritant (caries and subsequent restoration) and normal pulpal anatomy; third, a long-standing irritant (caries and subsequent restoration) with reparative dentin formation; and fourth, the effects of trauma (internal resorption and excessive reparative dentin formation) on the pulpal anatomy.

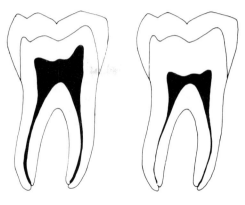

Figure 1–7 There is a decrease in the size of the pulp as the tooth ages.

surface. The radiograph of the bicuspids (Fig. 1–6) shows, left to right, a normal pulp anatomy in a young bicuspid with an intact crown. The second tooth has a recently placed amalgam restoration. Note that there has not been time for reparative dentin to form pulpal to it. The third tooth has a long-standing amalgam restoration. Note the abundance of reparative dentin pulpal to the alloy, causing a constriction of the pulp chamber. The fourth tooth is traumatized. The crown is intact, but note the ragged outline of the pulp chamber. This is caused by internal resorption, which often occurs following a traumatic incident. The constriction of the root canal, which is caused by excessive deposition of dentin along the walls of the root canal, is also common in traumatized teeth.

Age of Patients. There is a continuous deposition of secondary dentin in the chamber and root canals that reduces the size of the pulp as the patient ages (Fig. 1–7). The tooth on the left is younger than the tooth on the right and has a larger pulp chamber.

Reducing Posterior Teeth from Occlusion

Flatten the occlusal table of the crowns of posterior teeth to approximately the level of the central fossa and smooth any sharp edges. The patient will be more comfortable, and there will be a more consistent reference point and less chance of fracturing a cusp.

Patient Comfort. Frequently there is an inflammation of the periodontal ligament before and/or after endodontic treatment is started (Fig. 1–8). This can cause a swelling of the periodontal ligament, which in turn can slightly extrude the tooth into hyperocclusion, causing discomfort to the patient. Reducing the occlusion will minimize or eliminate this type of pain.

Consistent Reference Point. A flattened occlusal surface provides a more consistent reference point than a sloping occlusal surface does (Fig. 1–9). The difference in the height of a cusp from the cavo surface angle of the access cavity preparation to the tip of the cusp can easily exceed 1 mm. Unless you are consistent with your reference point, you can inadvertently instrument short or long by an amount equal to the height of the cusp. When you cannot reduce the occlusion or flatten the cusps, indicate in your records precisely where your reference point is — whether it is at the cusp

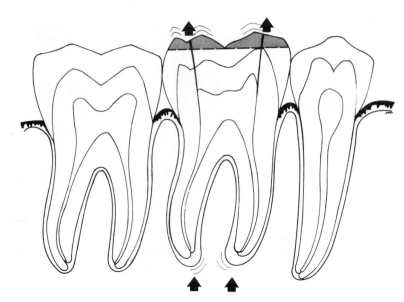

Figure 1–8 A mandibular molar is in hyperocclusion, caused by swelling of the apical periodontal ligament. Reducing the occlusion by the amount shown in the shaded area will help to prevent hyperocclusion.

tip, mid-incline, or at the cavo surface angle of the access cavity preparation.

Less Chance of Fracturing a Cusp. The access cavity preparation will slightly weaken the crown of the tooth structurally. This is particularly true if any of the cusps have been undermined by caries or restorations. Reducing the tooth from occlusion lessens the occlusal stress that this somewhat more fragile tooth must withstand and reduces the chance of cuspal or vertical fracture.

Tooth Strucure Not Sacrificed Unnecessarily. You will not be removing any tooth structure that would not be removed anyway during crown preparation. In Figure 1–10 the tooth on the left shows the amount of tooth structure that is removed for occlusal reduction. The tooth on the right shows the amount of tooth structure that is sacrificed during crown preparation. Since all posterior teeth require a crown or at least an onlay to restore the tooth following endodontic therapy, you can easily see that no tooth structure is being unnecessarily sacrificed.

Exceptions. Of course there are exceptions to reducing all posterior teeth from occlusion. Teeth with artificial cuspal coverage, such as a crown or onlay, obviously cannot be reduced from occlusion. Also, do not reduce the buccal cusps of maxillary posterior teeth that are to be restored with three-quarter crowns or onlays. However, the lingual incline of the buccal cusp and the lingual cusp can be reduced (Fig. 1–11).

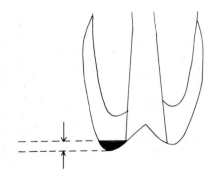

Figure 1–9 The height from the cavo surface angle of the access cavity preparation to the tip of the cusp is shown.

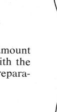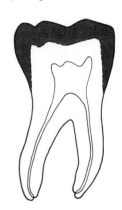

Figure 1–10 *Left:* The shaded area represents the amount of occlusal reduction on a lower molar. Compare this with the amount of reduction (*right*) that is necessary for crown preparation.

Removing Caries, Unsupported Enamel, and Unsound Restorations

All caries should be removed to eliminate a source of microorganisms, to be able to properly assess the amount of sound tooth structure remaining for restorative purposes, and to prevent loss of the seal between appointments. Unsupported enamel should be removed to prevent it from fracturing, which could cause a loss of the reference point or seal between appointments. Similarly, unsound restorations that may come loose should be removed to prevent loss of the reference point or seal between appointments.

Locating the Pulp Chamber

Many times it is useful to locate the pulp chamber before the rubber dam is placed. This is particularly true when the pulp chamber is difficult to locate owing to anatomic variation, excessive calcification of the chamber, or when the tooth is crowned. Without the rubber dam in place, you are able to see the entire arch, the root eminence, the neck of the crown, and any subtle changes in inclination or rotation of the tooth. This, in turn, will help you to visualize the pulpal anatomy and the long axis of the tooth. Once the pulp is located, place the rubber dam.

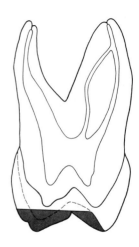

Figure 1–11 The shading indicates the amount of occlusal reduction that can be done on a maxillary first molar that will be restored with a three-quarter crown following endodontic therapy.

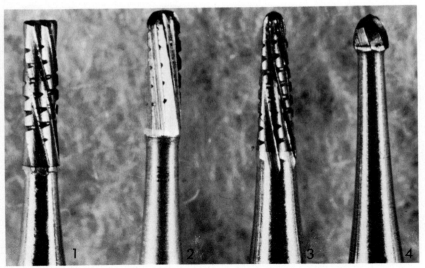

Figure 1–12 Left to right: (*1*) #557 bur, (*2*) #557R bur — note the rounded end, (*3*) 701R bur — again with a rounded end, and (*4*) #2 round bur.

Begin by cutting the approximate shape of the access cavity into the occlusal or lingual about 1 mm into the dentin and taper the preparation until you reach the pulp. In making this access cavity preparation, it is very helpful to use the high-speed round-ended fissure burs, such as #550R Series or #700R Series (Fig. 1–12). These burs combine the penetrating advantage of the round burs, yet keep to a minimum the tendency to gouge the walls, as often happens when using round burs and flat-end fissure burs.

Aim for the easiest place to locate the chamber (Fig. 1–13). With teeth that have large chambers, aim for the center of the chamber. In those teeth with small or calcified chambers, aim for the largest canal, such as the distal of mandibular molars and palatal canal of maxillary molars (Fig. 1–14). Even though the pulp has receded, be sure to cut the approximate shape of the final access cavity opening 1 mm into the dentin and then taper your opening toward the pulp. Do not reduce the size of your opening in an attempt to conserve tooth structure. Familiarity with the normal-sized opening will be an aid in locating the pulp. Also, a smaller opening limits the ability to see

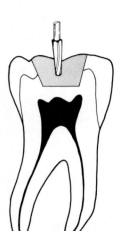

Figure 1–13 The initial tapered preparation used to locate the larger pulp chambers.

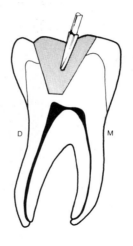
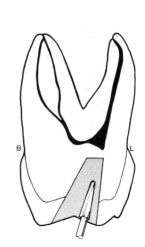

Figure 1–14 In lower molars with calcified chambers (*left*) the distal canal may be the largest and, therefore, it may be the easiest to find. In maxillary molars with calcified chambers (*right*) the palatal canal may be the easiest to locate.

the floor of the preparation. Once the chamber has been located, cut laterally to remove the roof of the pulp chamber (Fig. 1–15). A specially prepared 550R or 700R Series bur that has been made safe-ended is particularly useful, since this minimizes the chance of perforating the floor or gouging the walls (Fig. 1–16). The bur can be made by running the rounded end at high speed against the side of a heatless stone until the cutting end is round and smooth. In many molars there is an internal cervical collar of dentin just occlusal to the floor of the pulp chamber that causes a constriction of the chamber (Fig. 1–17). This cervical collar of dentin should be removed when the walls of the access cavity preparations are flared to allow for debridement of pulp tissue between the collar and the floor of the chamber; to allow easier location of the canals that may be tucked under the collar of dentin, particularly the mesial-lingual canals of maxillary molars; and to provide a more straight line access to the apical foramen.

When attempting to locate a receded pulp chamber, particularly in incisors, canines, and premolars, take sufficient radiographs to check the angulation of the preparation (Fig. 1–18). This should be done without the rubber dam in place, so that the rubber dam clamp is not superimposed on the access preparation in the radiographs. It is very easy to be headed in the

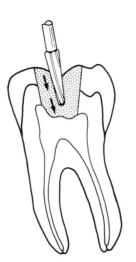
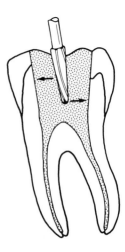

Figure 1–15 Locating the pulp chamber (*left*) and removing the entire roof of the chamber (*right*).

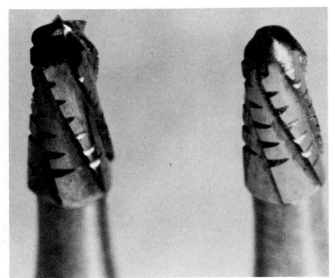

Figure 1–16 The bur before and after preparation of the safe end.

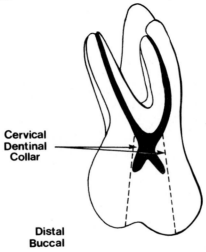

Figure 1–17 In maxillary and mandibular molars, there frequently is a collar of dentin around the walls of the chamber. It is necessary to remove this collar to debride the pulp tucked under it, to facilitate locating all the canals, and to provide better access to the apical foramen.

Cervical Dentinal Collar

Distal Buccal

Mesial Buccal

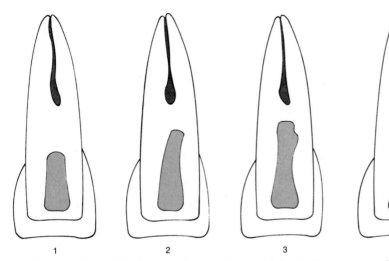

1   2   3   4

Figure 1–18 (1) This is approximately the normal depth of an access cavity preparation when the pulp is located. (2) The preparation is deeper, but headed toward the side of the tooth. (3) The preparation is slightly deeper, but once again it is headed in the right direction. (4) The pulp is finally located.

10

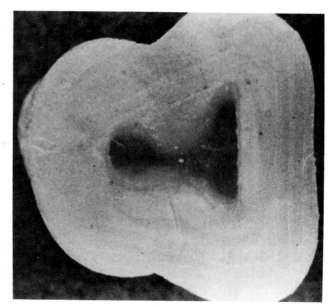

Figure 1–19 Maxillary molar sectioned just apical to the cemental enamel junction, illustrating the darker colored dentin lining the pulp chamber.

wrong direction. Radiographs will help show that you are headed for the pulp and not out the side of the tooth. Note the different shades of the dentin of the maxillary molar (Fig. 1–19) sectioned just apical to the cemental enamel junction. The dentin lining the pulp chamber is darker than the surrounding dentin. Therefore, as you approach the roof of the chamber, you will usually see the darker reparative dentin just before you penetrate into the chamber. Then once you are in the chamber, look for the root canals in the darker dentin. If you start to cut laterally from the floor of the chamber when looking for a canal and cut into the lighter dentin, you are headed in the wrong direction. Be sure to use a sharp endodontic explorer to punch through the roof of the chamber and to locate and trace the developmental grooves in the floor of the chamber that lead to the root canals. Dull, bent, or operative explorers are not suitable for this.

Removing the Entire Roof of the Pulp Chamber

The entire roof of the pulp chamber is removed so that all the pulp chamber, especially the pulp horns, can be debrided (Fig. 1–20). The walls are then slightly flared out toward the occlusal surface from the floor of the pulp chamber. This will allow you to see all the orifices of the root canals directly and prevents apical displacement of the temporary filling, which would cause a loss of the seal between the tooth and temporary filling (Figs. 1–21 and 1–22). Even more important, it allows straight-line access to the apical foramen (or as close to straight-line as root curvature will allow), so you can instrument and fill the root canals without being obstructed by the lateral walls. Guard against overpreparation by not gouging the lateral walls of the preparation, especially at the floor of the pulp chamber. Also remember that the lateral walls are only slightly flared out toward the occlusal surface. It is important to remember that in teeth with more than one root canal the shape of the access cavity is determined by the floor of the pulp chamber because the entire roof of the pulp chamber is removed and

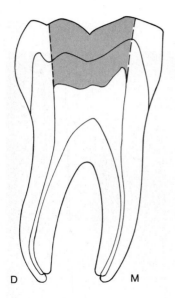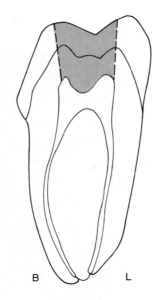

D   M   B   L

Figure 1–20 The mesio-distal view (*left*) and the buccal-lingual view (*right*) illustrating the flare of the walls of an access cavity preparation of a mandibular molar.

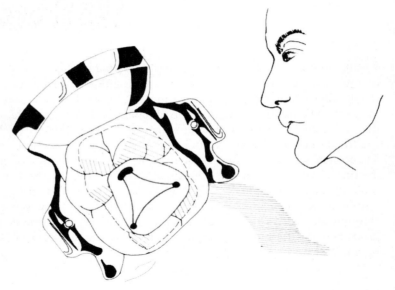

Figure 1–21 You should be able to see all the orifices of the root canals in a single line of sight. Then you can be reasonably certain that your access preparation is large enough to provide straight-line access to the apical foramen.

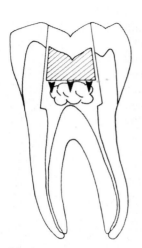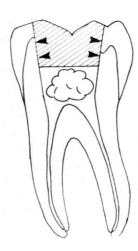

Figure 1–22 *Left:* Incorrect flaring resulting in apical displacement of the temporary filling and loss of the seal. *Right:* Correct flaring from the floor of the pulp chamber to the occlusal, which will prevent apical displacement of the temporary filling. Note how similar the incorrect flaring is to an amalgam preparation and how the correct preparation is slightly more flared than an inlay preparation.

12

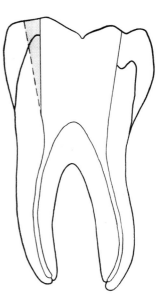

Figure 1–23 The mesial wall (shaded area) can be flared more for better access when the patient has limited opening.

the walls are flared out toward the occlusal surface. The shape, number, and location of the root canals also will affect the shape of the access cavity. Keeping this in mind will make it easier to prepare the access cavity, especially in teeth with an atypical anatomy.

The general outline of the access cavity can be modified to make it easier to instrument and fill the root canal without compromising the restorability of the tooth. It may be necessary to increase the flare of the mesial wall of molars to allow better access to the root canals, particularly when the patient has a limited opening or a small mouth (Fig. 1–23). In order to allow access to the apical foramen, it may be necessary to extend the preparation well into a cusp when the location of the orifice of a canal is under a cusp, as is often true in maxillary molars (see Fig. 1–3). Or it may be necessary to extend the preparation well into the mesial marginal ridge when the roots are sharply curved toward the distal (Fig. 1–24). The cavo surface angle can be beveled to allow more light into the access cavity in posterior teeth that are to be crowned (Fig. 1–25). Occasionally, it may be necessary to greatly reduce the occlusion when the patient has a very limited opening or when it is very difficult to locate a calcified root canal (Fig. 1–26). Under most circumstances, tooth structure that would be used to support the

Figure 1–24 The preparation is extended far to the mesial to provide better access to the apical foramen of this mandibular third molar with roots that are sharply curved to the distal. However, do not leave a thin wall of enamel on the mesial. If it is necessary to extend the preparation this far mesially, also reduce the marginal ridge so there is no chance of having it fracture between appointments.

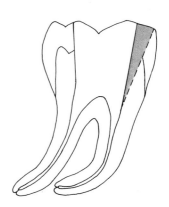

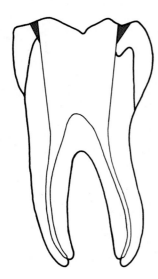

Figure 1–25 A 1 mm bevel of the cavo surface angle.

restoration of the tooth should not be sacrificed, but occasionally this is necessary. It is better to sacrifice coronal tooth structure that can be replaced with the restoration than to sacrifice the quality of the root canal filling because of an inadequate access cavity preparation.

Locating the Root Canal Orifices

The cardinal rule is to always assume that there are more root canals than are normally found in the tooth until they are ruled out. We are aided in locating the canals by the anatomy of the tooth, radiographs, developmental grooves, and changes in color of the dentin.

The shape and location of the root canals will be approximately the same as the shape and location of the roots. The preoperative radiographs will help to indicate the shape and number of the roots and root canals, the

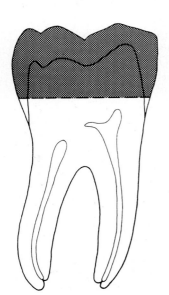

Figure 1–26 Substantial reduction of coronal tooth structure may be necessary to locate receded root canals.

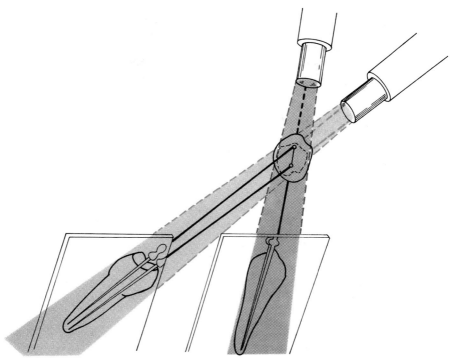

Figure 1–27 The projection in dark gray is a straight-on angle causing the buccal and lingual canals to be directly superimposed on each other. Then the radiograph is taken from a mesial or distal horizontal angle, as indicated on the left by the light gray area; the buccal and lingual objects are separated. If this light gray projection is taken from a mesial angle, the buccal canal will be projected distal to the lingual canal on the film. (From Weine, F. S. (ed.): Endodontic Therapy, 2nd Ed. St. Louis, The C.V. Mosby Co., 1976.)

relationship of the roots to the crown, and anatomic variations of the roots and root canals. However, the radiographs are only two dimensional; therefore, when the angle view is compared with the straight-on view, the buccal object rule states that when x-rays are projected onto a radiographic film, the object (root canal) that is farthest from the film (buccal) moves a greater distance than the object that is closer to the film (lingual) when the horizontal angle of the x-ray cone is changed (Fig. 1–27).[3] To check for multiple canals in a single root, it may be helpful to place a file in the root canal that has been located. Then, take a radiograph from a mesial or distal angle (Fig. 1–28). Unless the film is grossly distorted and there is only one canal, the instrument should be located relatively close to the center of the tooth, regardless of how extreme the mesial or distal angle of the radiograph. However, if the file appears off center, with one third of the tooth on one side of the file and two thirds of the tooth on the other side of the file, be very suspicious of another canal (Fig. 1–29). There may be just one elliptical canal and the file is against the wall at the buccal or lingual end of the canal, which then appears off center on the radiograph, but most of the time there will be another root canal. If another canal is suspected, use the buccal object rule to determine whether the suspected canal is buccal or lingual to the canal the file is in.

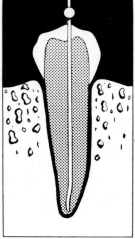
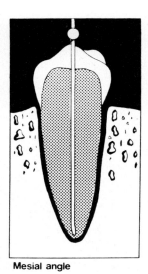

Straight on **Mesial angle**

Figure 1–28 If there is only one canal, no matter how distorted the root becomes on the radiograph with a wide mesial or distal angle, the endodontic instrument will be at or very near the center of the root.

In molars and in multi-canal bicuspids, the developmental grooves on the floor of the pulp chamber lead to the canals. Do not destroy these developmental grooves with the bur. Instead, using a sharp explorer, follow these grooves to the canals. This is especially helpful when there has been extensive calcification of the chamber and the canals are difficult to locate. In such difficult cases, when a canal is located, open or flare the orifice to the canal so that an image can be developed of where the remaining canal(s) should be located. Use a bur to remove a small amount of the developmental groove in the area where the remaining canal(s) are anticipated. A sharp explorer is then used to attempt to punch through any calcification and locate the orifice. If it is still not located, repeat by cutting a little deeper. This rather tedious and time-consuming procedure is repeated until the orifice to the canal is found. Do not cut deeper than the developmental groove because with the loss of this landmark it is easy to unintentionally cut laterally and perforate into the furcation. It will be necessary to use this technique frequently in maxillary molars to locate the mesio-lingual canal.

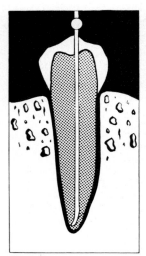
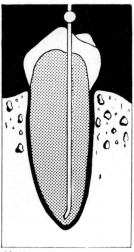

Straight on **Mesial angle**

Figure 1–29 The straight-on view may show the endodontic instrument in the center of the root, but if the mesial or distal view shows the insrument considerably off center, there probably are two canals in that root.

Look for the canal in the darker reparative dentin (see Fig. 1–19). If the floor of the chamber is cut laterally into the lighter dentin, a perforation may occur into the furcation or out the side of the tooth.

Checking for Total Debridement of the Chamber

Occasionally, there may be an exceptionally bulbous portion of the chamber. In such a case, flaring of the walls from the floor of the pulp, as is normally required, would result in unnecessary loss of tooth structure. Instead, flare the access cavity as is necessary to meet all the other requirements and use a #6 round slow speed bur to debride this bulbous portion. Check for any previously overlooked pulp horns.

Occasionally, the developmental grooves are very deep and should be removed with a bur. However, this is seldom necessary; the grooves should not be removed until all the root canals have been located, and the procedure should be done at a very slow speed. The #2 endodontic bur is useful here. These deep grooves are most often found in multi-canal bicuspids and joining the mesial canals of lower molars.

SPECIFIC EXAMPLES OF ACCESS CAVITY PREPARATION

Maxillary Incisors

Before the access cavity preparation is begun, visualize the internal anatomy of the tooth three dimensionally by forming a mental image not only of the mesio-distal dimension, but also of the buccal-lingual dimension (Figs. 1–30 to 1–33).

The access cavity preparation for the maxillary centrals and laterals is very similar. The outline is triangular, extending apically onto the cingulum and incisally to within 2 to 3 mm of the incisal edge (Fig. 1–34). It must extend incisally enough to (1) allow for debridement of the pulp horns and (2) minimize the lingual deflection of the endodontic instruments (Fig. 1–35). The outline must also extend apically onto the cingulum enough to allow access for cleaning and shaping of the lingual surface of the root canal and to minimize the buccal deflection of the endodontic instruments.

The bur should be directed toward the root canal beginning in the lingual fossa (Fig. 1–36). To do this the bur is held approximately parallel to the buccal surface, not perpendicular to it as is seen in many of the older texts that were printed prior to the widespread use of high speed.

The rough triangular outline of the access cavity is cut into the lingual dentin and should be kept slightly smaller than the anticipated final outline. The preparation is then cut toward the root canal from the lingual fossa area until the pulp is reached. If there is any question about the direction the preparation is going, stop and take a radiograph to confirm the location and angulation. Once the pulp chamber has been located, place the rubber dam. This is a good time to switch to a safe-ended 550R or 700R Series fissure bur (see Fig. 1–16). Using this type of bur further reduces the chance of gouging the walls or floor of the access cavity preparation. Then cut laterally to allow for complete debridement of the chamber and access to the apical

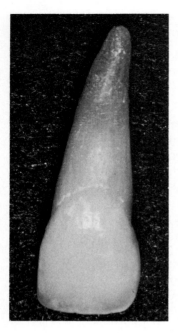

Figure 1–30 Mesial-distal view of a maxillary incisor.

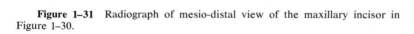

Figure 1–31 Radiograph of mesio-distal view of the maxillary incisor in Figure 1–30.

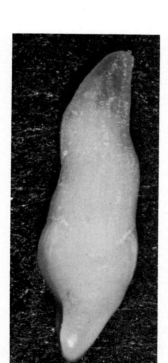

Figure 1–32 Buccal-lingual view of the maxillary incisor in Figure 1–30.

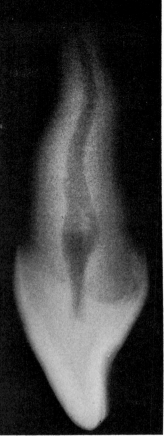

Figure 1–33 Radiograph of buccal-lingual view of the maxillary incisor in Figure 1–30.

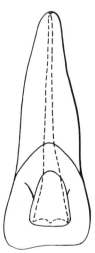

Figure 1–34 The outline of the access cavity preparations of a maxillary incisor.

Figure 1–35 (*1*) The correct access cavity preparation, allowing straight-line access to the apical foramen. (*2*) The access cavity preparation does not extend enough incisally. (*3*) The access cavity preparation does not extend down onto the cingulum.

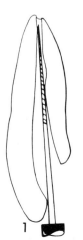

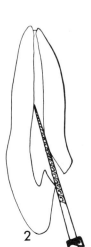

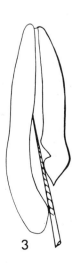

1　　2　　3

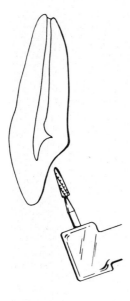

Figure 1–36 The inclination of the bur for access cavity preparation of a maxillary incisor.

foramen. The pencil line shown in Figure 1–37 delineates the cavo surface outline.

Once the access cavity outline has been completed and the chamber debrided, the lingual bulge of dentin found pulpal to the lingual-cemento-enamel junction must be removed (Fig. 1–38). This can be done very quickly with the smooth, round-ended fissure burs, Peeso reamers, or Gates-Glidden burs, but extreme caution must be used to prevent unnecessary loss of dentin. Another way this can be accomplished that is slower and a little safer is to use large endodontic reamers. The reamers are used sequentially, beginning with one that is small enough to get past this lingual bulge of dentin. In maxillary incisors a #50 reamer might be selected. Then use progressively larger reamers until this lingual bulge of dentin is entirely removed (Figs. 1–39 and 1–40). Note on the radiographs and the sagittal sections how the access cavity has opened the tooth to enable thorough

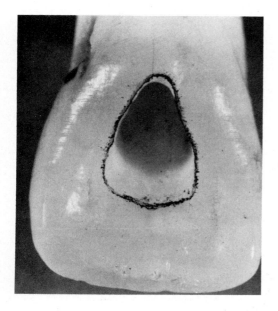

Figure 1–37 The outline of the access cavity preparation of a maxillary incisor.

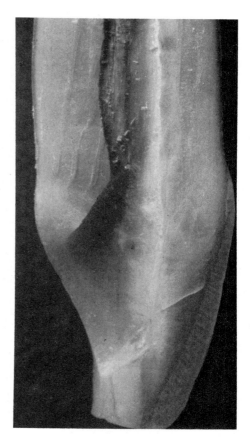

Figure 1–38 The lingual bulge of dentin found pulpal to lingual-cemento-enamel junction.

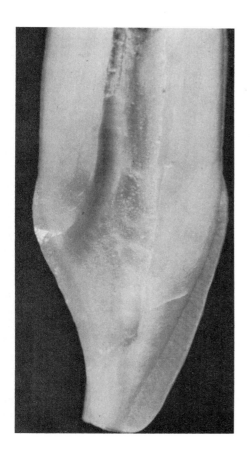

Figure 1–39 The lingual bulge is removed, providing access to the foramen and lingual surface of the root canal.

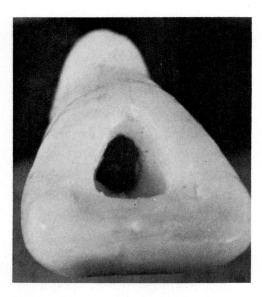

Figure 1–40 The access cavity preparation provides nearly straight-line access to the apical foramen.

debridement of the chamber and root canal (Figs. 1–41 to 1–45). When the roots are curved, as frequently occurs, it is impossible to achieve straight-line access to the portion apical to the curve. But it is easier to clean and shape the curved portion properly if the obstructions coronal to it have been removed. There are times when the incisal third of the crown is inclined too far to the lingual to allow straight-line access without unnecessary sacrifice

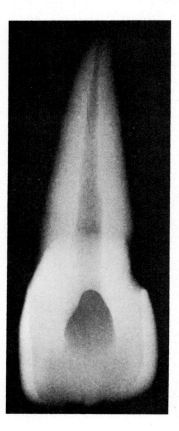

Figure 1–41 Radiograph showing the mesial-distal view of the maxillary incisor in Figure 1–30 with access cavity preparation completed.

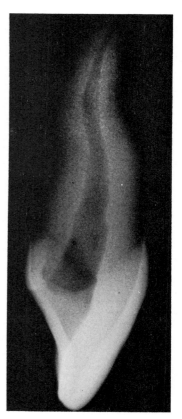

Figure 1–42 Radiograph showing the buccal-lingual view of the maxillary incisor in Figure 1–30 with access cavity preparation completed.

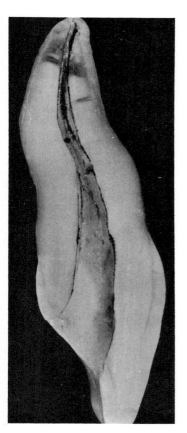

Figure 1–43 Buccal-lingual sagittal sections of the maxillary incisor in Figure 1–30 with the completed access cavity preparation. Note that there is near straight-line access to the apical foramen. However, at times it will be necessary to curve the endodontic instrument slightly to by-pass the lingual incisal.

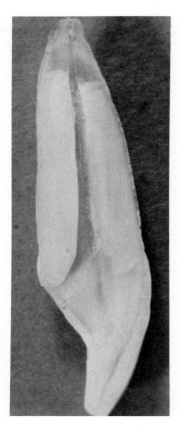

Figure 1–44 Buccal-lingual sagittal section of a maxillary incisor.

Figure 1–45 Buccal-lingual sagittal section of a maxillary incisor.

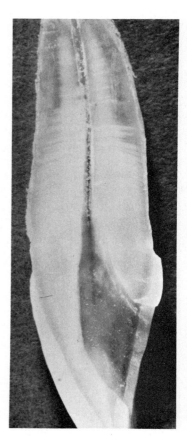

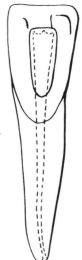

Figure 1–46 Diagram of the access cavity preparation for a mandibular incisor.

of the incisal lingual tooth structure. Instead, slightly curve the apical two thirds of the endodontic instruments to bypass this minor obstruction.

Occasionally, teeth will be encountered with substantial calcification of the pulp chamber and root canal. Rather than switching to a seldom used smaller oval access cavity outline, it is helpful to use the same triangular access cavity outline that is familiar. Even more important, by maintaining this normal-sized triangular opening, the changes in color of the dentin can be seen, which are so helpful in locating the calcified root canals.

Mandibular Incisors

The outline of the access cavity preparation for mandibular incisors is very similar to, but smaller than, the triangular outline form used for maxillary incisors (Fig. 1–46). However, because the mandibular incisor is so wide buccal-lingually compared with the mesio-distal width, the pulp is also going to be wide buccal-lingually and the access cavity preparation must be extended well down onto the cingulum to provide access to the lingual portions of the root canal (Fig. 1–47; see Fig. 1–1). With the access cavity preparation completed, note how the entire root canal is accessible to proper cleansing and shaping with nearly straight-line access to the apical foramen (Figs. 1–48 to 1–50).

Since the mandibular incisors are narrow mesio-distally, it is very easy to understand why there is a tendency to underprepare the access cavity (Fig. 1–51). The straight-on radiograph might make one think that this access cavity preparation meets all the requirements (Fig. 1–52). It even appears to provide straight-line access to the apical foramen (Fig. 1–53). But looking at the buccal-lingual radiograph, you can see that this access cavity is underprepared (Fig. 1–54). It fails to meet either of the two main objectives of an access cavity preparation. First, that portion of the chamber incisal to the opening cannot be debrided, and second, it would be nearly impossible to debride the lingual canal (Fig. 1–55). Even if there were only one canal, it would be very difficult to debride the lingual portion of that canal. If the

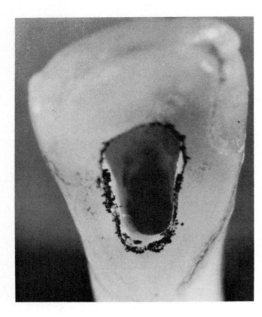

Figure 1–47 Completed access cavity preparation for a mandibular incisor. The cavo surface is outlined in pencil.

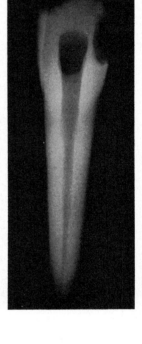

Figure 1–48 Radiograph showing the completed access cavity preparation for the mandibular incisor in Figure 1–47. The radiolucent area on the mesial (*right*) is a plastic restoration.

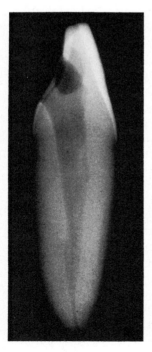

Figure 1–49 Radiograph showing the buccal-lingual view of the completed access cavity preparation of the mandibular incisor in Figure 1–47. Note that the mesial plastic restoration, which appears radiolucent, is superimposed on the access cavity preparation.

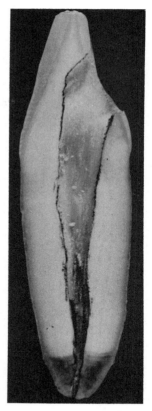

Figure 1–50 Sagittal section of mandibular incisor with completed access cavity preparation and root canal outlined in pencil.

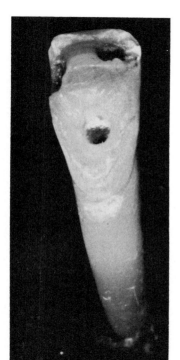

Figure 1–51 Underprepared access cavity.

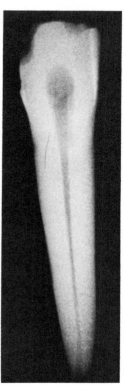

Figure 1–52 Straight-on radiograph of underprepared access cavity of mandibular incisor in Figure 1–51 causes the preparation to appear normal.

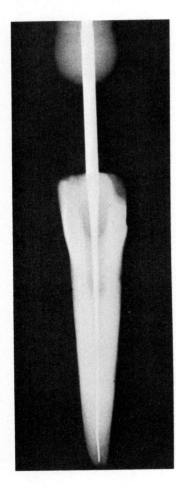

Figure 1–53 Straight-on radiograph of underprepared access cavity of mandibular incisor in Figure 1–51 incorrectly appears to provide straight-line access to apical foramen.

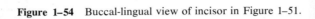

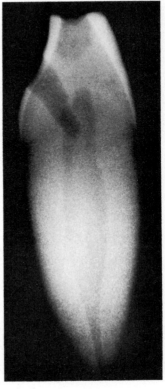

Figure 1–54 Buccal-lingual view of incisor in Figure 1–51.

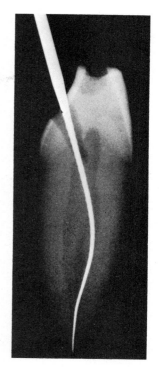

Figure 1–55 Buccal-lingual view of incisor in Figure 1–53.

access cavity is properly extended incisally and onto the cingulum, the chamber can now be adequately debrided and there is access to the lingual canal as well as to the buccal canal (Figs. 1–56 and 1–57).

Maxillary and Mandibular Canines

The maxillary and mandibular canines have a very similar access cavity preparation (Fig. 1–58). Again, it is important to visualize the shape of the pulp. The tooth is wider buccal-lingually than it is mesio-distally. Also, since the internal anatomy roughly approximates the external anatomy, the pulp will be wider buccal-lingually than it is mesio-distally (Figs. 1–59 and 1–60). The outline is oval, extending incisally to include the pulp horn and extending onto the cingulum to provide access to the lingual surface of the root canal. Remember that mandibular canines occasionally have two roots.

Premolars

The anatomy of the pulp chamber of all the premolars is similar, with a greater buccal-lingual dimension than mesio-distal dimension (Figs. 1–61 and 1–62). Consequently, the outline for the access cavity preparation is oval in order to provide for adequate debridement of the chamber and access to the apical foramen (Fig. 1–63). This outline form is used whether there is one canal or two. Occasionally a premolar will have three canals and then the outline is modified slightly to accommodate this third canal by becoming more triangular, similar to the access cavity outline form used in maxillary canals.

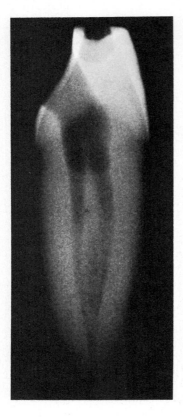

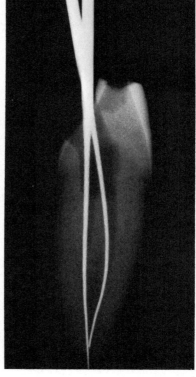

Figure 1–56 Buccal-lingual view of completed access cavity preparation. Compare with Figure 1–54.

Figure 1–57 Buccal-lingual view with access to both the buccal and the lingual canals. Compare with Figure 1–55.

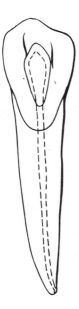
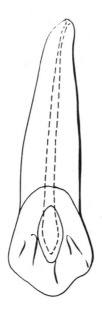

Figure 1–58 Outline of access cavity preparation for a maxillary and mandibular canine.

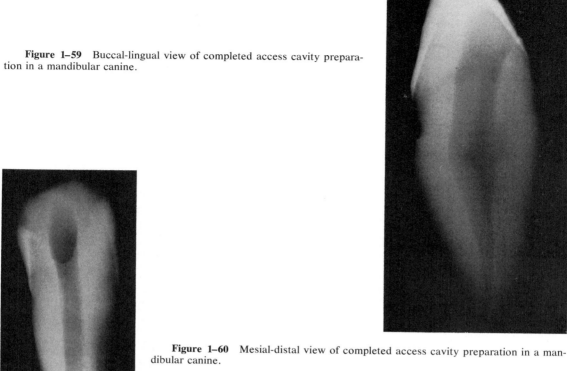

Figure 1–59 Buccal-lingual view of completed access cavity preparation in a mandibular canine.

Figure 1–60 Mesial-distal view of completed access cavity preparation in a mandibular canine.

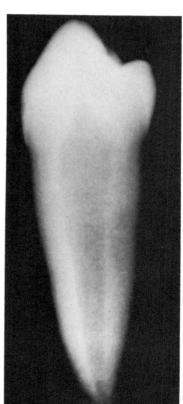

Figure 1–61 Buccal-lingual view of mandibular premolar.

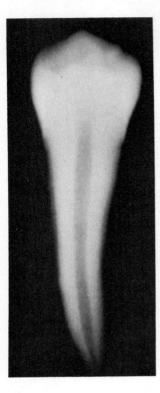

Figure 1–62 Mesial-distal view of mandibular premolar.

Prior to beginning the access cavity preparation, visualize the shape of the pulp in three dimensions. Also take note of any rotation, abnormal anatomy, or abnormal inclination to the tooth that would affect the shape of the outline form and the direction of the long axis of the tooth. It is not uncommon to have a rather wide occlusal table with a narrow neck to the crown. This widened occlusal table may not be symmetrical. That is, it may

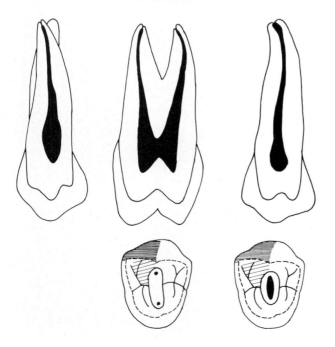

Figure 1–63 Oval outline normally used for access cavity preparation for maxillary and mandibular premolars.

extend more to the mesial than to the distal, as is often found in maxillary first premolars. When this occurs, be sure to shift the occlusal opening over to the long axis. It is important to constantly be aware of the long axis of the tooth because penetration toward the pulp is always in the long axis.

Once there is a good visual image of the shape of the pulp and the long axis of the tooth, reduce the tooth from occlusion. Then remove any caries, unsupported enamel, and unsound restorations. Begin by cutting the oval outline form into the occlusal dentin approximately 1 mm but stay slightly smaller than the anticipated final outline. Continue to cut pulpally in the long axis of the tooth, aiming for the part of the pulp easiest to find, which is usually the center of the pulp chamber. However, if the chamber has excessive reparative dentin formation caused by caries, restoration, abrasion, erosion, attrition, or trauma, it may be easier to locate the pulp buccal or lingual to center. If there has been excessive calcification of the chamber, take frequent radiographs to confirm the location and angulation of the access cavity preparation. The reparative dentin is darker than the primary dentin, so look for the chamber in the darker dentin. As you cut toward the chamber, also make frequent checks with a sharp endodontic explorer to try to punch through the roof of the chamber. The reason for proceeding so cautiously is to attempt to prevent a perforation through the side of the tooth or into the furcation of a multi-rooted tooth. Should a perforation occur, it usually will be small enough to be repaired with alloy or other suitable material.

Once the pulp chamber is located, place the rubber dam and switch to the safe-ended #557R or #701R fissure bur. Remove the entire roof of the pulp chamber, which allows for total debridement of the chamber and an unobstructed straight-line access to the apical foramen or as close to it as the curvature of the root permits (Figs. 1–64 to 1–66). The walls are flared toward the occlusal surface to allow better visibility of the root canal(s) and help prevent apical displacement of the temporary filling. The outline can be modified by placing a 1 mm bevel around the cavo surface margin to allow for more light and better visibility (Fig. 1–67).

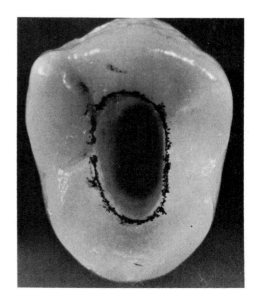

Figure 1–64 Completed access cavity of mandibular premolar. The cavo surface angle is outlined in pencil.

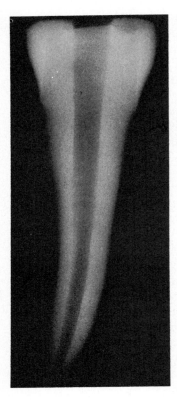

Figure 1–65 Mesial-distal view of completed access cavity preparation of the mandibular premolar. Compare with Figure 1–62. Note that the occlusal surface has been reduced from occlusion.

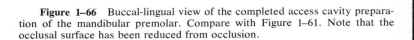

Figure 1–66 Buccal-lingual view of the completed access cavity preparation of the mandibular premolar. Compare with Figure 1–61. Note that the occlusal surface has been reduced from occlusion.

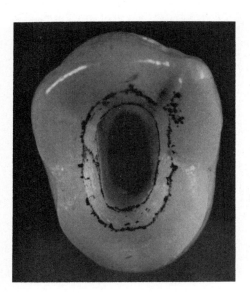

Figure 1–67 A 1 mm bevel on cavo surface margin outlined with pencil.

Maxillary Molars

When visualizing the internal anatomy of the maxillary molars, it is a common mistake to see the three roots and assume that there are only three canals. It is important to remember that even though the mesio-buccal root is about the same size as the disto-buccal root when viewing the tooth directly from the buccal, which is the common way the tooth is viewed radiographically, the mesio-buccal root is often much larger than the disto-buccal root when viewed from the side of the tooth (Figs. 1–68 and 1–69). When the mesio-buccal root is substantially larger than the disto-buccal root, it will usually have two root canals, a mesio-buccal canal and a mesio-lingual canal. The incidence of having four canals in maxillary first molars has been reported as approximately 60 per cent[4] and in second molars, 35 per cent.[5]

Two canals cannot always be seen in the mesio-buccal root on the preoperative radiographs, even when the radiograph is taken from a distal angle. But, if it is always assumed that there are two canals present in the mesio-buccal root of all the maxillary molars until the second canal is ruled out, their locations will be easier to find and fewer root canals will be missed.

One important anatomic landmark, which can be seen before the access cavity preparation is begun, is the bulbous mesio-buccal surface of the crown (Fig. 1–70). Note how the mesio-buccal surface is larger and extends more to the buccal than to the disto-buccal surface. The pulp chamber extends up into this bulbous portion, and a very high percentage of teeth with this anatomy have four canals.

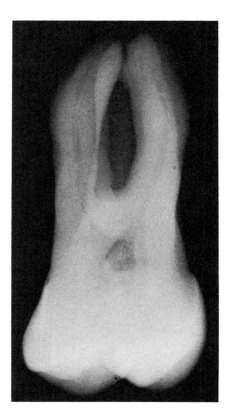

Figure 1–68 Mesial-distal radiograph of maxillary first molar.

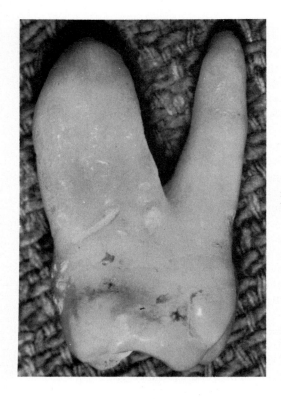

Figure 1–69 Buccal-lingual view showing how large the mesio-buccal root (*left*) is in this dimension. This is the same tooth as in Figure 1–68. The smaller root is the palatal.

Now visualize the anatomy of the chamber and location of the canals, assuming there will be four canals present. Looking at the occlusal surface, the pulp chamber generally has a triangular shape and tends to be slightly mesial of center (Fig. 1–71). There are three very common modifications:

1. Those teeth that have a bulbous mesio-buccal surface will have the pulp chamber extending into that portion (see Fig. 1–3).

2. There may be large pulp horns mesial and distal to the lingual canal, requiring the access cavity preparation to be extended mesially and distally to debride these pulp horns properly. When that happens, the apex of the triangle becomes rather flattened, changing the outline to trapezoidal or even rectangular.[6]

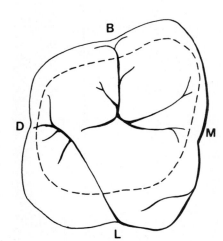

Figure 1–70 Occlusal view of a maxillary molar with bulbous mesial-buccal crown.

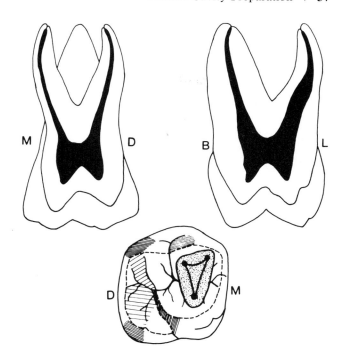

Figure 1–71 Buccal-lingual and mesial-distal anatomy and access cavity outline for a maxillary first molar.

3. The mesio-distal dimension often becomes narrower in second and third molars.

Reduce the tooth from occlusion. Remove any unsupported enamel, caries, and unsound restorations to prevent loss of the coronal seal. Locate the pulp chamber by cutting the anticipated shape of the access cavity opening approximately 1 mm into the dentin, staying slightly smaller than the final preparation. Then cut deeper toward the pulp, aiming for the easiest place to locate the pulp.

Remove the entire roof of the pulp chamber and flare the walls. Remove the internal cervical collar of dentin that is present in most maxillary and mandibular molars (see Fig. 1–17). Locate the canals and make any modification of the outline that is necessary.

The mesio-lingual canal is usually the most difficult to find. It is located directly lingual to the mesio-buccal canal (Fig. 1–72). Many times there will be a small developmental groove on the floor of the chamber leading lingually from the mesio-buccal canal to the mesio-lingual canal. Using a sharp endodontic explorer, probe along this developmental groove until the mesio-lingual canal is located. Frequently it is necessary to carefully remove a small amount of dentin (0.25 mm) from the mesial wall of the access cavity preparation, starting at the mesio-buccal canal and extending directly lingually for 2 to 3 mm along the floor of the pulp chamber. When this occurs, the outline of the access cavity preparation is modified to accommodate this mesio-lingual canal (Figs. 1–72 to 1–74; see also Fig. 1–3).

Once all the canals have been located, check to see that you have straight-line access to the canals, that the walls are flared, and that the chamber has been completely debrided.

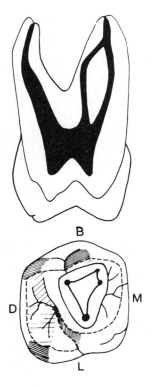

Figure 1–72 Buccal-lingual view of the mesial-buccal and palatal roots. The outline of the access cavity is modified to provide access to the mesial-lingual canal.

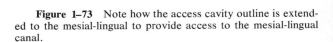

Figure 1–73 Note how the access cavity outline is extended to the mesial-lingual to provide access to the mesial-lingual canal.

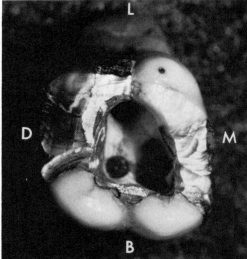

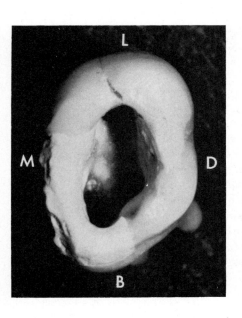

Figure 1–74 Note how the access cavity outline is extended to the mesial-lingual to provide access to the mesial-lingual canal.

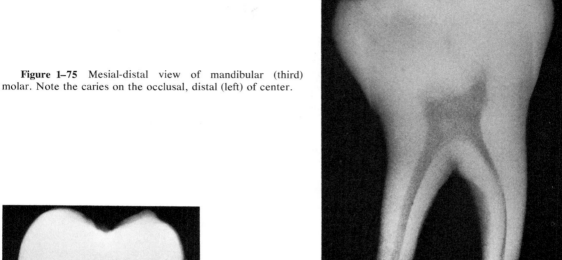

Figure 1–75 Mesial-distal view of mandibular (third) molar. Note the caries on the occlusal, distal (left) of center.

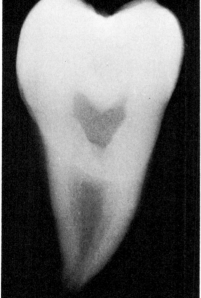

Figure 1–76 Buccal-lingual view of the mandibular (left) third molar in Figure 1–75.

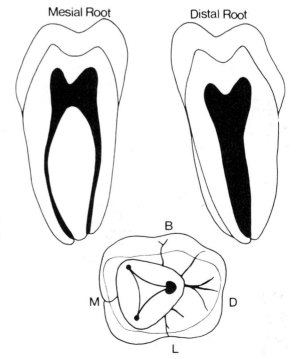

Mesial Root   Distal Root

B

M   D

L

Figure 1–77 Buccal-lingual illustrations of the mesial and distal roots with the shape of the access cavity when three canals are present.

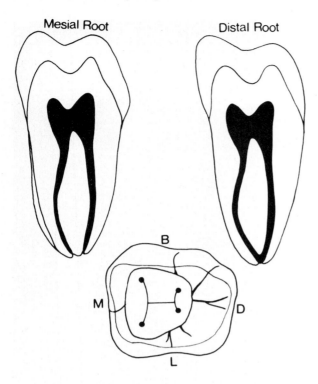

Figure 1–78 Buccal-lingual illustrations of the mesial and distal roots with the shape of the access cavity when four canals are present.

Mandibular Molars

Begin by visualizing the internal anatomy of the mandibular molars, which usually have two conical roots with one elliptical or two separate root canals in each root (Figs. 1–75 and 1–76). The most common arrangement is two canals in the mesial root and one elliptical canal in the distal root, but frequently there are two canals in each root. Again, it is important to always

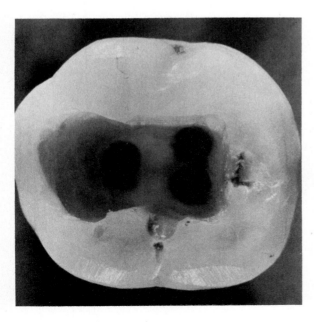

Figure 1–79 Occlusal view of the mandibular third molar in Figure 1–75 with good access to the canals. Note that the caries has been removed from the distal (left) portion of the access cavity preparation.

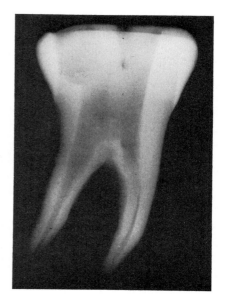

Figure 1–80 Access cavity preparation of the mandibular third molar in Figure 1–75, allowing straight-line access as close to the apical foramen as root curvature will allow. Note where the caries was removed from the distal (left) portion of the access cavity preparation.

assume that there are four canals present until you can rule out any of them.

The outline of the access cavity preparation is usually trapezoidal (Fig. 1–77). This is particularly true if there are only three root canals. If there are four canals, the distal portion of the preparation is wider (Fig. 1–78). In some cases it may be so wide that the shape of the preparation becomes rectangular.

When the access cavity preparation has been completed, there will be straight-line access as far apical as root curvature will allow (Figs. 1–79 and 1–80). Note that the cusps were flattened when the tooth was taken out of occlusion. The occlusal caries has been removed, the entire roof of the chamber has been removed, and the walls have been flared. Also note the unobstructed view of the three canals.

All the mandibular molars are basically the same. Certainly, anatomic variations will be encountered and there are so many variations among the anteriors, premolars, and molars that it would be difficult to list them all. But, if the principles of access cavity preparation are followed for all the teeth treated, there will be no difficulty in managing the access cavity preparation in any of them.

REFERENCES

1. Vertuci, F. J.: Root canal anatomy of the mandibular anterior teeth. JADA 89:369, August 1974.
2. Benjamin, K. A., and Dowson, J.: Incidence of two root canals — human mandibular incisor teeth. Oral Surg. 38:122, July 1974.
3. Weine, F. S.: Endodontic Therapy, 2nd Ed. St. Louis, The C. V. Mosby Co., 1976.
4. Pineda, F.: Roentgenographic investigation of the mesiobuccal root of the maxillary first molar. Oral Surg. 36:253, August 1973.
5. Ingle, J. I., and Beueridge, E. E.: Endodontics, 2nd Ed. Philadelphia, Lea and Febiger, 1976.
6. Acosta Vigouroux, S. A., and Trugeda, S. A.: Anatomy of the pulp chamber floor of the permanent maxillary first molar. J. Endo. 4:214, July 1978.

2

Preparation of Root Canals and Filling by Lateral Condensation Techniques

SAMUEL S PATTERSON, D.D.S., M.S.D.
CARL W. NEWTON, D.D.S., M.S.D.

The term "lateral condensation" of gutta percha is somewhat misleading. In its true meaning, lateral condensation of gutta percha would refer to compression of gutta percha against tapering side walls of the prepared root canal. However, when compressing gutta percha, it is impossible to compress against the side walls of the root canal without compressing apically. Condensation therefore is both vertical and horizontal. With this in mind, the term "lateral condensation" as used here will refer to a compression of gutta percha toward the apex of the tooth as well as toward the lateral tapering walls of the root canal — in other words, compression in all directions.

Gutta percha, when analyzed under magnification, is a mass of material composed of about 19 to 30 per cent gutta percha with fillers of zinc oxide, barium salts, resins, and waxes and dyes.[1,2] Under magnification, these materials combine into a solid mass (Fig. 2–1) with macro- and microscopic voids throughout the mass. There are numerous air spaces throughout the content of a gutta percha master cone when viewed under high magnification. In the process of filling a root canal, gutta percha is compacted as it is compressed (Fig. 2–2).

The process of filling a root canal with gutta percha and sealer is analogous to filling a bottle with water. No matter how much pressure one places on the volume of liquid, there is little displacement of this volume other than eliminating air bubble inclusions. Therefore, if gutta percha is softened by heat, it will assume some of the physical characteristics of a liquid. The voids between the master gutta percha cone and auxiliary cones will be displaced by the softened gutta percha or the sealer substance and the microscopic inclusion of air spaces will become displaced with root canal filling material (Fig. 2–3).

CROWN "TEMPORIZATION" PRIOR TO ACCESS OPENING

Prior to treating a tooth for endodontic reasons, it is frequently necessary to "temporize" the crown so that a leakproof rubber dam can be

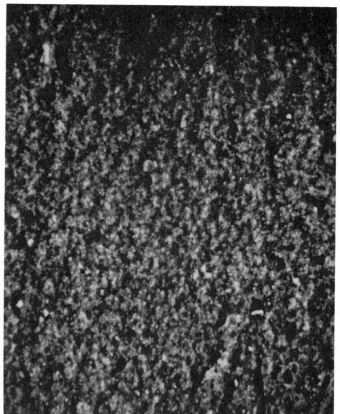

Figure 2–1 Scanning electron microscope photograph (SEM) of a cross section through a size 140 gutta percha point separated after quick freezing with nitrogen (× 320). Premier.

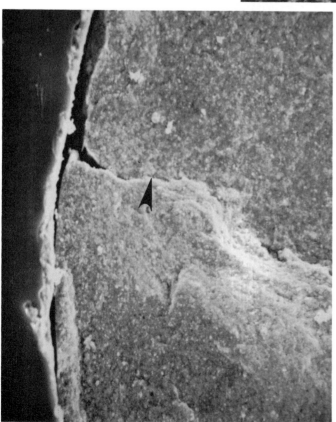

Figure 2–2 Scanning electron microscope photograph of a gutta percha–filled root canal after lateral condensation with thermoplasticizing technique (× 320). Arrow indicates voids.

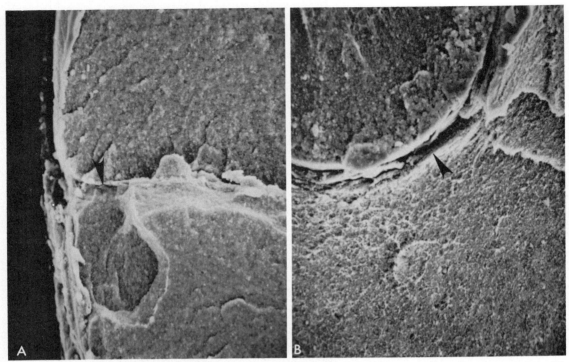

Figure 2-3 These scanning electron microscopic photographs show a closer adaptation of accessory points with less sealer to compensate for voids when heat (*A*) is used compared with cold gutta percha (*B*) techniques (× 320). Arrows indicate voids.

placed over the tooth requiring endodontic therapy. If a lateral wall is missing, it should be replaced by some temporary filling material or band.

Supporting the crown by placing an alloy restoration or banding the tooth will accomplish the following:

1. A leakproof rubber dam.
2. Better retention of the interappointment temporary seal.
3. A likely means of preventing further crown fracture between appointments.
4. Temporary restoration of function during the interim between completion of the endodontic treatment and restoration of the treated tooth.

A simple method of banding is illustrated in Figure 2-4.

The easiest means of temporizing a tooth is to use the band portion or the lateral wall portion of an anodized aluminum crown form. Most posterior teeth require full crowns if they have caries or extensive restorations or occlusal coverage following endodontic therapy. This prevents crown fracture resulting from post-treatment brittleness.

Since crown preparation requires reduction of the proximal contact points and occlusal reduction, these processes can be started to facilitate placement of a band. Occlusal reduction will not only provide a flat cuspal area for accurate file length determination, but it will also reduce the possibility of cuspal interference if apical periodontitis occurs following treatment.

After gross coronal reduction, an anodized aluminum crown is trial fitted. The occlusal area is removed from the anodized aluminum crown

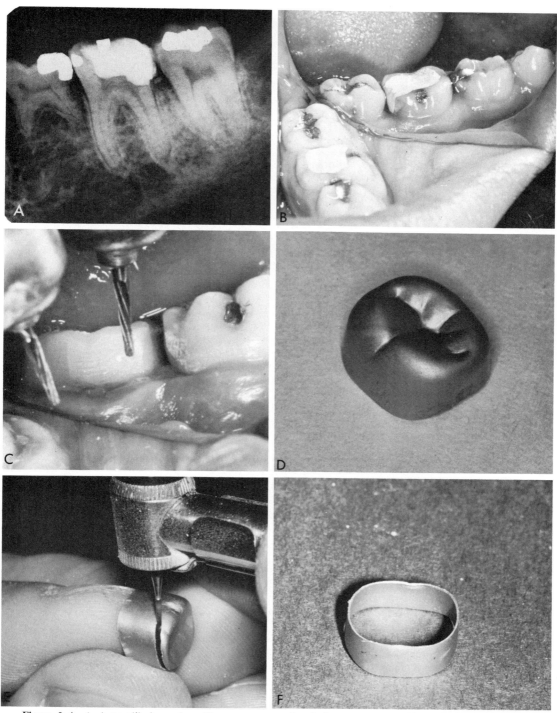

Figure 2–4 *A*, A mandibular molar with one or more walls missing presents a problem with rubber dam isolation and interappointment seal. *B*, Gross caries is removed and roughly restored to contour with temporary cement to reduce contamination prior to band fabrication. *C*, Proximal contacts are reduced to facilitate placement of the band. Occlusal reduction helps prevent periodontitis secondary to treatment and loss of seal through loss of temporary cement during masticatory forces. Parallelism should be maintained to increase retention and reduce undercuts. *D*, Select an anodized aluminum crown that most closely fits the preparation. Adjustments in the tooth preparation may be necessary for optimal fit. *E*, Separate the occlusal surface with a high speed bur or separating disc to fabricate a band from the crown. The patient's and operator's eyes should be shielded to prevent injury. *F*, Refit the band and contour the cervical and occlusal margins with scissors.

Illustration continued on following page

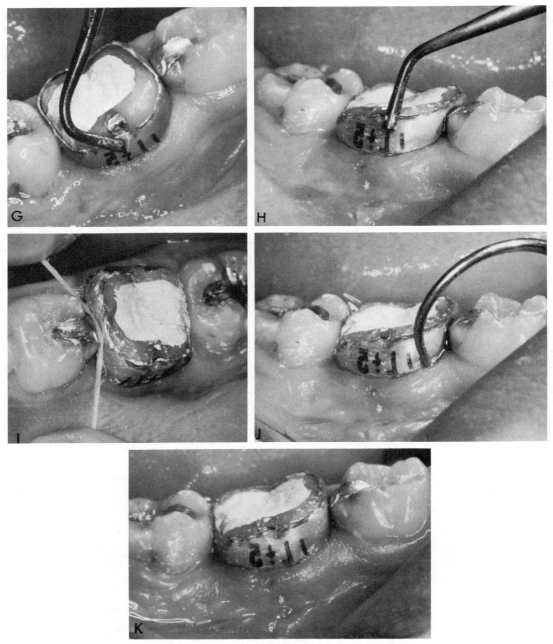

Figure 2–4 *Continued G,* Cervical and occlusal margins are crimped to fit closely and be nonirritating to the gingiva, buccal mucosa, and tongue. *H,* The band is cemented in place and the margins are burnished before the cement fully sets. *I,* Contacts are checked with floss for normal contours and excess cement removed. *J,* The sulcus is probed to prevent leaving a rough margin or any cement to serve as an irritant. *K,* Completed temporary band is checked for occlusal interference and is ready for isolation.

form with a fissure bur at high speed and the rough margins are smoothed. The band is again trial fitted to see that it does not extrude beyond the height of the marginal ridges to interfere with occlusion. The band must fit snugly at the cervical aspect and cover the cervical extent of the missing tooth structure. With a curved beaked contouring pliers the cervical aspect of the crown is crimped slightly toward the tooth structure to facilitate a tighter cervical fit. The occlusal aspect of the band is treated in a similar manner.

Prior to cementation, all the caries and overhanging unsupported tooth structure should be removed. If this is done before the band is prepared, it is impossible to fit or contour a band properly owing to the lack of tooth structure. Of course, during caries excavation the operating site should be protected from salivary contamination with cotton rolls and a saliva aspirator.

After all the caries has been excavated, the band is ready for cementation. A generous supply of zinc oxyphosphate is now mixed, and the band is inverted on the index finger and filled with a very loose mix of cement. The pad of the finger is used to direct the band to its location and force the cement into the excavated areas. As soon as the band has been placed, a band pusher is used to thoroughly seat the band cervically. Once the band is seated, it is good practice to compress the cement, because frequently the cement will not flow into the deep crevices and between the band and the tooth. Compression of the liquefied cement can be accomplished by saturating a No. 3 cotton pledget with alcohol and then holding the pledget with a treatment forceps and tamping it against the soft cement, forcing the cement cervically. When the cement has hardened and the excess has been removed, the interproximal space is examined with dental floss to insure space for the thickness of the rubber dam material between the band and the adjacent tooth. It is also important that no excess cement be left in the gingival crevice area to irritate this tissue. Articulating paper is used to double-check the occlusal contact, and when it has been determined that the tooth is not in premature occlusion, the rough edges of the band are smoothed with an abrasive rubber wheel so there will be no irritation to the tongue or gingiva. The tooth is now ready for the rubber dam application.

PLACEMENT OF RUBBER DAM

In endodontics it is generally necessary to isolate only the one tooth or the few teeth that are being treated at a particular visit.

The rubber dam is placed with the appropriate clamp to give the maximum viewing area and the maximum space for digital manipulation in and around the tooth. There are a great variety of rubber dam clamps, and any clamp that the operator finds comfortable can be used.

Three types of rubber dam material are recommended for endodontic therapy:

1. A light-colored rubber material, in three thicknesses and 5 and 6 inch squares. (This type is somewhat transparent, and the reflection of the x-ray packet when placing the film for a ''working'' radiograph can be seen.)

2. Same as (1), but in a dark color for greater contrast. (This type facilitates photographic techniques.)

3. A new green, mint-flavored rubber dam material. (This type causes less eyestrain, and patients respond favorably to the ''wintergreen'' flavor and odor of the rubber material.)

The tooth and dam are disinfected by swabbing with a solution of povidone iodine or hydrogen peroxide.[3] A blast of warm air dries the disinfectant and inverts the rubber dam material into the gingival sulcus. The operator is now ready to start an access opening. Access opening will be discussed only in generalities, since Chapter 1 has described the shape and function of specific access openings.

ACCESS OPENINGS

A sterile bur in an air turbine handpiece is used to penetrate the enamel and roughly shape the outline of the access opening for the tooth being treated. After penetrating the dentin short of the pulp chamber roof, a slow-speed, long-shank, surgical-length round bur of appropriate size is used to remove the overlying dentin and the roof of the pulp chamber. The access opening is extended to the limits of free accessibility to the root canals. All debris, pulp tissue, and dust should be removed to provide clear vision of the floor of the access preparation. In young teeth, the access opening has a larger occlusal extension, since the pulp chamber is usually larger. Diffusely calcified pulp chambers require careful occlusal access to avoid perforating some aspect of the crown when searching for small root canal orifice(s).

USE OF THE FIBER OPTIC LIGHT

The fiber optic light is helpful when attempting to locate the canal orifice of a diffusely calcified pulp canal (Fig. 2–5). The tip of the light source should be held at a right angle to the cervical area of the tooth (Fig. 2–6). The overhead light should be reduced to increase the concentration of light that will emanate from the pulp chamber. If the fiber optic tip is properly placed, the pulp chamber will glow with a reddish-orange hue. The root canal orifice appears as a dark speck (Fig. 2–7). At this stage of exploration the tip of a No. 8 or 10 file is directed into the newly located canal, and, working with probing motion, the instrument is "walked" to the apical aspect of the root canal.

Many teeth that appear inoperable from the two-dimensional view of an intraoral radiograph frequently are manageable when manipulation is per-

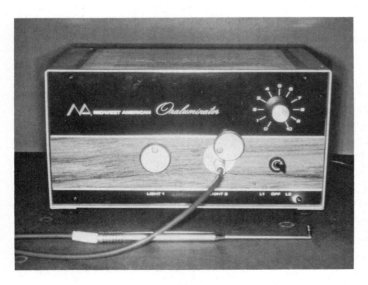

Figure 2–5 This fiber optic instrument has jacks for two optical probes and a rheostat to control intensity on a scale from one to ten. This demonstrates a right angle source of light (Midwest American Oraluminator)

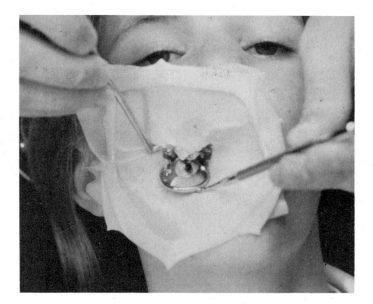

Figure 2–6 Illuminator tip is held at right angle at the cervical margin overlying the root. Reducing any outside light adds to the contrast.

formed. The radiograph most often indicates a condition that appears to be far more difficult to operate than acutally exists when operating in three dimensions.

USE OF LUBRICANTS, CHELATES, AND IRRIGANTS

Once a small diameter file has reached the apical extent of the root canal and this length has been verified with a radiograph, the file is moved in an up-and-down filing motion for a distance of 1 to 2 mm. Care must be

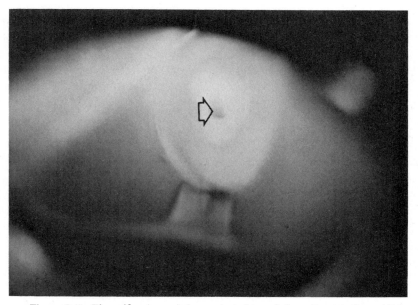

Figure 2–7 The orifice (*arrow*) demonstrated here is in contrast to the reddish-orange hue of dentin. Black and white photographs prevent an accurate illustration of this contrast.

exercised not to thrust the file beyond its apical termination. A few drops of surgical soap* are placed in the access opening with an irrigating syringe. The soap is carried to the depth of the canal with a fine root canal instrument. Not only does this lubricate the instrument, making subsequent rasping of the canal wall easier, but it also dissolves necrotic pulp canal residue and tissue. The canal is liberally scrubbed in a manner that washes necrotic tissue and debrides a surface wound. Wider diameter instruments are introduced into the root canal as the instruments meet decreasing resistance against the dentinal wall. The antiseptic ingredient in the soap is a very effective dentin disinfectant.[4]

Chelates are used by many operators in a similar manner; however, ethylenediamine tetraacetate has a tendency to soften the prepared dentinal walls of the root canal preparation and leave a less desirable or softer canal periphery to condense against.[5] *Caution* — Chelates should never be used to try to advance a small instrument into a tight canal, hoping to advance the instrument through a blockage. The instrument may create a new canal rather than follow the natural blocked canal and result in root perforation.

Neither should a chelate be left in a root canal as an interappointment medicament. Often the inorganic component of dentin will be removed, leaving a soft, decalcified dentin. The alteration of the root canal walls may produce a poor root canal filling, since the filling will be packed against a softer wall of dentin. This decalcified, softened dentin may shrink in time, producing a void between the canal wall and the filling material.

Irrigants should be used freely while preparing the root canal. They also lubricate the root canal instruments and facilitate removal of vital and necrotic tissue.

When treating a tooth for pulpitis, the use of sterile normal saline or distilled water reduces the inflammatory effect of instrumentation on the severed vital pulp stump left in the cemental canal.†

Root canals with necrotic tissue should be irrigated with sodium hypochlorite U.S.P. (NaOCl). Commercial chlorine bleach has been recommended for this purpose; however, we prefer the purer U.S.P. solution.

A 2.5 per cent solution of sodium hypochlorite U.S.P. is recommended as a root canal irrigant, since at this concentration it rapidly dissolves tissue. It is somewhat cytotoxic,[6] but less so than the 5 per cent solution; however, it should never in any dilution be forced beyond the dentocemental constriction, since it is extremely irritating and can cause excruciating pain.

CANAL EXPLORATION

The technique of canal exploration is very important, particularly in small canals of molars and premolars, as well as canals of other diffusely calcified teeth. Fortunately, the future holds great promise for better cutting

---

*Septisol — hexachlorophene 0.75%, soap, and coloring agent — Vestal Laboratories, St. Louis, Mo.; Hibiclens — chlorhexidine gluconate 4%, isopropyl alcohol 4%, soap, coloring agent, and perfume — Stuart Pharmaceuticals, Wilmington, Del.

†The cemental canal is the short inverted ("morning glory") funnel starting at the dentino-cemental junction and ending at the surface of the cementum. This term was introduced by Dr. Y. Kuttler.

instruments and for greater flexibility in instruments to facilitate the exploration and preparation of the root canal. At present, we have available No. 8 and 10 files, which are extremely fine and sometimes useful in exploring the very fine canals. Improvement in their quality is in the offing. Few root canals are straight, even if the radiograph gives the illusion of straightness. Upper lateral incisors, lower incisors, and the palatal roots of upper molars are most deceptive in their radiographic interpretation. Usually, in addition to distal curvatures, the incisors have a lingual inclination and the palatal roots of upper molars curve to the buccal in the apical one third. If attempts are made to explore or instrument these teeth with straight, stiff files, the wall of the root canal may be perforated, creating a condition that may necessitate apical surgery or extraction. At its best, the apical seal is most questionable. Therefore, the file must be preshaped prior to entering the root canal.

PRESHAPING ROOT CANAL INSTRUMENTS

There are two general types of bends that can be placed in a file (Fig. 2–8). The most common bend is a gradual curvature estimated to resemble the curvature of the root in the radiograph. In a second type of bend, which must be performed with extreme caution, the apical 2 to 3 mm of the root canal file is abruptly changed to a 15 or 20 degree sharp bend. A bend sharper than 20 degrees is more apt to cause apical file fragmentation.

If a file handle does not have a reference relating to the direction of bend in the root, some indentation or notation should be made on the handle to demonstrate the direction of the bend or dilaceration of the root canal (Fig. 2–9). Some operators prefer to use heart-shaped rubber or plastic stops. The apex of the heart-shaped stop points in the direction of the root canal deflection. By removing the instrument with the long axis of the root canal, buccal and lingual curvatures can be detected.

Caution should be used when entering a fine curved root canal with reaming action. Reaming action is a rotating or twisting motion with the root canal instrument that can result in transportation of the root canal (that is, creating a canal outline where it previously did not exist) or can cause

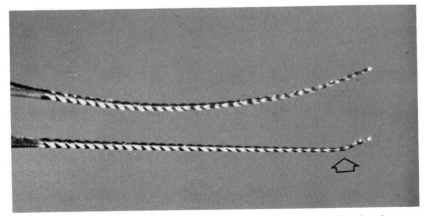

Figure 2–8 The upper file demonstrates a gradual curve approximating that seen on the preoperative radiograph. The sharp bend in the lower file (*arrow*) is referred to as a ''pathfinder.''

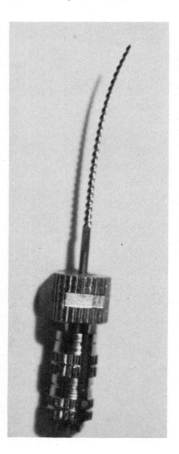

Figure 2–9 The curvature of this file is in the same direction as the slot in the handle. The operator can determine the direction of the instrument during preparation by observing the handle alone.

possible perforation of the root canal in the apical one third. There is also the risk of screwing the file against the tight walls of the root canal. If the instrument is forcibly turned or twisted counterclockwise after binding and partially unwinding, it is more likely to separate.

Most endodontic instruments are made by twisting an instrument blank in a clockwise direction. If the instrument binds in a tight canal, counterclockwise movement of the instrument handle beyond two complete turns will frequently cause fragmentation. The easiest way to penetrate a diffusely calcified small root canal is to vibrate the instrument handle between the thumb and forefinger in an arc of about 5 degrees back and forth. With a constant and moderate pressure, the instrument is then forced to the predetermined depth, which is verified with a diagnostic radiograph. If the diagnostic file is more than plus or minus 2 mm from the desired working length of the root canal, the necessary adjustment is made and rechecked with a radiograph.

TERMINATION OF APICAL DEPTH OF CANAL PREPARATION

Kuttler[7] has demonstrated that there are two parts to the root canal: the dentinal canal, which extends from the floor of the pulp chamber to the dentino-cemental junction, and the cemental canal. The dentino-cemental junction is the narrowest portion of the canal and should therefore be the farthest extent of the preparation. The blood vessels are smallest at this point and produce the least injury with pulp extirpation; likewise, the tissue growing in the greater diameter of the apical foramen is periodontal membrane (Fig. 2–10). This narrow waist also provides a matrix to condense root canal filling against and minimizes changes of overextending or underfilling. Kuttler showed that in young patients this is about 0.05 mm from the external surface of the cementum. In older persons it may be 1 mm or more, depending on the deposition of cementum over the root (Fig. 2–10).

Viewing the apical aspect of the tooth, the root canal constricts to the dentino-cemental junction and then seems to open in the shape of a decided flare. This frequently is not at the very apex of the tooth (Fig. 2–11). In some persons, Palmer et al.[8] found that the apical foramen exited as much as 3 mm from the radiographic apex of the tooth. If the root canal deflects either mesially or distally, the apical opening of the canal is generally slightly coronal to the apex of the tooth but on the side of the root deflection.

MANAGEMENT OF STRAIGHT CANALS

The management of straight canals needs very little special consideration. A reaming action can be used; that is, the type of movement in which the file is rotated on its axis, eventually to 360 degrees. This cuts the dentin much like a carpenter's plane. When reaming action is desired, the instrument should be rotated 10 or 15 degrees, then withdrawn, cleansed, and reinserted to the working length. This time rotate the instrument approximately 30 to 45 degrees, withdraw, cleanse, irrigate, lubricate, and possibly turn the instrument three fourths of a complete turn. On the next insertion to the desired preparation depth, the instrument can be rotated the full 360 degrees. Files or reamers of progressively larger diameter can be used carefully. This motion can be used only to full length straight canals. This type of rotation in a curved canal can cause the apical aspect of the root canal to be prepared to a greater diameter than the middle portion of the root canal, and a helix form is cut in the dentinal walls of the root canal. As the apical preparation increases and the width of apical root structure decreases because of

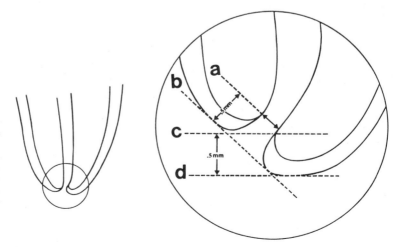

Figure 2–10 The cemental canal has been measured to be approximately 0.5 mm in length. The distance from the minor diameter (cementinodental junction) and the major diameter is measured from line *a* to line *b*. The point at which this canal exits has also been measured to be approximately 0.5 mm from the radiographic apex (measured between lines *c* and *d*). Therefore, the point at which the preparation is terminated (dentino-cemental junction) varies 0.5 to 1.0 mm from the radiographic apex and is determined by these clinical variables.

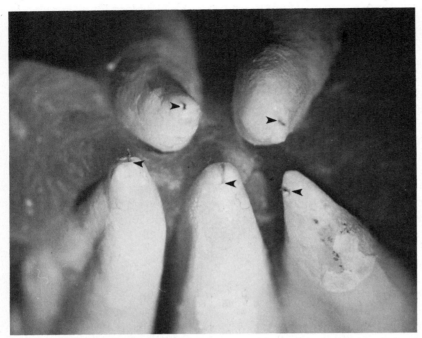

Figure 2–11 This apical view of six maxillary canines shows variation in the level and root surface each canal exits. Number 10 files can be seen protruding from the apex.

the tapering anatomy of human roots, reaming action is likely to cause a root perforation (Fig. 2–12). This undesirable condition is referred to by Weine et al.[9] as a "zip." In other words, the root canal can be opened to a helix shape somewhat like a figure 8, wide at the floor of the pulp chamber, narrow in the middle of the root canal, and wide at the apical termination. It is difficult to fill such a canal successfully (Fig. 2–13), particularly if the root canal instruments have caused an elliptical perforation at the apex. The perforation is ovoid-shaped, and since the master cone filling materials are round shaped, it is difficult to obtain a seal. Ideally the central core will stop at the surface of the root, and sealer will fill the rest of the ovoid space. This is

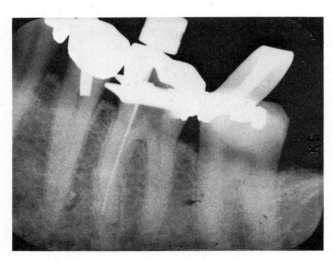

Figure 2–12 Perforation resulting from reaming action in a curved canal and violating the curvature with a straight instrument.

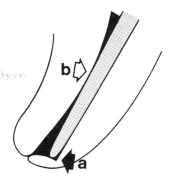

Figure 2–13 Lateral condensation requires a tapered preparation with the narrowest point at the apex. Condensers and pluggers are unable to compensate for the void left between the master point and "zip" (*a*) beyond the constriction (*b*).

wishful thinking, however, and these root perforations account for a great number of the root canal failures.

MANAGEMENT OF CURVED CANALS

As stated previously, most root canals are curved in some manner, some more acutely than others. A thorough knowledge of the management of curved canals is one of the keys to endodontic success. Certain rules stand out when treating curved canals: (1) The instruments used in preparing the curved canal must all terminate at the same place in the root canal preparation; (2) reaming action must never be employed in preparing canals that are curved; (3) curved canals require curved instruments; and (4) the final preparation must include the shape of the original canal.

Bear in mind that as a curved canal is prepared, much of the curvature is reduced and it is often necessary to shorten the working length of the instrument being used (Fig. 2–14). If the canal is straightened and the original instrument length is adhered to, the instruments that are the same length of the curved canal are now longer than the new preparation, which is straighter. The instruments will now extend beyond the predetermined depth of the canal and frequently perforate the apical foramen.

It is frequently desirable to radiograph a larger diameter instrument that has been readjusted to compensate for the new shorter length of the less curved root canal preparation. "Back-up" is the error of allowing dentin chips to pack the root canal far short of the original preparation length.

Figure 2–14 The final preparation (*a*) should completely encompass the original canal (*b*). The inside wall of the curved canal will be slightly straighter and the length of the instrument should be shortened accordingly.

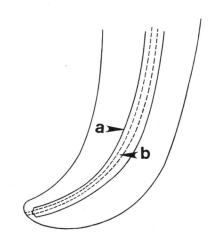

INSTRUMENT STOPS

One of the advantages of instruments that can be accurately measured and set in a handle, such as the "Test File, Ostby, or Kruger Stop," is the ability to prepare a very accurate matrix preparation within the confines of the root canal. This type of preparation terminates in a sharp apical triangle or the shape of the apical 1 mm of the last instrument used. Such a preparation creates a firm wall of dentin that can withstand considerable condensation pressure and avoids escape of the filling material into the periodontal ligament space. This type of instrument prepares a sharp matrix form within the confines of the root canal, which has been referred to by Glick as the "Washington Monument" shape.

With a rigid instrument stop, the operator can manipulate by feel. When the handle butts against the coronal landmark, the instrument stops. The operator prepares the canal by feel and can manipulate with a greater sense of security so that the instrument will not extend beyond the precise apical destination. When using unreliable movable stops, the operator must constantly watch the stopping point of the instrument. This requires closer visual observation and more tactile sense. When treating posterior teeth, the physical discomfort of constantly watching for possible displacement of the stop adds greatly to the operator's fatigue.

One disadvantage of the Test File Control instrument is the increased time that is necessary to set and lock the instruments accurately. This disadvantage can be offset by having a number of preset instruments in a convenient holder. Another disadvantage arises in manipulating teeth that have a working length longer than 28 mm, since 28 mm is the maximum length at which the instrument can be adjusted. Some cuspids may measure as much as 35 mm or more.

USE OF MECHANICAL INSTRUMENTS

Mechanical instruments such as the Gyromatic contra angle, the Kerr "Endolift," and long shank burs such as Gates-Glidden burs and Peeso reamers have been suggested from time to time to facilitate canal preparation.

The advantage of placing root canal preparation instruments in a mechanical device seems to be a saving of operative time. This is indeed an important factor; however, the accuracy of canal preparation with most of these devices can usually be challenged. Most mechanical devices have a tendency to transport at least part of the root canal, particularly in curved canals. As indicated earlier, transportation means creating a canal outline where it previously did not exist. Often a portion of the orginal root canal has not been touched by the mechanical device, and residual tissue remains to further contaminate the root canal.[10] Likewise, some operators have found it advantageous to combine the mechanical devices with hand instruments. Hand instrumentation is followed by mechanical instrumentation. Dentists are understandably handpiece-oriented, and this will provide stimulus for continued experimentation with these techniques.

Regardless of the type of instrument used in preparing the root canal, if a proper access opening has not been established and principles of canal preparation followed, the canal may be transported and poorly prepared with any type of instrument, mechanical or hand.

Many curved canals are difficult to manipulate because of the curve that occurs in the root canal from the junction with the floor of the pulp chamber, extending as far as 4 to 6 mm apically. The curvature in the pulp chamber root canal portion of the canal can be eliminated by rotating a canal orifice opener into the junction at the pulp canal floor and the root canal. A Gates-Glidden bur, size No. 2 or 3, can be carefully rotated in a contra-angle to a depth of 4 to 6 mm (Fig. 2–15). A Gates-Glidden bur should freely follow the canal and should never be forced. The bur should resolve before insertion and cut only on retraction. It is advisable to open the canal to at least a #25 file before attempting to use the Gates-Glidden instrument.

This procedure, properly performed, will straighten the root canal in its beginning third and leave only an apical curvature (Fig. 2–16). Root canal instruments can now be reshaped with a slight apical curvature and the tactile sense thus increased. The instrument enters the straight aspect of the canal and, since it bends only in the gradual apical curvature, larger instruments can be used with little problem of binding and subsequent fragmentation. The instrument action must be a filing motion, that is, an up-and-down circumferential movement. The cutting effect is mostly on the upstroke; however, some excess packing of dentin filings can occur if the instrument is not returned to the predertermined apical depth each time it is introduced.

When preparing a root canal, smaller instruments should be used

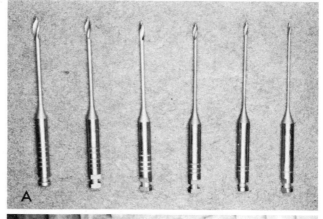

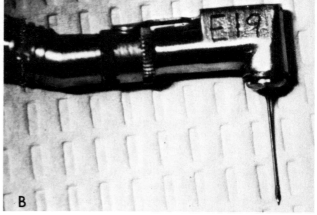

Figure 2–15 *A*, Gates-Glidden burs are available in sizes 2 to 6 and coded with rings on the shaft. *B*, The distance from the cutting tip to the handpiece is usually 19 mm.

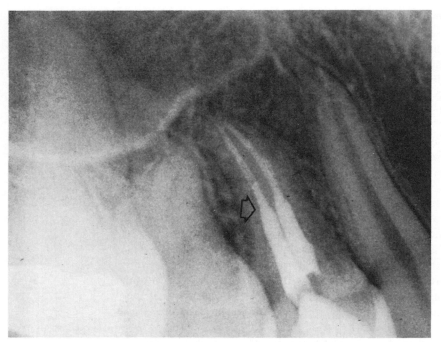

Figure 2–16 Use of Gates-Glidden burs has flared the coronal portion of the root canal (*arrow*) and facilitated apical preparation and condensation.

generously along with copious irrigation and lubrication. K-type files, rather than the Hedstrom files, are recommended in these small sizes.

Advantages of K-type Files Over Hedstrom Files. Hedstrom files are manufactured by a method in which the instruments are turned on a lathe. If the blades of the instrument are accidentally wedged in tight sections of the root canal, they are more apt to fragment than is the K-type file. In the larger sizes, beyond #40, fragmentation of the Hedstrom file is not as common. It should also be noted that Hedstrom files cut into dentin more rapidly than will the K-type file. They also cut only on the pull stroke. The K-type files can be used in a circumferential, up-and-down motion with rasping action to the periphery of the pulp canal. Files are better for this purpose than reamers, since reamers have a planing action and are most effective when twisted. If the canal is straight, it is safe to use the reamer; however, reamers should not be used in curved canals.

When the K-type file is used in extremely tight or calcified canals, the instrument has a tendency to unwind. This can easily be detected, since a shiny area will appear in the file where the flutes begin to separate (Fig. 2–17). Instruments should be examined often, and as soon as this shiny area is observed, the instrument should be discarded and a new sterile instrument used in its place.

PROPER DIAMETER OF THE PREPARED ROOT CANAL

The question is frequently asked, "How wide should a root canal be prepared?" The answer depends upon the technical procedures that are going to be used in attempting to obliterate and fill the root canal space. The

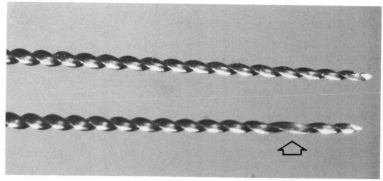

Figure 2–17 This illustration compared a normal #30 K-type file and one that is beginning to unwind (*arrow*). Close examination of instruments during usage is necessary so that they can be replaced as required before they separate completely.

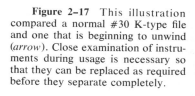

preparation should be of a diameter wherein all the soft or necrotic tissue has been removed, and the canal is widened to a diameter in which a sufficient bulk of gutta percha can easily be placed and condensed to the apical extent of the preparation. A properly prepared root canal will (1) include the outline of the original canal, (2) be shaped in such a manner as to accept a bulk of filling material, (3) terminate with a matrix form as the narrowest aspect of the dentinal canal, (4) allow sufficient thickness of dentin along the length of the root canal to give maximum strength to the remaining tooth structure, (5) contain no residual tissue, and (6) have smooth tapering walls. Canals in mature molars should be opened to a size 30 or 35 apical diameter if possible. Beyond #35, instruments lose their flexibility and have a tendency to recover the straight characteristics of the original metal blank.

STEP BACK OR FLARE PREPARATION

If the curved canal has been prepared to the apical depth with a size #30 file, the #35 file is set 1 mm short of the #30 length. For example, if the #30 instrument length was 21 mm, the #35 file should be set at 20 mm. After the #35 file seems passive with no resistance, the #30 instrument, set at 21 mm, is reintroduced to assure that the canal is patent to its length of 21 mm.

Each subsequent larger-diameter instrument is reduced 1 mm; however, before the next larger size is used, the #30 instrument is reintroduced into the canal to the original length. Copious amounts of irrigant should be used through the instrument preparation of the root canal in order to float or force the canal contents and dentinal dust from the prepared space. In this manner, the canal can be widened progressively and also kept patent and not blocked short with dentin chips. If the treated tooth has a straight canal, the canal can frequently be enlarged to a greater diameter. Straight canals are easier to enlarge since reaming (twisting) action can be used. Diffusion techniques for filling root canals usually do not require the extreme canal diameter that the vertical condensation procedure does because of the flow property given gutta percha by solvents.

Upper central incisors, cuspids, distal-buccal roots of upper molars, and distal roots of lower molars can usually be opened to a greater diameter because there is a greater tendency to straight pulp canal anatomy in these roots. However, unseen in the radiograph is the buccal curvature of the apical portion of the upper lingual roots and the buccal or lingual curvature of the apical portion of the roots of all lower teeth. If this is recognized early

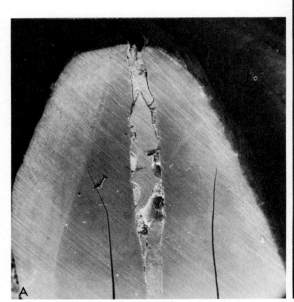

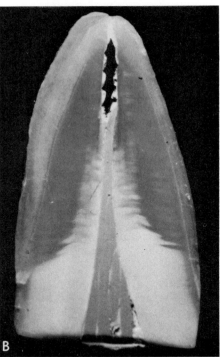

Figure 2–18 This specimen has a plug of dentinal fillings apical to a size 35 file segment. *A*, The scanning electron microscope photograph demonstrates the flutes of the file embedded slightly into the dentin wall (original magnification × 60). *B*, Photomicrograph of same specimen shows the file in place 1 mm from the apical foramen (original magnification × 10).

in the canal preparation, filing action of the root canal instruments should take precedence over reaming action.

APICAL DENTIN "PLUG"

As stated earlier, the termination of the root canal is at the dentino-cemental junction and beyond this dentino-cemental junction is the so-called flaring cemental canal with the major canal diameter. In spite of all attempts of irrigation to remove dental chips, some chips or dentin shavings are inadvertently packed at the junction of the dentinal and cemental canals. These chips are matted together by the irrigating solution into an impervious dentinal plug, referred to by some as dentin "mud." Experimental procedures performed by Adams et al.[11] on broken endodontic instruments have shown that it is almost impossible to prevent the filling of the narrow apical constriction with dentin chips if the root canal preparation did not open through the major canal constriction (Fig. 2–18). Teeth prepared in this manner were found to be resistant to radioactive calcium-45 leakage penetration, even if a fragmented file was used as the filling. When root canals were viewed under the electron scanning microscope, the dentinal plug could be seen filling the diameter of the apical aspect of the root canal preparation. In essence, the dentin chips blocked the root canal and acted as a physical barrier. This dentin chip barrier in itself, without root canal filling, was impervious to apical leakage. Whenever the apical aspect of the root canal was left patent by instrumentation through the apical foramen, calcium-45 isotopes showed leakage into the root canal (Fig. 2–19). The apical plug cannot be adequately demonstrated in young teeth with large or immature root canal development.

METHODS OF TREATING OVERPREPARED ROOT CANALS

Sometimes a root canal may be inadvertently overinstrumented. In other words, the instrument used in preparing the root canal will protrude through the apical aspect of the root.

With the patient properly anesthetized at the first visit, all viable tissue should be removed, root canal lengths properly determined, and all canals preliminarily prepared to two sizes larger than the original measurement file diameter.

At the second appointment, approximately 1 week later, it should not be necessary to use local anesthesia. If the patient feels a sharp pain when the root canal instrument is placed at its predetermined depth, a new radiograph should be made. Most likely it will show the file penetrating beyond the length of the root or extending through the external surface of the root. Readjusting the file will allow further comfortable root canal manipulation. If the patient insists on having the tooth anesthetized, there will, of course, be no sensitivity to file manipulation; but if the file length is longer than the root length, blood will exude from the root canal. The bloody exudate will indi-

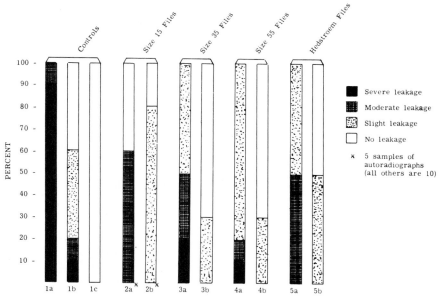

Figure 2–19 Bar graph showing leakage results. Each bar represents ten autoradiographs. (Bars 2a and 2b are representing only five samples each.) (From Patterson, S. S et al.: J. Endo. 5:142, 1979. Copyright by the American Dental Association. Reprinted by permission.) *Bar 1a,* No dentinal plugs, no filling. *Bar 1b,* No dentinal plugs, gutta percha filling. *Bar 1c,* Dentinal plugs, gutta percha filling. *Bar 2a,* Five specimens without dentinal debris, size 15 files. *Bar 2b,* Five specimens with dentinal debris, size 15 files. *Bar 3a,* No dentinal plugs, size 35 files. *Bar 3b,* Dentinal plugs, size 35 files. *Bar 4a,* No dentinal plugs, size 55 files. *Bar 4b,* Dentinal plugs, size 55 files. *Bar 5a,* No dentinal plugs, Hedstrom files. *Bar 5b,* Dentinal plugs, Hedstrom files.

cate that (1) the instrument has violated the apical terminal depth or (2) not all viable tissue was removed at the first visit. A radiograph will inform the operator as to the cause of hemorrhage. A file adjusted considerably short of the radiographic apex may mean retention of viable tissue.

If there is chronic apical periodontitis due to residual apical inflammation, continued canal preparation should be delayed until the tooth is completely asymptomatic. Apical periodontitis is usually due to (1) residual pulp tissue in the root canal, (2) overinstrumentation through the apical foramen of the root canal, (3) inoculation of the apical investing tissue caused by forcing infected tissue and bacteria from the root canal through the apical foramen, or (4) overmedication or forcible irrigation. If there is an area of pathosis around the apical aspect of the tooth, the patient may not have pain, but frequently blood may be detected on the end of the root canal instruments. Areas of apical rarefaction usually have very rich blood supplies, and it is not uncommon for granulation tissue to grow into the root canal. Perhaps the root canal had been prepared to a size 25, 30, or 35 before the overextended file error was discovered. To correct this, the preparation should be modified with the "back-up" technique (Fig. 2–20).

Back-up Preparation. In this technique, a new measurement control is made and a readjusted canal length is determined, which is shorter than the original and within the confines of the root canal. It is now necessary to prepare the root canal to a much larger size than originally anticipated, creating a new terminal point for a larger gutta percha master cone.

The newly prepared back-up preparation now has a firm apical wall that will permit apical condensation of gutta percha. Since the apical foramen has previously been violated, some sealer substance may exude through this artificially enlarged apical opening. The less foreign body compressed into the apical periodontium, the better the investing tissue will respond to the endodontic therapy.

INSTRUMENT FRAGMENTATION

Instrument fragmentation may occur in spite of all precautions by the operator. If the fragmentation occurs in the confines of the root canal after a fully matured root canal has been prepared to a size 30 or larger, there is an excellent chance that the apical aspect of the root canal preparation was filled with a so-called dentinal plug and fragmentation will not alter the seal of the root canal.[9] If the instrument is fragmented in a small size (8, 10, 15, or

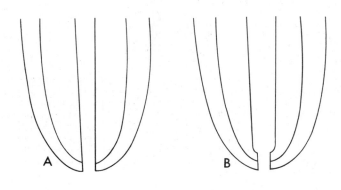

Figure 2–20 Overpreparation has destroyed the constriction necessary to serve as a matrix to resist condensation pressure (*A*). By reducing the file length, a limited matrix can be prepared to help contain the filling material (*B*).

20) during the initial canal curettage stage of preparation, the chances of leakage are great, and successful endodontic therapy is highly questionable. Fragmentation may eventually require an apicoectomy to remove the unfilled portion of the root canal if the fragmented instrument cannot be dislodged. If the fragmented instrument protrudes through the apical aspect of the root canal into the periapical investing tissues, again either apical surgery must be instituted to remove the foreign body or the tooth must be removed. Sometimes, with ideal health of the patient and good quality of the treated tooth, intentional replantation can be considered after removing the questionable segment of the tooth, but documentation supporting a favorable prognosis for such replantation is lacking. Fragmentation is not to be condoned; however, it does occur. Fox et al.[12] and Crump and Natkin[13] have shown that in spite of the fragmentation, the tooth and investing tissues remained normal and apical pathosis, when present preoperatively, also healed (Fig. 2–21).

FITTING OF MASTER GUTTA PERCHA CONE

There are two ways to fit a master gutta percha cone in a properly prepared, curved root canal. If the root canal has been prepared with an apical stop, tug-back with the fit of the master gutta percha cone is not necessary. When canals are being prepared in buccal roots of upper molars, first premolars, and mesial canals of lower molars, a No. 25, 30, or 35 gutta percha cone is used as a master point. With these small diameters, it is often difficult to get enough compression to feel tug-back. Good lateral condensation with vertical and apical pressure will obliterate the apical root canal space nonetheless.

When it is possible to prepare the root canal to a large diameter, a gutta

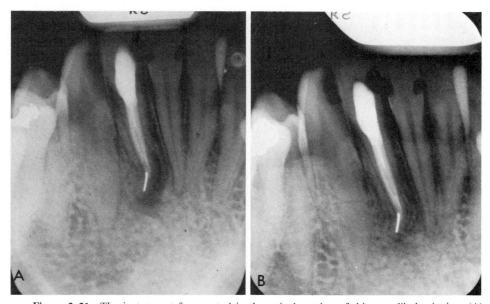

Figure 2–21 The instrument fragmented in the apical portion of this mandibular incisor (A) occurred after considerable preparation, resulting in a filling approximating the CDJ and a healed periapex on recall (B).

percha cone can be fitted with "tug-back." This requires having a master cone of almost the same size as the last root canal instrument used to prepare the apical segment of the canal.

CUSTOMIZATION OF MASTER GUTTA PERCHA CONES

When dealing with a large diameter root canal and particularly one that may have an immature apical foramen, it is possible to customize the apical fit of the master cone (Fig. 2–22). There are two commonly accepted methods to customize gutta percha cones.

The first requires the use of chemical solvents such as chloroform or eucalyptol to chemically alter the shape of the master gutta percha point. To

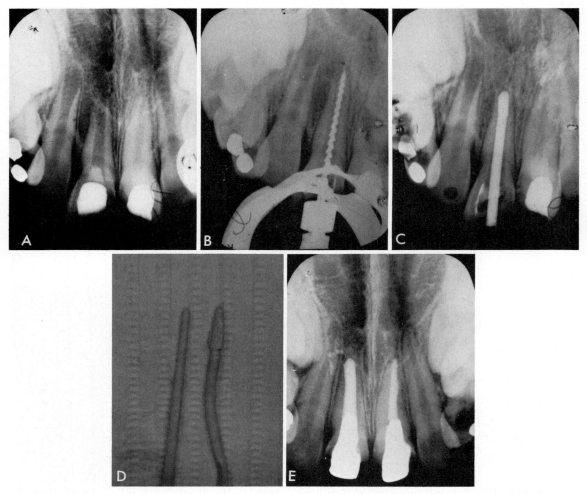

Figure 2–22 *A,* Open canals with parallel or flaring canal walls make the fitting of masterpoints and obtaining an apical seal most difficult. *B,* Canal walls are planned and the canal thoroughly cleansed with a large Hedstrom file. *C,* Master gutta percha point is customized to give an impression of the apex and close adaptation at the apical 3 to 4 mm to resist condensation. *D,* Chemically softened gutta percha should be filled immediately, whereas heat customized points may be stored without dimensional change. *Left,* unaltered gutta percha. *Right,* After customizing. *E,* Canal filled and post and core in place.

perform the chemical customizing of gutta percha, place a few drops of the solvent in the bottom of a sterile dappen dish. The master cone should be slightly oversized as compared with the last diameter of the root canal instrument. This size cone will bind against the canal walls about 2 to 4 mm short of the apical preparation. The apical 2 to 3 mm of the cone is placed in the solvent for a few seconds, then removed, and introduced into the root canal as deep as it will go. The master gutta percha point is reintroduced into the solvent and then back into the root canal in the same line of insertion until the altered gutta percha cone reaches the depth of the last file used to prepare the root canal. If a locking groove endodontic pliers is used to secure the master cone at the determined preparation depth, the chemically treated gutta percha cone can be trial fitted until the beaks of the pliers touch the incisial or occlusal landmark at the premeasured length. The customized cone should have good tug-back and be an impression of the apical termination of the canal preparation. It is always best to have the canal walls coated with irrigant when customizing techniques are used, so that chemically softened gutta percha does not stick to the walls of the root canal preparation. This is not a serious problem, but it does take time to reintroduce the files to remove the gutta percha that clings to the canal surface before proceeding to customize another gutta percha point. Properly handled, the oversized master gutta percha cone is gradually forced apically and takes on the shape of the apical aspect of the root canal.

After the customized gutta percha master cone has been properly fitted and checked, it is necessary to identify the path of reinsertion of the master cone. An indentation can be made on the lingual of the master cone at the height of the access preparation with a warmed explorer tip. This dot or indentation in the master point indicates that the point must be properly oriented to the lingual on reinsertion.

After the master cone has been checked radiographically, it should be removed and thoroughly irrigated with sterile water to eliminate any residual solvent. The point can also be dipped in an alcohol solution to remove the excess chloroform or eucalyptol.

The root canal should be filled at the customization appointment, since shrinkage[14] most likely will occur if the gutta percha cone is stored for use at a subsequent appointment.

The disadvantages of this technique are: (1) most solvents such as chloroform are cytotoxic to some degree;[15, 16] (2) there is some shrinkage to the chemically treated gutta percha after the solvent has dried; (3) the flow of material is hard to control and overfilling may be the end result; and (4) the chemically treated gutta percha is more porous[14] and more subject to fragmentation during trial fitting.

The second method of customization involves altering the master gutta percha point by physical means, such as heating the end of the gutta percha to a temperature that makes it soft and pliable. This type of customization of the master point can be done by taking a gutta percha point that is slightly smaller in diameter than the root canal preparation or one that will butt against the apex of the root canal preparation matrix form. Since gutta percha softens when heated, the apical 2 to 3 mm of a master gutta percha can be dipped in sterile water that has been heated and introduced into the canal preparation. The bulk of the master cone remains cold and acts as a plunger against the softer 2 to 3 mm apical segment. Weisman[17] has suggested placing distilled water in a thimble or inverted anodized crown form and sinking it in a heated bead sterilizer. The water is quickly warmed to temperatures in excess of the softening temperature of gutta percha. The apical 2 to 3 mm of the master point is inserted into the hot water, and the gutta percha is softened by conduction. A locking forceps is used to hold the gutta percha cone, which is now inserted in the prepared root canal matrix form. This process is repeated as often as necessary in order to get the prepared cone to assume the shape and diameter of the apical preparation of the root canal. If the operator is adept at using an electric heating device or a Bunsen burner, just the apical 2 to 3 mm segment can be softened and then introduced into the root canal. In this way the soft gutta percha flows under the thrust of the colder bulk of gutta percha cone, taking an impression of the root canal preparation in the same manner as with the chemically treated gutta percha. Under these circumstances, excellent tug-back can be obtained, and the gutta percha point is customized individually for that root canal preparation.

Once the gutta percha points have been properly fitted, either by customization or by using a standard-sized gutta percha point that has tug-back, the point or points should be radiographed for verification. If the root canal has an excellent apical stop and the preparation of the root canal corresponds to the adjusted length of the last file used, the gutta percha point can be measured against the length of the file. If both are the same length, the radiographic verification of the master gutta percha point can be eliminated. However, for the operator with less experience, it is best to check the fit radiographically. If the canal is not going to be filled at this appointment, the master cone can be stored for future use. The master cone thus prepared should remain unchanged after customization. To complete the preparation appointment if the canal is not to be filled at this visit, Cavit-G is placed over a medicated cotton pledget and covered with oxyphosphate cement. The intertreatment seal should always be checked for premature occlusion.

More importance seems to be placed on single appointment versus multi-appointment therapy. However, it is our opinion that postoperative pain can be minimized if the canal is filled at a period after the root canal(s) have been prepared. Preparation of the root canal 0.5 to 1.0 mm short of the dentino-cemental junction frequently is accompanied by a very moderate degree of discomfort due to periodontitis. In the interest of patient comfort, it is preferable to prepare the canal(s), fit the master cone(s), and subsequently, about 1 week later, fill the root canal. If a root canal can be filled after a delay between the preparation phase and the filling phase, the patient will experience little or no postoperative discomfort.

INTERAPPOINTMENT ANTISEPTIC TREATMENT

There is some question as to the validity of placing treatment medication in root canals between appointments. Some operators use no medication other than an irrigant together with instrumental cleansing of the canal. They actually depend upon thorough preparation of the root canal to remove the plaques of bacterial growth, the necrotic tissue, and the infected dentin. Without placing any other type of medicament, the tooth is closed so that the trauma of instrumentation will heal prior to filling the root canal. The cytotoxic effect[18] of medicaments on tissue is weighed against their antimicrobial effects. Marosky et al.[19] have found that all treatment cements have some degree of microleakage (Fig. 2–23). Introducing an antiseptic material on a pledget of cotton into the pulp chamber between appointments helps compensate for the microleakage that will occur through the treatment cement restoration. A double seal of cement will reduce microleakage. For example, if Cavit-G is placed over the medicated cotton pledget in the pulp chamber and then enough room (2 to 3 mm) is left for placement of zinc oxyphosphate cement, IRM, or any other cement that is resistant to abrasion, there is less opportunity for bacterial contamination in the pulp chamber and root canal due to temporary cement marginal microleakage between appointments (Fig. 2–24). The cytotoxic effect on the severed pulp stump or the apical periodontal investing tissues of any medicament sealed in the root canal should be a determining factor in the selection and handling of drugs.

It is not the intent of this chapter to enter into the controversy of culturing root canals versus nonculturing. However, if the philosophy of culturing is followed, it is necessary to have a time lag between taking the culture and the second or third visit of the patient. Seven days will normally allow enough time for bacterial growth in the culture medium in order to detect the possibility of bacteria in the root canal. Newer methods of culturing, as described by Griffee[20] and Sundqvist,[21] may be more accurate in detecting a wider spectrum of microorganisms in canals, but an easily adaptable clinical application is not yet available.

ONE-APPOINTMENT VERSUS MULTI-APPOINTMENTS

In a study by Flatley et al.,[22] in which symptomatic pulpitis was treated in both single and multiple appointments, the following conclusion was reached: "The unpredictability of the one-appointment visit and the use of analgesics only to relieve the painful episodes preclude one-appointment

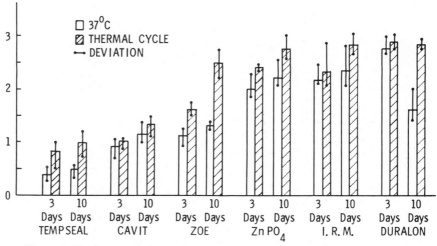

Figure 2–23 Bar graph demonstrating the average leakage values given for various temporary materials that are used clinically. (From Patterson, S. S et al.: J. Endo. 3:113, 1977. Copyright by the American Dental Association. Reprinted by permission.)

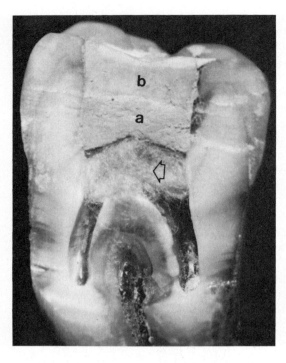

Figure 2–24 A longitudinal section through a mandibular molar demonstrates a medicated cotton pellet (*arrow*), double sealed Cavit-G (*a*) and zinc phosphate cement (*b*).

endodontics. Multiple appointments allow the operator to assess the health of the tissue at the time of filling and to treat it locally by intercanal medication if necessary."

REMOVAL OF MOISTURE PRIOR TO FILLING ROOT CANAL

Since there is some residual moisture in the root canal from previous irrigation, medicaments or exudation from the severed pulp stump, and ingress of tissue fluids, it is necessary to dehydrate the root canal before

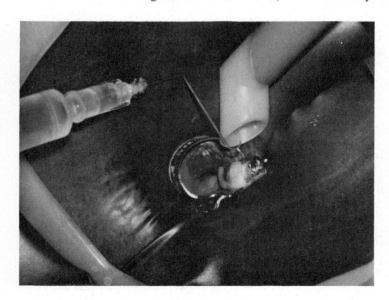

Figure 2–25 Alcohol is introduced with a disposable syringe, and the canals are dried with sterile paper points.

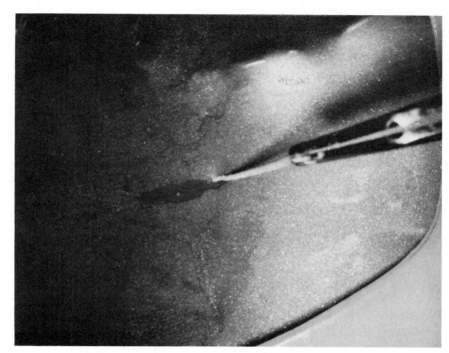

Figure 2–26   The paper point can be streaked across the rubber dam to determine if moisture is present. (A moist paper absorbent point will leave a "trail" of moisture on the rubber dam.)

filling. Moisture resulting from the aforementioned causes should first be removed with sterile absorbent points. The canal is then irrigated with either 95 per cent ethyl alcohol or 99 per cent isopropyl alcohol; both have great affinity for moisture. Two ml of alcohol is placed in an irrigating syringe and flushed into the root canal system (Fig. 2–25). Make sure that the needle fits loosely. A root canal file is set at the proper length and is inserted in a churning manner to force the alcohol to the apical depth of the preparation. The alcohol is allowed to remain for approximately 2 or 3 minutes and then removed with sterile absorbent points. Frequently, it is difficult to determine whether the absorbent point is wet with alcohol or dry. If the point has moisture, it can be streaked on the rubber dam and will make a visible moist mark (Fig. 2–26). If all the moisture and alcohol have been removed from the root canal system, the paper point will be dry and will not streak. At this point the operator is ready to fill the root canal spaces.

FILLING OF ROOT CANAL

The master point, auxiliary points, and root canal sealing material should all be prepared and arranged for convenience prior to filling the root canal. The type of root canal sealer used may vary according to the operator's ability to manipulate a specific type of sealer or his preference for specific qualities inherent in specific sealers. The use of Kerr's Tubi-seal* root canal sealing cement will be described here. The choice of this sealer stems from some of its physical properties. When the base and the accelerator are properly spatulated, a thick, creamy, sticky, white paste

---

*Kerr Tubi-seal. Sybron/Kerr, Romulis, Mich.

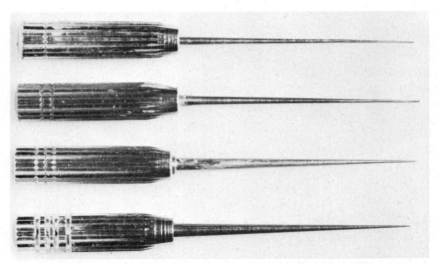

Figure 2–27   Finger spreaders of incrementally larger sizes (coded with rings on the handle) are arranged in order and premeasured in the canal to prevent binding.

will be produced, which has excellent properties of flow and will not stain the tooth structure it contacts. If Tubliseal should exude through a poorly prepared root canal of a tooth with normal apical periodontal tissues, it can cause a painful response that sometimes lasts for 5 or 6 days. However, if the root canal has been properly prepared, none of the sealer should escape through the apical foramen but may flow into the auxiliary and lateral canals. If in the case of necrosis with apical pathosis, some of the sealer escapes into the pre-existing lesion, the excess usually resorbs and causes little if any postoperative discomfort.

The root canal sealer is spatulated for 15 to 20 seconds, until it is a homogeneous mass of a light creamy color. The setting time of the sealer can be controlled by the amount of accelerator placed in the mix. It is now ready to be introduced into the root canal. This can be accomplished in one of three ways: (1) the last file used in preparing the root canal introduces the sealer by turning counterclockwise; (2) rotary instruments such as lentula paste fillers may be used, although there is always the risk of fragmentation of this type of instrument; or (3) the paste sealer can be introduced into the root canal with the fitted master point. Sufficient sealer should be introduced into the root canal to insure that all the walls of the root canal preparation are covered with sealer. As the file, lentula paste filler, or master point is withdrawn, some of the sealer is also removed from the surface of the wall. Reintroducing sealer two or three times may be necessary. As the gutta percha and sealer are introduced into the canal, the excess will exude from the coronal access opening. After the sealer has been thoroughly applied to the walls of the root canal preparation, the master point is seated and locked by turning the gutta percha cone with pressure directed apically. A #1, #2, and #3 finger spreader of the Luks* type (Fig. 2–27) should be readily available. As soon as the master point has been properly seated, a #1 finger spreader is placed between the wall of the root canal preparation and the master point, with an attempt to force the master point against the lateral

*Finger spreader as per Dr. S. Luks, Union Broach Co., Long Island, N.Y.

wall and apical termination of the root canal (Fig. 2–28). When the #1 spreader has been removed, a #2 spreader is inserted and worked in a rotary or circumferential manner, thus creating space for an auxiliary point. As soon as the #2 spreader has been removed, a #3 root canal spreader is introduced. Each size enlarges the space for the auxiliary point to a greater diameter. A medium fine auxiliary point lightly coated with sealer is introduced into this space (Fig. 2–29). Auxiliary cones come in various sizes — fine fine, medium fine, and so on. They have a taper that comes to a fine point. Selection of the desired size depends on the inherent strength of the gutta percha cone and the size of condenser or plugger used.

The size selected must have the tensile strength to allow insertion without folding back. Usually the medium fine auxiliary point meets this qualification. One or two points are placed in this manner to further wedge the master point into the root canal so that subsequent spreading and pressure with heat will not dislodge the master point or cause it to be withdrawn from its nesting place in the root canal preparation. The finger

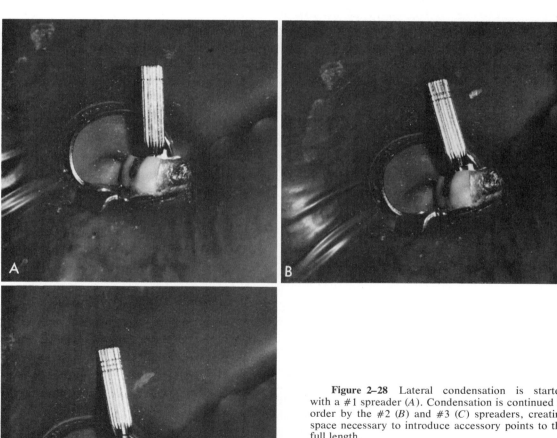

Figure 2–28 Lateral condensation is started with a #1 spreader (*A*). Condensation is continued in order by the #2 (*B*) and #3 (*C*) spreaders, creating space necessary to introduce accessory points to the full length.

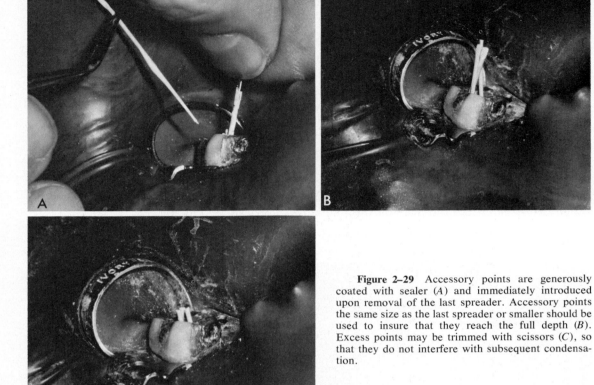

Figure 2–29 Accessory points are generously coated with sealer (*A*) and immediately introduced upon removal of the last spreader. Accessory points the same size as the last spreader or smaller should be used to insure that they reach the full depth (*B*). Excess points may be trimmed with scissors (*C*), so that they do not interfere with subsequent condensation.

spreaders are now placed in the bead sterilizer, not to sterilize them, but merely to allow them to warm sufficiently to displace the previously placed gutta percha (Fig. 2–30).

The gutta percha in the root canal is now subjected to a thermoplasticizing technique. Since most bead sterilizers operate at temperatures in the range of 425°F, the #1, #2, and #3 Luks finger spreaders are placed in these sterilizers and are heated by conduction. When a spreader is introduced into the root canal immediately after removal from the sterilizer, there is an exchange of heat. As the spreader reaches the depth of the root canal preparation alongside the previously placed auxiliary points and master point, it has a tendency to warm and soften those cones of gutta percha. The spreader is then turned 360 degrees and moved back and forth. If the spreader is smooth and clean, the gutta percha in the canal should not cling to it and become dislodged. Subsequently, the heated #2 spreader is placed, then the #3 spreader. Another tapering auxiliary gutta percha point is then coated with sealer and introduced into the space left by the #3 finger spreader. This process is continued until the spreaders will not reach more than 1 or 2 mm beyond the junction of the pulp chamber and the opening of the canal orifice. At this time, the root canal should be filled thoroughly (Fig. 2–31).

In the process of filling the root canal, the master and auxiliary points

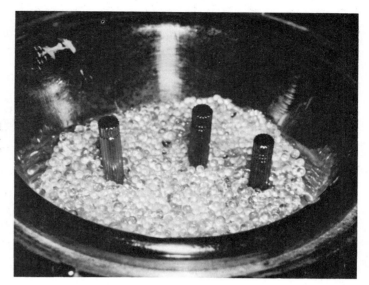

Figure 2–30 The spreaders are heated in the bead sterilizer after preliminary condensation, and the technique is continued by thermoplasticizing the gutta percha.

have been warmed and are compressed upon each other with an intermediary layer of sealer between each pair of gutta percha cones placed into the root canal. This produces a homogenized mass of gutta percha and sealer. In the process the auxiliary points have been forced apically as well as laterally, but they can go only as far apically as the matrix of the preparation of the root canal. In the very apical 1 mm segment or in the vicinity of minor canal constriction, dentinal chips that were loosened during the preparation of the root canal and could not be removed by irrigation may have become impacted into a leak-resistant seal. In theory there are two root canal fillings: (1) the plug of dentinal chips in the minor constriction at the preparation terminus and (2) the guttta percha and sealer filling in the dentinal canal. We frequently have a double-sealed root canal. If there are lateral or auxiliary canals, these will become filled with root canal sealer that has been forced laterally under pressure during the lateral condensation.

Hopefully, the sodium hypochlorite used for irrigation has dissolved the contents of these lateral or auxiliary canals. There is some conjecture as to whether this really happens. Most likely, the forces exerted during the compression procedures mechanically push all debris ahead of the sealer or softened gutta percha and displace this undesirable tissue. The lateral canal

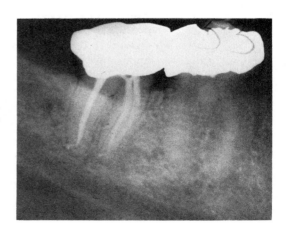

Figure 2–31 Final radiograph reveals the tapered preparation and sealer, demonstrating the major and minor diameters of the cemental canal at the apex.

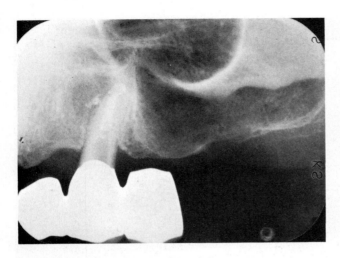

Figure 2–32 Evidence of a lateral canal is demonstrated by extruded sealer. This lateral radiolucency is very characteristic of a lateral canal, and the filling of this canal was an expected result.

tissue is pushed into the periodontal ligament space, and this reaction often accounts for postoperative discomfort following root canal filling. This can be seen as little puffs of sealer or little lines of a radiopaque material radiating from the main root canal system (Fig. 2–32).

During the process of lateral condensation, attention should be given to the size of the root canal spreader used for laterally condensing the gutta percha. If the root canal spreader has too great a taper, it may bind against the walls of the dentin near the entrance to the pulp canal, rather than create a space between the gutta percha and the dentin for an auxiliary cone. If binding occurs, it is not uncommon to produce a root fracture. Usually the root will fracture vertically, and this necessitates the removal of the tooth or root if the fracture involves one root of a multi-rooted tooth. If the instruments used for lateral condensation are smaller than the prepared canal, fracture will not occur.

Following condensation of the gutta percha, the excess root canal filling material and sealer must be removed from the coronal aspect of the tooth. A large bur rotating at slow speed will greatly facilitate removal of the excess material from the pulp chamber. Care must be taken, however, not to remove additional tooth structure, but only gutta percha and sealer. With the aid of high volume aspiration, the tooth can be kept clear of debris and the operator can see exactly what he is doing. If the sealer and filling are left in the coronal aspect of an anterior tooth, even though the sealer has a white appearance, the gutta percha contains dyes and causes a discoloration at the cervical aspect of the crown. Discoloration should be avoided and if the tooth is to be restored with merely a lingual restoration, as in the case of an upper anterior tooth, it can be placed at this time. If, however, dowel space is required, the dowel space should be prepared after removal of the excess gutta percha from the pulp chamber. All root canals requiring dowel space should first be thoroughly filled. This requires filling lateral canals so that percolation from an open lateral canal cannot occur in the prepared dowel space.

A temporary seal is placed in the coronal access preparation, and plans should be made to complete the crown restoration of the tooth. If the tooth has been properly treated, any area of pathosis should heal. There is a risk of crown fracture if the operator elects to wait 4 to 6 months for a bony heal to show on a postoperative radiograph. If periodontitis due to the canal filling placement is present, this should subside in less than a week. The comfort of the treated tooth is an indication that healing is taking place. Thus we now are able to return the tooth to health and function, the goal with every endodontically treated tooth.

REFERENCES

1. Friedman, C. M., Sandrik, J. L., Heuer, M. A., and Rapp, G. W.: Composition and mechanical properties of gutta-percha endodontic points. J. Dent. Res. 54:921, September–October 1975.
2. Friedman, C. M., Sandrik, J. L., Heuer, M. A., and Rapp, G. W.: Composition and physical properties of gutta-percha endodontic filling materials. J. Endo. 3:304, August 1977.
3. Moller, A. J. R.: Microbiological Examination of Root Canals and Periapical Tissues of Human Teeth. Goteborg, Elanders Boktrycker, Aktiebolag, 1966, pp. 30–33.
4. Parsons, G. J., Patterson, S. S, Miller, C. H., Katz, S., Kafrawy, A. H., and Newton, C. W.: Uptake and release of chlorhexidine by bovine pulp and dentin specimens and their subsequent acquisition of antibacterial properties. Oral Surg. Oral Med. Oral Pathol. 49:455, May 1980.
5. Patterson, S. S: In vivo and in vitro studies of the effect of the disodium salt of ethylenediamine tetraacetate on human dentine and its endodontic implications. Oral. Surg. 18:83, 1963.
6. Spangberg, L., Engstrom, B., and Langeland, K.: Biologic effects of dental materials. 3. Toxicity and antimicrobial effect of endodontic antiseptics in vitro. Oral Surg. Oral Med. Oral Pathol. 36:856, December 1973.
7. Kuttler, Y.: Microscopic investigation of root apices. JADA 50:544, May 1955.
8. Palmer, M. J., Weine, F. S., and Healey, H. J.: Position of the apical foramen in relation to endodontic therapy. J. Can. Dent. Assoc. 37:305, August 1971.
9. Weine, F. S., Kelly, R. F., and Lio, P. J.: The effect of preparation procedures on original canal shape and on apical foramen shape. J. Endo. 1:255, August 1975.
10. Klayman, S. M., and Brilliant, D. J.: A comparison of the efficiency of serial preparation versus Giromatic preparation. J. Endo. 1:344, 1975.
11. Adams, W. R., Patterson, S. S, and Swartz, M. L.: The effect of the apical dentinal plug on broken endodontic instruments. JOE 5:121, April 1979.
12. Fox, J., et al.: Filling root canals with files: Radiographic evaluation of 304 cases. N.Y. State Dent. J. 38:154, March 1972.
13. Crump, M. C., and Natkin, E.: Relationship of broken root canal instruments to endodontic case diagnosis: a clinical investigation. JADA 80:1341, June 1970.
14. McElroy, D. L.: Physical properties of root canal filling materials. JADA 50:433, 1955.
15. Food and Drug Administration: Memorandum to State Drug Officials, Washington, D.C., U. S. Government Printing Office, 1974.
16. Spangberg, L., and Langeland, K.: Biologic effects of dental materials. I. Toxicity of root canal filling materials on HeLa cells in vitro. Oral Surg. 35:402, 1973.
17. Weisman, M. I.: Warm-water impression technique for sealing large canals. JOE 2:124, May 1976.
18. Spangberg, L.: Cellular reaction to intracanal medicaments. Transactions of the Fifth International Conference of Endodontics. 1973, pp. 108–123.
19. Marosky, J. E., Patterson, S. S, and Swartz, M.: Marginal leakage of temporary sealing materials used between endodontic appointments and assessed by calcium 45 — an in vitro study. JOE 3:110, March 1977.
20. Griffee, M., Patterson, S. S, Miller, C. H., Kafruiry, A. H., and Newton, C. W.: The relationship of *Bacteroides melaninogenicus* to symptoms associated with pulp necrosis. Oral Surg. Oral Med. Oral Pathol. 50:457, November 1980.
21. Sundqvist, G.: Bacterial studies of necrotic pulps. Umea University Odontological Dissertations, No. 7, Umea Sweden, 1976.
22. Flatly, C. J.: Incidence of post-operative pain following one-appointment treatment of painful pulpitis without apical radiographic involvement. Thesis, Indiana School of Dentistry, 1975.

3

Vertical Compaction of Warm Gutta Percha

HERBERT SCHILDER, B.A., D.D.S.

The objective of nonsurgical endodontic treatment is the total debridement of the root canal system followed by three-dimensional obturation of the remaining endodontic space. Numerous clinical and histologic studies confirm the frequent existence of side branching, delta formation, and multiple canals in individual roots.[1-3] Clinical success is enhanced by adopting techniques that maximize the potential for debriding and totally obturating root canal systems effectively and consistently.

Most reliable endodontic techniques have been built upon the triad of root canal *instrumentation, sterilization,* and *filling.* Modern endodontics, recognizing to a greater extent the biologic and anatomic problems to be dealt with, has gradually modified the triad to *cleaning and shaping, mechanical sterilization,* and *three-dimensional obturation.*[4, 5] This more sophisticated appreciation of the biologic and mechanical issues involved in endodontic treatment has produced increasingly more satisfactory treatment results.

Improved success rates in endodontic treatment resulting from better cleaning and shaping and more effective obturation of root canal systems have, indeed, altered the dental profession's entire view of periapical pathosis and the healing capacity of lesions of endodontic origin.

Apical lesions of endodontic origin, which in past years would be treated surgically, are now being treated successfully nonsurgically. The misguided fear of apical epithelium, chronic lesions, fistulous tracts, and so on has receded during the past two decades with gradual improvement in clinical techniques.

Cleaning and shaping are perhaps the sine qua non of good endodontic technique. The concept embodies two important objectives. *Cleaning* requires the removal of all organic substrate from the root canal system. This includes necrotic tissue, pulp remnants, and associated microbes. *Shaping* requires the development of a logical cavity form that any dental practitioner can fill effectively. Equally important, when properly accomplished, shaping facilitates cleaning. It is impossible to thoroughly debride an unshaped canal.[4, 5]

When thorough debridement is achieved, mechanical sterilization is concomitantly accomplished by the physical removal of microbes along with the underlying organic substrate. This greatly reduces the need for drugs in modern endodontics.

Essentially, therefore, after proper diagnosis and treatment planning, clinical endodontics can be thought of as a rather precise extension of operative dentistry. It may be viewed as a cavity concept with certain biologically and anatomically imposed modifications. In restorative dentistry, dentists seek to clean out carious lesions and to prepare logical cavity forms (see G. V. Black[6]) to receive three-dimensional, hopefully hermetically sealed, restorations. The carious lesions are most often located in the coronal part of the tooth, and the process of caries removal hopefully removes all organisms related to the process of decay. It follows that most dental restorations are also coronal or at the cervical part of root surfaces.

It should take little adjustment for the dental profession to shed the limitations imposed by earlier endodontic concepts and techniques and to sense the parallel with operative dentistry. In endodontics, the major problem is necrotic and/or potentially necrotic material in roots and root canal systems.

CLEANING AND SHAPING OF THE ROOT CANAL

The cavity form required, therefore, for effective removal of substrate and for predictable three-dimensional obturation is one that extends from the apical foramen to the coronal access cavity. For the purpose of describing the technique of vertical compaction of warm gutta percha, a few of the more salient mechanical objectives of this root canal cavity design should be recalled. The exact techniques recommended by the author for cleaning and shaping have been described in detail elsewhere.[4, 5]

A well-shaped root canal is one that presents a gradually tapering cone, the narrowest part of which is directed apically and the widest part of which is directed coronally. The development of the cone will require the operator to carefully prepare the apical few millimeters so as to ensure that each internal cross-section of the prepared canal is wider as one withdraws from the apex into the canal itself.

Additionally, respect must be maintained for the natural curvatures of roots and root canals. A well-shaped canal will take into account these normal and frequent turns and will exhibit *flow*. That is, the prepared conical shape will occur in multiple planes, depending upon the normal curvature of the original canal. The lesson here is to learn to shape around canals in such a way that they then are straightened in their coronal and middle thirds but *never* in their apical third. This is easily learned. A well-shaped canal requires that its apical foramina not be transported by tearing, ripping, perforating, or blocking — all common mistakes when "instrumentation" alone is considered.

Lastly, the apical foramen should be kept as small as is practical and not be enlarged needlessly beyond its original size. For purposes of compacting warm gutta percha, 0.2 to 0.25 mm might be considered a minimal dimension for easily practicing the technique.[4, 5]

At this point a word should be said about the instruments used for the cleaning and shaping of the root canal system. Complete cleaning and shaping are achieved with three hand instruments — barbed broaches, reamers, and files — aided at times by engine-driven Gates-Glidden drills. All cleaning and shaping procedures are accompanied by copious irrigation.

Barbed broaches are made by gouging or cutting spurs from the round shaft of the instrument. Because of the inherent fragility of this instrument, it must be used with extreme caution and must be discarded after use. Since the function of the broach is to remove pulp tissue, and not merely to rearrange it, a broach of the proper size should be selected. This would mean that the broach would be wide enough to engage and remove the pulp, but not so wide as to make binding contact with the walls of the canal. A barbed broach should not be used in calcified canals or around curves. A broach should not be used more than two thirds into the canal.

Reamers and files are manufactured by twisting square or triangular shafts of metal on their long axes, thereby translating the vertical "edges" into partially horizontal cutting blades. The cutting edges of files are oriented in a more horizontal direction and are closer together than the cutting edges of reamers, so files are most effective when used in a push-pull motion in the canal. To accomplish thorough cleaning and shaping with a file, this must be done around the entire circumference of the canal wall and throughout the entire length. The reamer, on the other hand, has cutting edges that are oriented more vertically, so it is used in a rotary motion. Because of this rotary motion used with reamers and because the edges are spaced farther apart than files, reamers tend to remove debris upon withdrawal and therefore do not build up the accumulation of dentinal filings in a canal that files do. Because of the rotary motion employed with reamers, they should not be used around curves since they will tend to straighten a curve, creating a "whiplash" effect.

Gates-Glidden drills are small, flame-shaped rotary cutting instruments with long shafts for use with contra-angles. They are designed to cut without pressure, on the belly of the instrument, and to break near the contra-angle if unwarranted force is applied during use. This allows for easy removal from the canal in the event of breakage. Gates-Glidden drills are not used as pathfinders and are used only to enlarge the orifice of the canal. They are not used in canals that do not accept them freely and are not for use in the body of the canal itself.

The point of termination of the root canal filling has been the subject of discussion for decades. The so-called apical foramen rarely ends at the geometric apex of the root. Nor, on the other hand, is it routinely located far from the root apex. In the clinical descriptions to follow, instrumentation to the "apex" signifies placement of reamers and/or files to the radiographic apex or to a point only a fraction of a millimeter short of the radiographic apex.

The following descriptions presuppose appropriate pretreatment when necessary, proper placement of the rubber dam, sterilization of the field and of all instruments to be placed in the canal, and normal access cavity development.

Cleaning and shaping of the root canal system for the warm gutta percha technique are accomplished by serial reaming and filing and constant recapitulation rather than by sequential placement of all instruments to the apical end of the canal preparation. Serial reaming and filing connote the fact that instruments of greater width are used short of the apex in series to make room for reception and directed use of finer instruments apically. Recapitulation refers to the repeated reintroduction and reapplication of instruments previously used throughout the cleaning and shaping process in order to create well-designed, smooth, unclogged, evenly tapered, and unstepped root canal preparations.

After access preparation, the chamber is irrigated with sodium hypochlorite and a barbed broach is used to remove additional debris or remaining pulp tissue. The canal is irrigated after using the broach, prior to probing to the apex with the initial trial instrument. A #1 file is most routinely used for the trial length determination radiograph. An appropriately larger instrument may be employed if a #1 file would be so loose as to be displaced while the radiograph is being taken. If the initial instrument is at the radiographic apex, this length is recorded and transferred to the next several instruments. If the initial instrument is short of the apex, the canal is irrigated, appropriate adjustment is made on the length, a #1 instrument is inserted to the new length, and another radiograph is taken. If the initial instrument is beyond the apex, a new length is determined, the canal is again irrigated, and a #2 file is placed to the new length. A radiograph is taken to confirm the accuracy of this length.

A word about "working length" is in order at this point. As the body of the canal is enlarged to accept larger instruments, the canal becomes less curved and therefore the actual length between the point of reference and the apex will tend to become shorter. This must be remembered throughout the cleaning and shaping procedure and adjustments made. This can be accomplished only by taking additional radiographs during the shaping of the canal to confirm the accuracy of the distance to the apex.

The #1 file will act as much as a pathfinder as a file and will rarely produce enough shavings to require the use of a reamer to remove debris. The #2 file, with appropriate intentional deflection, is advanced apically and worked in and out repeatedly with 0.5 mm strokes until it fits loosely in the canal. After irrigation it is followed by a #2 reamer to remove debris. Owing to the rotary motion used with reamers, they must not be used around sharp curves. When the #2 instrument fits loosely, a suitably deflected #3 file is positioned apically, and is used in a push-pull motion until it fits loosely. A #3 reamer is used after irrigation to remove the shavings left by the file. This process is continued with increasingly larger instruments and frequent irrigation until the apical portion of the canal has been satisfactorily cleaned.

A film is taken of the last file that was placed to the apex, and the length is adjusted accordingly. The next size reamer is inserted and is given only a half turn when it first makes contact with the canal walls. This should occur before the full "working length" is reached. The reamer is withdrawn without any attempt to force it further apically. The stop on the instrument should be adjusted to this depth of penetration for future reference. The canal is irrigated, the next larger reamer is inserted to the point where it first contacts the walls, and the procedure is repeated. This is repeated with the next size reamer, each time adjusting the stop on the instrument to indicate the point of penetration, as this will occur short of the working length. The funneling procedure has now begun as the body of the canal is being tapered and widened so that it neither restricts nor directs advancing instruments in paths unrelated to the critical apical portion of the canal.

After irrigation, recapitulate for the first time. Replace to the apex the last instrument that was radiographed at the apex. Irrigate and reapply every reamer in the series previously used. In most cases, without additional pressure, each reamer can be advanced closer to the apex before contacting the walls of the canal and receiving its half turn. After initial recapitulation and additional irrigation, the use of a Gates-Glidden drill at the entrance to the root canal will unify the access preparation with the canal walls shaped by the serial reaming and filing, allowing the operator to place instruments in the canal without misdirection or interference from coronal tooth structure or from coronal or middle third canal walls. The elimination of such interference is critical to successful manipulation of the apical instruments. The Gates-Glidden drill is inserted only a few millimeters into the canal and never into the middle third of the canal. The point of the drill makes no contact whatsoever, as the cutting is done entirely at the belly of the drill. This must be followed by copious irrigation. Additional recapitulation is done, as described previously, and at this point the operator may decide to increase the size of the apex by one file. An additional film is taken to confirm accurate length and the canal is copiously irrigated, dried, and sealed.

When skill has been developed in properly shaping root canals, obturation becomes a relatively simple and satisfying experience.

OBTURATION TECHNIQUES

The objective of obturation in endodontics should be to seal permanently as much of the cleaned and shaped root canal system as is possible. Ample evidence exists that the thoroughness with which the root canal system is sealed is a major determinant in endodontic success.[7] Generally, it has been accepted that the most desirable root canal filling consists of a dimensionally stable, nonresorbable solid cone assisted by a sealer or cement.[8] Ideally, the sealer should constitute only a small fraction of the obturating material in order to reduce the possibility of dissolution and dimensional instability associated with most pastes and polymer fillings.[9]

Miscellaneous Techniques

Many techniques have been employed to meet these objectives. They can all be expected to produce a certain degree of clinical success. Euchopercha, chloropercha, and chlororosen techniques utilize the solubility of gutta percha in chloroform and in certain essential oils to produce a physically plastic mixture that, with lateral condensation, can be expected to replicate reasonably well the internal anatomy of the root canal system. Indeed, when these techniques are carried out faithfully, it may be demonstrated that a number of accessory canals are filled as well. Several problems of the technique include the difficulty of curtailing the apical movement of the chemically softened material, the potential irritant effects of the chloroform on the periapical tissues, and the measurable shrinkage that occurs when the chloroform or essential oil volatilizes after treatment.[4]

Silver points in conjunction with sealer have in the past enjoyed great popularity as a root canal filling material. Silver points have the advantage of being able to negotiate narrow and severely curved canals. Their radiopacity is impressive, and when handled well, they are able to seal the apices of many root canals. Unfortunately, because silver points are pre-formed, they are unable to adapt to the intricacies of most root canal systems. Also, when apical foramina are ovoid, it is impossible to seal canals without relying

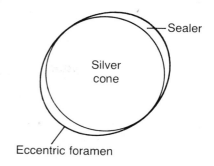

Figure 3–1 Variation in shape between round silver cone and eccentric foramen. The apical seal in such a case depends more on the sealer than on the silver cone itself. Dissolution of sealer may, over a period of time, lead to leakage and clinical failure of the case.

heavily on cement, since a round silver cone may bind on two points only, without completely obturating an eccentrically shaped foramen (Fig. 3–1). Experience over a number of years has demonstrated a large number of failures when cement has washed out, resulting in seepage not only apically but also along the entire body of the silver cone as well.

Lateral condensation of gutta percha in conjunction with nonsolvent cement has long been taught and utilized for root canal filling. The objective is to press gutta percha cones laterally against each other and against the dentinal walls of the canal so as to produce a dense and well-adapted filling. Tactilely, the illusion of a homogeneous mass is created. Unfortunately, the gutta percha cones never merge into a homogeneous mass after this technique (as does occur with gutta percha solvent techniques).[7] Rather, the cones glide and slip over each other until they are frozen in a sea of cement as the sealer sets in the later stages of the condensation procedure (Fig. 3–2).

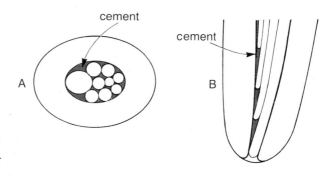

Figure 3–2 *A*, Cross-section of middle third of root demonstrating primary and auxiliary cones. Gutta percha cones frozen in a sea of cement. *B*, Longitudinal section of apical portion of root demonstrating primary and auxiliary cones. Gutta percha cones never merge into a homogeneous mass. *C*, Warm gutta percha with vertical compaction. Gutta percha becomes a homogeneous mass, filling prepared root canal from wall to wall with only a microfilm of intervening sealer.

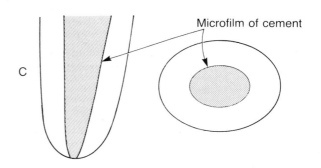

This leads to undesirably large amounts of cement in the final filling. Also, little improvement over the initial fit of the master gutta percha cone apically is possible if condensation is, *in fact*, lateral and primarily in the middle and cervical thirds of the canal. Recent evidence indicates that an apical seal with "lateral condensation" is enhanced when the spreader is utilized very close to the apex. In these instances, the spreader is acting essentially as a vertical compactor.[10]

In reality, heat transfer instruments are rarely carried very deeply into canals except in anterior teeth. Most molar root canals presumably filled by lateral condensation have actually been filled by the method of a single gutta percha cone generously engulfed in sealer. The introduction of finger pluggers provides a reasonable means for operators to try to deal with this problem.

Root canal fillings consisting solely of pastes have been used for over a century and persist to this day. Their appeal is twofold. First, they may be vehicles for pharmacologic agents or they may be pharmacologic agents themselves. Examples would be Sargenti's paraformaldehyde paste and Wycoff's iodoform paste. The list is endless, and pastes with exotic chemical potentiality are still being introduced today. The second appeal of these materials, a deceptive one that is shared by a plethora of newly introduced techniques and materials, is that they can be extruded into canals that have been inadequately cleaned and shaped or that have not been cleaned and shaped at all.

Although a certain degree of success can be achieved with paste fillings, no amount of chemical disinfection will neutralize a grossly contaminated root canal system. On the other hand, modern endodontics shows that a thoroughly debrided canal requires little in the way of pharmacologic assistance. Pharmacologic pastes are an anachronism whose promise of simplicity assures their retention in the dental armamentarium in spite of the unpredictability of the results they provide.

Technique of Vertical Compaction of Warm Gutta Percha

Vertical compaction of warm gutta percha combines reasonable ease with maximal effectiveness in consistently sealing simple root canals and complex root canal systems. Fortunately, gutta percha can be softened not only by chemical action, but also by heat. This fact, combined with improved methods of cleaning and shaping, permits root canal systems to be filled more rationally than was previously possible.

The method of vertical compaction of warm gutta percha depends, to a considerable extent, on the ability to place vertical compactors directly into root canals, much as amalgam pluggers can be placed into coronal cavity preparations. Gradual changes in the shape of prepared root canals make this possible.[4, 5] These changes in canal preparation, however, were at least as much a response to the need for total cleaning and substrate removal as to the requirements of vertical compaction.

A happy solution has occurred. Better prepared canals are cleaner; cleaner canals contain fewer microbes and less toxic substrate[11]; better shaping has led to better cleaning and fortuitously now allows for the facile placement of instruments to easily compact the slightly softened gutta percha directly into the deepest part of root canal preparations.

In essence, one accomplishes an accurate penetration into the root canal system, including significant accessory canals. With this technique, accessory canals are routinely observed to be filled in the cervical and middle thirds of roots as well as in apical bifidities, trifidities, and delta formations.[7] On occasion, auxiliary canals leading to the base of infrabony pockets and into previously resistant bifurcation and trifurcation lesions are also filled. In a sample of more than 10,000 patients treated with this technique in the Endodontic Clinic of the Goldman School of Graduate Dentistry at Boston University, *40 per cent of the patients* exhibited demonstrably filled accessory canals on postoperative radiographic examination.[12] These figures are consistent and have been repeated year after year with only minor variation by many operators accurately employing the technique.

The technique involves the prefitting of appropriate gutta percha pluggers into the prepared root canal, the selection and preparation of a master gutta percha cone, the placement of the master cone into the canal with a small amount of sealer, the controlled softening of the gutta percha with a heat transfer instrument, and the gradual vertical compaction of the softened gutta percha into the space of the cleaned and shaped root canal system. Ideally, a microfilm of cement should surround the final gutta percha filling.[9] Vertical compaction produces dense homogeneous gutta percha fillings with minimal cement content. All significant portals of exit are permanently sealed.[7]

The technique is predicated on capturing the maximum cushion of softened gutta percha with appropriate pluggers and moving the entrapped material toward the apex. At no time in this technique do the pluggers contact the dentin walls of the canal preparation. To do so is directly antithetical to the basis of the technique because a plugger wedged into the canal preparation *cannot possibly compact the gutta percha* apical to it (or ahead of it, or apically, or in the apical part of the canal). Vertical pressure is also essential to compaction of the mass in order to compensate for potential contraction as the material returns to body temperature. Any thermoplastic technique that does not include vertical compaction will result in gradual reduction in volume of the original root canal filling.[13]

The technique is quite simple but should be carried out exactly if optimum results are to be achieved in each case. The armamentarium consists of a series of pluggers, or compactors, and a heat transfer instrument. The pluggers are marked with 5 mm serrations so that the depth at which they are used within the prepared root canal can be known to the operator at all times. Two lengths are available. The shorter instruments have approximately 23 mm of working length and were designed primarily for use in anterior teeth. In clinical practice, however, most root canal systems can be obturated effectively with the shorter series of pluggers, the longer ones being reserved for unusually long cuspids or incisors. The angle of the plugging end to the shaft is the same for all instruments and has been designed so that the shorter series fits equally well into posterior and anterior teeth.

Heat transfer instruments resemble spreaders in that they are slender and taper to a point. However, they are *never* used with pressure or placed in contact with dentin. They are designed to deliver heat to gutta percha in the root canal. The metal in the working ends has been carefully adjusted so that the instruments can be used repeatedly for up to a year without oxidation.

When necessary, the working end can be unscrewed from the shaft and inexpensively replaced.

The pluggers (both the short series and the long series) are available in a graded series of working end diameters, ranging from 0.4 to 1.5 mm.* The instruments are also labeled in conventional numerology from #8 to #12 by half sizes so that a #8 corresponds to 0.4 mm, #8½ corresponds to 0.5 mm, and so on. Thus, a wide variety of plugging diameters is available to accommodate to root canals of any width. It should be understood, however, that no more than two to four pluggers are necessary for effective obturation of any one canal.

The gutta percha cones that are most suitable for this technique are those in the tapered series (fine, medium-fine, medium and so on) rather than those in the so-called standardized series (20, 25, 30, and so on) (Fig. 3–3).

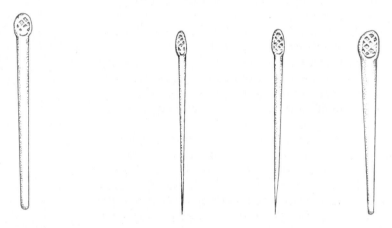

Standardized gutta percha cone

Tapered series of gutta percha cones

Figure 3–3 Standardized gutta percha cone, and tapered series of gutta percha cones.

Although the quality of the compounded gutta percha is the same for both the tapered and standardized series of gutta percha cones in any brand, the standardized series is inconvenient to use because it does not provide sufficient bulk of gutta percha to effectively obtain an impression of the root canal system. The author prefers to use Mynol gutta percha cones† with this technique, but Healthco‡ and Hygienic gutta percha cones§ are acceptable substitutes.

As has been suggested above, a minimal amount of cement is desirable to ensure maximum sealing of the canal system. Scanning electron microscopic evidence shows that, in spite of the wall-to-wall nature of gutta percha in a three-dimensionally obturated canal, the gutta percha is at no time chemically bound to the dentin surface. The amount of cement used should be kept to a minimum because previous investigations have demonstrated that excessive amounts of cement are prone both to dissolution and to shrinkage over a period of time.[11] For a variety of reasons, the author

*Ransom and Randolph, Toledo, Ohio.
†Mynol Chemical Co., Broomall, Pa.
‡Healthco Inc., Boston, Mass.
§Hygienic Dental Manufacturing Co., Akron, Ohio.

prefers to use Kerr Sealer* with this technique. Any one of a wide number of nonirritating sealers with which the operator feels comfortable may be used with this technique since the cement will constitute only a microfilm around the completed gutta percha filling when the technique is carried out properly.

The small amount of cement that is used in this technique is placed into the prepared canal with a lentulo paste filler. Although these instruments have been designed to fit into contra-angles, they should be used only by hand in this technique. It is dangerous and inadvisable to spin any cement into a prepared root canal by means of a dental engine.

Until recently, the heat for this technique was provided with a heat transfer instrument and a Bunsen burner flame. This remains a convenient means for obtaining heat for those dentists who have safely mounted natural gas Bunsen burners. Alcohol burners provide inadequate heat, and portable ''butane'' heaters burn excessively hot and can be a risk when employed in a dental office. Presently, a number of cleverly designed flameless heat sources are available that effectively heat a heat transfer instrument. The author prefers to use the metal point heater distributed by the Analytic Technology Corporation, Redmond, Wash. This device heats the tip of a heat transfer instrument to cherry red in a second, while the device itself stays at room temperature, producing no heat whatsoever in itself or in the dental operatory. In addition, electrically controlled heat transfer instruments are available, but wires are required from the electric source to the back of the instrument. The technique is essentially the same regardless of the operator's choice of heat source.

The master gutta percha cone should be selected carefully. Preparation of the cone is the starting point for a good root canal system obturation. Most gutta percha cones that appear to bind on initial placement into the root canal system *do not* bind apically but, in reality, bind laterally somewhere short of the root apex. This well-known fact makes it desirable, therefore, to cut off an appropriate portion of the original cone in order to maximize apical gutta percha bulk (Fig. 3–4). It also requires that apical gutta percha be compacted effectively to fully seal the canal, an objective that is more easily achieved with vertical compaction than with lateral condensation.

The gutta percha cones most frequently used as master cones for well-prepared canals are usually fine-medium, medium, or large for anterior teeth and fine-medium and medium for posterior teeth. Any choice, of course, may be suitable in any individual canal, and it should be borne in mind that canals that have been well-cleaned and well-shaped will easily receive these cones. Fine gutta percha cones are rarely required, and

---

*Kerr Co., Romulus, Mich.

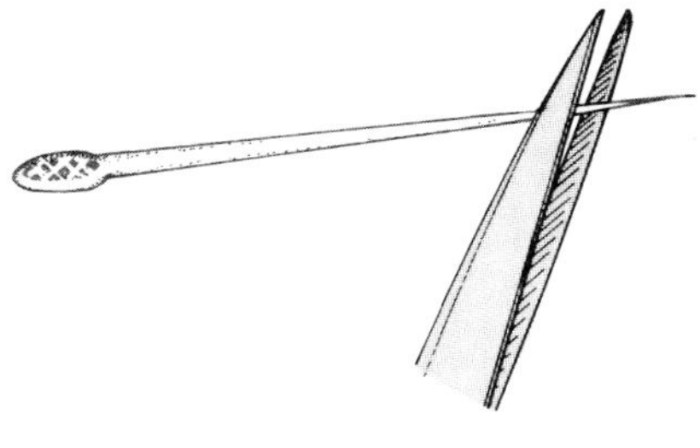

Figure 3–4 Removal of tip of gutta percha cone. This serves to maximize bulk; to secure apical, rather than mid-root, lateral binding; and to facilitate the ultimate hermetic seal of the apical foramen.

fine-fine cones are never used. When large anterior canals must be filled, it is often desirable to special-roll large or extra-large gutta percha cones in order to reduce their taper slightly.

In all instances, the apical portion of the gutta percha cone should be cut back so that the narrow-pointed end is rejected. This portion of any gutta percha cone is of little value in effectively sealing the canal. By selective removal of varying amounts of the apical tip of a gutta percha cone, any size cone can be easily adjusted to provide a great variety of master cones. During adjustment, the tips of the gutta percha cones are cut off with sterile dental scissors, and the fit is assisted by radiographic control.

The adjusted master cone should be fitted approximately 0.5 to 1 mm short of the radiographic terminus of the canal, should exhibit apical "tug-back," and should provide sufficient bulk for subsequent compaction. "Tug-back" refers to the tactile sensation of apical snugness. (At this time, in tapered canals and ovoid canals, it is sometimes desirable to fit a supplemental cone laterally for added bulk before compaction is begun [Fig. 3–5].) A supplemental cone is usually medium, not fine-fine as in lateral condensation.) The objective of the technique is to compact gutta percha apically rather than to compress cement hydrostatically.

The few pluggers to be used in any individual case are now prefitted into the canal (Fig. 3–6). As has been stated above, the essence of the technique is to capture a maximum cushion of softened gutta percha and to compact it vertically. Accordingly, using a narrow plugger in the wide portion of a canal preparation is ineffective, since such a plugger will penetrate the gutta percha without compacting it effectively (Fig. 3–7). It is equally senseless to use a wide plugger in the narrow portion of a canal preparation, since the plugger will bind against the dentinal walls and be unable to compact the softened material.

For example, it may be determined that #10½, #10, and #9½ pluggers are suitable for obturating a certain prepared root canal system. Accordingly, the instruments should be prefitted into the canal so that the operator becomes familiar and comfortable with each instrument at each level of the canal preparation. Prefitting may indicate to the operator that the #10½

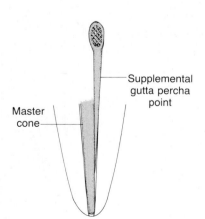

Master cone

Supplemental gutta percha point

Figure 3–5 Placement of supplemental cone after cementation of master cone but before start of compaction. This is done occasionally, but only when additional bulk of gutta percha is required in the middle and cervical portions of the canal to assure effective obturation of the entire root canal system.

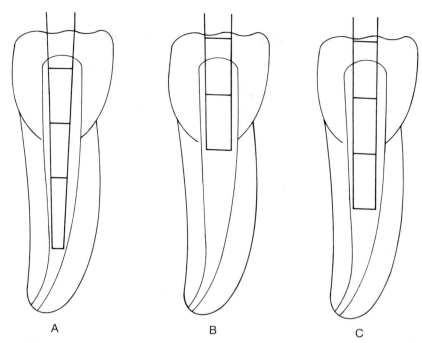

Figure 3–6 Prefitting of pluggers. *A*, The #9½ fits conveniently to the depth of 20 mm. *B*, The #10 fits conveniently to the depth of 15 mm. *C*, The #10½ fits conveniently to the depth of 10 mm.

Figure 3–7 *A*, Small plugger pierces warm gutta percha with little compaction. *B*, Large plugger captures maximum cushion of warm gutta percha, compacting it not only apically, but, without effort, laterally as well.

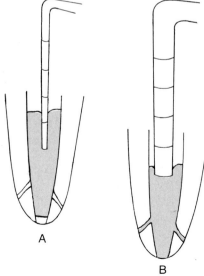
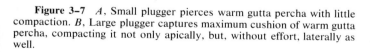

plugger fits conveniently to the depth of 10 mm, the #10 fits conveniently to the depth of 15 mm, and the #9½ fits conveniently to the depth of 20 mm. In this case, the operator would know that when compaction is being carried out, the #10½ plugger will not be used deeper than 8 mm, the #10 not deeper than 13 mm, and the #9½ not deeper than 18 mm so that good compaction can occur with each instrument. All of these numbers are given for example only and naturally vary from case to case.

The heat transfer instrument of appropriate width is also selected at this time.

The prefitted pluggers and the heat transfer instrument are now arranged conveniently on the dental tray near the selected heat source while the root canal sealer is mixed. Bear in mind, however, that in this technique only the heat transfer instrument is intentionally heated; the pluggers are used at room temperature throughout the compaction procedure. Heating the pluggers intentionally at any time is unnecessary and detrimental to their carefully designed metallurgic properties.

The cement should be mixed routinely according to the directions of the manufacturer and/or any special requirements perceived by the operator. Under most circumstances, the author prefers to increase the powder/liquid ratio of Kerr Sealer slightly to obtain a mixture that, while still fluid, is somewhat denser than the manufacturer's recommendation.

The technique will now be carried out by means of a series of compactions of softened gutta percha with pluggers, reheating by means of a heat transfer instrument, additional compaction with pluggers, reheating, and compaction deeper into the canal. With this process, an exact impres-

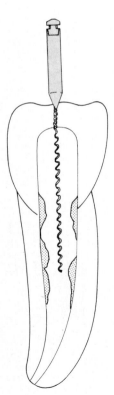

Figure 3–8 A small amount of sealer is placed along walls of canal with hand-held lentulo spiral. The lentulo is placed little more than halfway into the prepared canal.

sion can be taken of the apical half or apical one third of the root canal system.

A small amount of sealer is introduced into the prepared canal by hand with a lentulo spiral filler (Fig. 3–8). Care should be taken to apply the cement evenly along the length of the canal without using too much of the material. The objective is to attain a true gutta percha filling and not one that consists primarily of cement. The apical third of the prepared master cone is coated with cement and is gently reinserted into the root canal until maximum depth has been achieved.

A radiograph taken at this point should indicate that this seemingly tight gutta percha cone is still 0.5 to 1 mm short of the radiographic terminus of the canal. An indication of radiopacity beyond this point, although not serious, signifies either that the master cone was not well fitted originally or that excessive cement has been used.

The portion of the cemented master cone that extends into the access cavity is now removed with a hot spoon excavator. The excavator may be heated with either a Bunsen burner or a metal point heater. The widest prefitted plugger, in this instance the #10½ plugger, is now used to compact the gutta percha into the cervical portion of the canal preparation with a series of 2 or 3 mm vertical strokes (Fig. 3–9).

Compacting strokes in this technique are always short ones, with pressure being applied from the fingers and wrist, never from the arm and shoulder. It is worth repeating that the objective at all times is to capture the maximum cushion of softened material and to gradually move this forward.

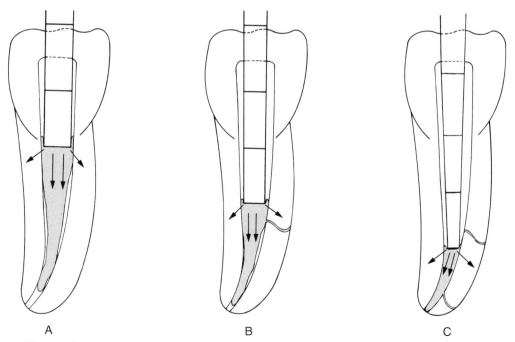

A   B   C

Figure 3–9 Compaction of gutta percha. *A*, The widest prefit plugger, the #10½, compacting the gutta percha into the cervical portion of the canal. *B*, The #10 plugger capturing the maximal cushion of softened gutta percha in the middle portion of the canal. *C*, The #9½ plugger molding gutta percha into the apical portion of the canal preparation. Note the automatic obturation of significant accessory canals.

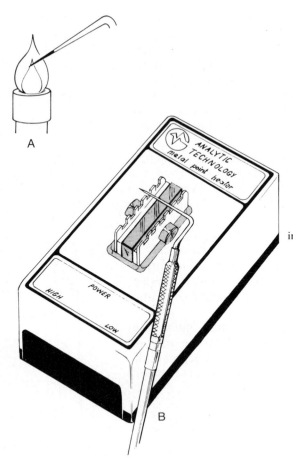

Figure 3–10 *A*, Heat carrier tip is heated to cherry red in flame. *B*, Heat carrier is heated with metal point heater.

In actual practice, the plugger is compressed centrally into the mass, moved 2 or 3 mm apically, withdrawn slightly, and reinserted so as to capture any material that has been bypassed by the previous stroke. This process is repeated one or two times before additional heat is added to the gutta percha.

The rhythmic use of the heat transfer instrument and the pluggers is now begun (Fig. 3–10). The heat transfer instrument is heated to cherry red, inserted directly into the central portion of the gutta percha to a depth of 3 or 4 mm only, and quickly withdrawn (Fig. 3–11). It is important that each time the heat transfer instrument is used, it is hot enough to transfer heat to the gutta percha mass and to be withdrawn easily from the gutta percha before it "freezes" on the heat transfer instrument, resulting in inadvertent removal of the gutta percha cone at an early stage of the compaction process. Once compaction has proceeded more deeply into the canal, it is impossible to remove the gutta percha involuntarily in this way.

As the heat transfer instrument is withdrawn, the temperature of the gutta percha is elevated only in the zone immediately surrounding it and apically to the extent of an additional 3 or 4 mm. Gutta percha is not a conductor of heat, but is an insulating material. The elevation of temperature in the apical third of the canal occurs only gradually over a period of several minutes as the cycles of heating and compaction are continued. It is

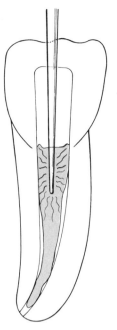

Figure 3–11 Warming the gutta percha with the heat transfer instrument. The heat transfer instrument is heated cherry red, inserted 3 to 4 mm into the central mass of gutta percha, and withdrawn quickly. The temperature of the gutta percha is elevated only in the zone immediately surrounding the heat transfer instrument and apically, approximately 3 to 4 mm.

erroneous to believe that the temperature of gutta percha in the entire root canal preparation is instantaneously elevated with the first or second application of heat or that the temperature of the gutta percha in the apical third is ever elevated as much as in the cervical and middle thirds of the canal.[14]

Thermocouple studies have indicated that the apical gutta percha is moldable at 40 to 44° C. In fact, it is impossible to elevate the temperature in the apical 2 mm more than 9° C above body temperature, even if one attempted to do so deliberately.[14] To return to our example, the heat transfer instrument is removed, and immediately the #10½ plugger repeats the vertical compaction process, being compressed first centrally into the softened mass, brought out slightly to recapture the softened material, and compacting it again once or twice. The plugger is removed; the heat transfer instrument is reheated, reapplied to the approximate depth of 3 or 4 mm, and withdrawn; and compaction with the #10½ plugger is repeated.

Two important things are happening now, which should be noted. One is that the working level of the gutta percha in the root canal preparation seems automatically to be moving deeper into the canal. The other is that the temperature of the apical gutta percha is slowly being elevated a few degrees above body temperature. The apical gutta percha will soon become moldable.

The working level of the gutta percha moves progressively deeper for two reasons. The first is that the softened gutta percha mass, which is being compacted vertically into the conically shaped canal preparation, automatically assumes a lateral component of force. This follows routine laws of physics and requires no lateral direction of the instrument on the part of the operator. The second reason is that, as the process continues and the gutta percha is tightly compressed in the preparation, the dentist may periodically and selectively remove small portions of gutta percha when withdrawing the heat transfer instrument. In very little time, the compaction process approaches the middle third of the canal preparation.

It soon becomes appropriate to select a plugger of slightly smaller diameter as the narrower portion of the preparation is approached. In the example being used above, the operator would switch from the #10½ plugger to the #10 plugger as the compaction process approaches a depth of 8 mm into the canal. It will be recalled that the #10½ plugger had been prefitted to a maximal depth of 10 mm, a depth at which it was indicated that additional effective compaction would be impossible. The #10 plugger is now best suited for capturing the maximal cushion of softened gutta percha in order to proceed with the effective obturation of the root canal system. The procedure of heating and compacting the gutta percha is repeated as above.

In this process, it is useful to clear as much gutta percha as possible from the sides of the preparation, so that the working level is kept relatively even at the end of each series of vertical compressions. This ensures good compaction of the mass. Also, it will be seen later that there may be minor inconveniences in completing the procedure with total satisfaction if significant amounts of gutta percha and/or cement are bypassed at this stage.

As the rhythmic heating and compaction proceed more deeply into the preparation, the temperature of the gutta percha at the apical end rises slightly above body temperature. Thermocouple studies have identified with precision the levels of temperature encountered at each stage of the technique and at each level in the canal. Thermal profiles may be obtained that accurately describe the manner and rate at which the apical gutta percha is transformed into a semi-rigid and then moldable state (Fig. 3–12). Although these measurements are of considerable interest to researchers, it is important clinically to know three things: (1) the transformation is gradual, (2) the apical gutta percha need be elevated only 3 to 8° C above body temperature in order to be moved, and (3) if additional heat is not intentionally added, the compacted gutta percha will effectively seal the terminus of the root canal preparation, quickly return to body temperature, and resist further movement beyond the terminus of the preparation.[14] Previous correct shaping of the canal preparation makes apical sealing of the root canal system quite simple.

In most instances, the apical portion of the preparation is sealed when compaction is occurring 5 to 7 mm from the apex.[14] This, of course, is an approximation, but provides a clinically useful range for operators who are new to the technique. It is not normally expected that apical movement of the gutta percha will occur when compaction is taking place in the cervical third of the canal, nor should it be necessary to work closer than 5 mm from the apex in routine cases. Somewhere in the 5 to 7 mm +/− range, the apical portion of the canal will be sealed along with, in many cases, one or more accessory canals.

As has been indicated, sealing or "corkage" of the terminus of the canal preparation is most effective in this technique. This is true even when the canal preparation may be inadvertently ovoid or eccentric. Because the apical gutta percha is never molten, apical control is excellent. Variations of this technique that employ overheated and excessively plasticized gutta percha increase the probability of gutta percha extrusion beyond the terminus of the preparation. Likewise, variations of the warm gutta percha technique that do not apply vertical compaction to the softened mass as it

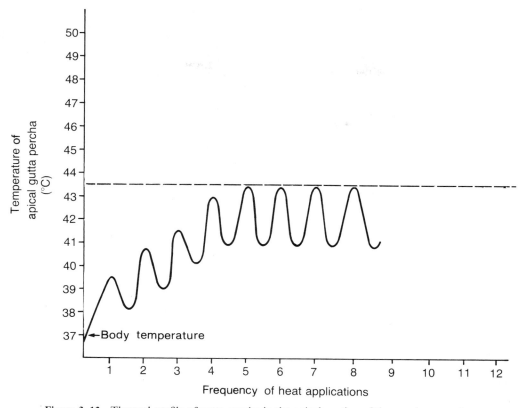

Figure 3–12 Thermal profile of gutta percha in the apical portion of the canal preparation.

cools to body temperature encourage loss of volume of the material in the final filling.[14]

When properly employed, the technique may or may not demonstrate radiographically a small amount of cement in apical contact with the periodontal ligament. This is observed more frequently opposite significant accessory canals in the root canal system than at the end of the main canal preparation itself. This material is innocuous. The reader is reminded of the previously reported and now well-known distinction between overfilling and vertical overextension of underfilled root canals.[15] That is, material (silver cones, gutta percha, pastes) may be overextended or extruded beyond a root canal system that has not been filled three-dimensionally or sealed by the material. This constitutes vertical overextension of a root canal system that may nevertheless be both uncleaned and *underfilled*. Under such conditions, seepage of bacterial toxins and proteolytic enzymes from residual organic substrate may be expected to lead to clinical failure. Overfilling, on the other hand, signifies a condition in which the *entire* root canal system has been obturated in three dimensions and surplus material is placed beyond the confines of the root canal system. Human histologic studies and countless clinical cases demonstrate that the excess material is innocuous under these conditions.[4] What is desirable is three-dimensional filling of the root canal system, a condition infrequently achieved in the past. When three-dimensional obturation is obtained, excess is irrelevant.

To return to our example, with either the #10 plugger or a moment or two later with the #9½ plugger, the apical portion of the gutta percha will be molded into the terminus of the canal preparation. This, of course, varies from case to case, depending basically upon the length and shape of the preparation. It it were necessary to compact deeper into the canal, in this case deeper than 13 mm, the operator would switch to the #9½ plugger in accordance with the information obtained when the pluggers were prefitted under the principles outlined above.

Dentists learning this technique quickly sense the similarity of compacting gutta percha vertically with condensation of amalgam. Except for the necessity of rhythmically transferring heat to the gutta percha as the compaction proceeds, the two techniques are remarkably similar as far as digital perception is concerned.

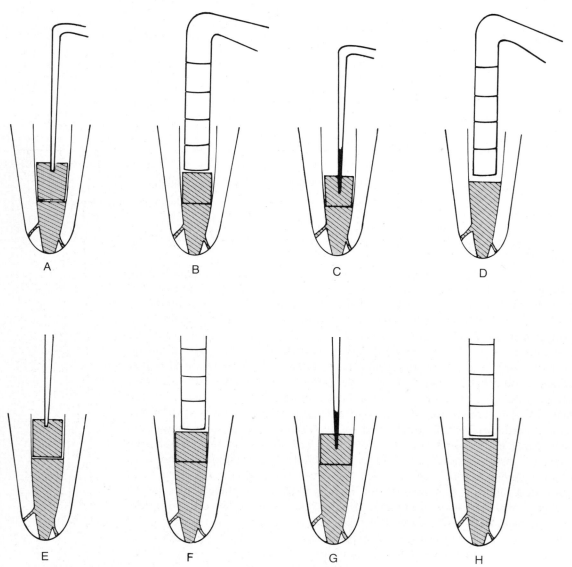

Figure 3–13 Back-packing. *A*, Carrying gutta percha segment to canal. *B*, "Cold welding" segment to main mass. *C*, Heat application. *D*, Compaction into uniform mass. *E*, Carrying second gutta percha segment. *F*, Cold welding. *G*, Heat application. *H*, Compaction into uniform mass.

Once the apical portion of the root canal system has been three-dimensionally sealed, the remainder of the canal preparation is obturated quickly by a process known as back-packing.

Back-packing consists of inserting 3 to 4 mm +/− segments of gutta percha, softening them with the heat transfer instrument, and compacting them in a manner similar to that described above (Fig. 3–13). The gutta percha segments are obtained by cutting ordinary gutta percha cones. Anyone interested in practicing this technique should always have available scores of precut gutta percha segments of varying width, although only two to four segments may actually be used for the compaction in any given case. In effect, a wave of heat application and compaction has been rhythmically carried apically into the canal preparation and is now repeated cervically until the preparation is entirely filled.

To facilitate back-packing, it is wise to lay out a selection of these 3 to 4 mm gutta percha segments of varying diameters (Fig. 3–14). Naturally, it is most effective to use relatively narrow segments in the deeper portion of the preparation and wider ones in the wider portion of the preparation. Use of wide gutta percha segments in the deeper portion of the preparation may lead to voids in the final filling that, although of little significance, indicate lack of facility with the technique. Voids may also occur if cement or gutta percha was carelessly left on the walls of the preparation during down-packing (Fig. 3–15). The gutta percha segments may adhere to this lateral residual material before union is established with the mass of gutta percha in

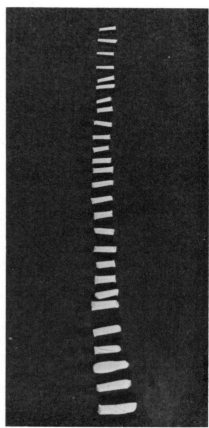

Figure 3–14 Gutta percha segments of varying diameters cut from auxiliary gutta percha cones. Only a *few* are needed in back-packing any single canal.

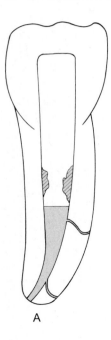

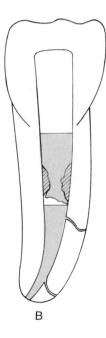

A

B

Figure 3-15 *A*, Cement or gutta percha inadvertently left on walls of preparation during down-packing. *B*, Possible resulting void.

the deeper portion of the preparation, interfering with the evenness of what should be a quick and smooth back-packing process.

In cases in which post spaces are desired, the operator has the option of terminating the procedure at the point of deepest down-packing or at any point during back-packing. Because of the frequency with which significant accessory canals are observed in the middle and cervical thirds of root canal systems, many operators prefer the second opportunity to obturate these auxiliary canals by completing the back-packing process cervically and removing gutta percha for the post space with a passively rotated Gates-Glidden drill.* Since a vertical wave of compaction has initially occurred along the entire length of the root canal, the ultimate selection of post space preparation in single-canal teeth is optional.

In multi-canal teeth, it is desirable to complete back-packing procedures in all instances so that warm gutta percha may be compacted into the flow of the pulp chamber with appropriately sized amalgam pluggers. This provides an opportunity for filling significant accessory canals in the floors of pulp chambers, leading to bifurcation and trifurcation areas. Heating and compaction are performed as outlined above, but, because of the bulk of the gutta percha involved, hot spoon excavators serve more conveniently as heat transfer instruments. The spoon excavators are heated either in a Bunsen burner flame or with the metal point heater. Therefore, when post spaces are desired in multi-canal teeth, the method of gutta percha removal with the passively rotated Gates-Glidden drill should be employed (Fig. 3-16). In either case, the final result is a root canal preparation filled wall-to-wall with dimensionally stable gutta percha. Recent studies demonstrate the absolute integrity of the remaining gutta percha regardless of what type of post preparation technique is employed.

The techniques described above have been used in clinical practice for

*Union Broach Co., Long Island City, N. Y.

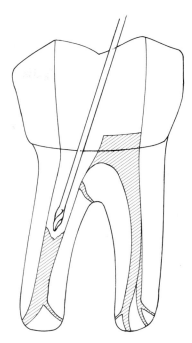

Figure 3–16 Passive rotation of Gates-Glidden drill to provide post space in posterior teeth. Post space is provided in anterior teeth simply by limiting or eliminating back-packing after apical obturation is achieved.

almost two decades. During this time, these techniques have been subjected to exhaustive study, including studies of the thermophysical properties of gutta percha;[14, 16] scanning electron microscopic studies of uncleaned, cleaned, and obturated root canal systems;[11, 17] microbiologic and biochemical assays of the organic substrate in uncleaned root canal systems;[18-20] serial sectioning of the roots of hundreds of teeth to develop hundreds of thousands of sections for studying the anatomy of root canal systems;[21, 22] studies of the pressures applied to plugging instruments and to the walls of canal preparations in both lateral condensation and vertical compaction;[13] studies of dimensional stability of a wide variety of root canal sealers;[23] as well as permeability studies of obturated root canal systems and extensive observation of teeth that were clinically treated in vivo and subsequently extracted for direct observation of the effectiveness of three-dimensional filling, both by scanning electron microscopy and by cleaning processes that allow direct observation of the effectiveness of the obturation procedures.[7]

What one achieves in this technique is an accurate duplication of the prepared root canal with uniformly compacted gutta percha. The amount of root canal sealer used should be minimal, should constitute no more than a microfilm, and should be evenly dispersed around the gutta percha fillings. "Lakes" of sealer, common in lateral condensation procedures, are avoided in this technique. The microfilm of sealer is measurable only in Angstrom units along most of the canal preparation.[9]

Accessory canals are either cleaned by direct entry with reamers and files or debrided by dissolution of substrate with sodium hypochlorite (previously described).[12] They are filled with gutta percha, with a combination of gutta percha and sealer, or with sealer alone.[7] The accessory canals are effectively filled with gutta percha more often than can be fully appreciated by those unfamiliar with the technique.

Acknowledgments

David A. Allison, D.M.D., and David L. Broweleit, D.D.S., assisted with the art work.

Richard Knopf, D.D.S., assisted with the manuscript preparation.

REFERENCES

1. Hess, W.: The Anatomy of the Root Canals of the Teeth of the Permanent Dentition, Part I. New York, Wm. Wood and Co., 1925.
2. Kuttler, Y.: Microscopic investigation of root apexes. J.A.D.A. 50:544, 1955.
3. Seltzer, S., Soltanoff, W., Bender, I. B., and Ziontz, M.: Biologic aspects of endodontics. Oral Surg. 22:375, 1966.
4. Cohen, S., and Burns, R.: Pathways of the Pulp, 2nd ed. St. Louis, The C. V. Mosby Co., 1980.
5. Schilder, H.: Cleaning and shaping the root canal. Dent. Clin. North Am. 18:269, 1974.
6. Black, G. V.: Operative Dentistry, 8th ed. Woodstock, Ill., Medico-Dental Publ., 1948.
7. West, J.: The Relationship between the three-dimensional Endodontic Seal and Endodontic Failures. Thesis, Boston University, 1975.
8. Grossman, L. I.: Endodontic Practice, 9th ed. Philadelphia, Lea and Febiger, 1978.
9. Casanova, F.: Understanding of Some Clinically Significant Physical Properties of Kerr Sealer through Investigation. Thesis, Boston University, 1975.
10. Allison, D., Weber, C., and Walton, R.: The influence of the method of canal preparation on the quality of apical and coronal obturation. J. Endo. 5:298, October, 1979.
11. Lifschitz, J.: Scanning Electron Microscope Study of the Warm Gutta Percha Technique. Thesis, Boston University, 1976.
12. Grey, G.: The Capabilities of Sodium Hypochlorite to Digest Organic Debris from Root Canals with Emphasis on Accessory Canals. Thesis, Boston University, 1970.
13. Cohen, J.: A Quantitative Analysis of the Forces and Pressures Generated Within the Root Canal System During Vertical Condensation of Warm Gutta Percha. Thesis, Boston University, 1974.
14. Goodman, A.: Thermo-Mechanical Properties of Gutta Percha. Thesis, Boston University, 1973.
15. Schilder, H.: Filling root canals in three dimensions. Dent. Clin. North Am. 11:723, 1967.
16. Shelton, W.: Thermo-Mechanical Properties of Trans-1,4 Polyisoprene. Thesis, Boston University, 1975.
17. Daughenbaugh, J.: A Scanning Electron Microscopic Evaluation of Sodium Hypochlorite in the Cleaning and Shaping of Human Root Canal Systems. Thesis, Boston University, 1980.
18. Auerbach, M.: The Systemic Use of Erythromycin to Prophylactically Control Endodontic Flare-Ups and the Anaerobic Status of the Exudate after Cleaning and Shaping. Thesis, Boston University, 1978.
19. Moskowitz, M.: Hydrolytic Enzymes in Endodontic Exudates, Thesis, Boston University, 1975.
20. Schein, B.: Endotoxins in Pulpal and Periapical Disease, Thesis, Boston University, 1973.
21. Fabio, M.: Root Canal Morphology of the Mandibular Second Premolar. Thesis, Boston University, 1980.
22. Smith, B.: Root Canal Morphology of the Maxillary First Molar: The Mesiobuccal Root. Thesis, Boston University, 1977.
23. Weiner, B.: A Comparative Study of Important Physical Properties of Various Root Canal Sealers. Thesis, Boston University, 1969.

4

Diffusion

DIFFUSION UPDATE

JAMES H. SHERARD JR., D.D.S.

INTRODUCTION AND HISTORY

The diffusion technique for preparing and filling of root canals has been advocated in varying forms for close to a century. Space does not permit a review of this history, which is very interesting. The history of endodontics alone is quite a compliment to the dental profession as a whole because of its conservative efforts at prevention and its determination to assist patients in retaining their natural dentition.

John R. Callahan,[1] who practiced around the turn of the century, was one of the early advocates of diffusion and felt strongly that sealing of the accessory canals was of utmost importance to the success of treatment. Callahan and others used a diluted solution of sulfuric acid, flushed with sodium bicarbonate solution, thus utilizing the natural law of the diffusion of liquids to debride the entire root canal network. According to Harry B. Johnston, Sr.,[2] the law of diffusion states, "When two or more liquids capable of being mixed are placed together, a spontaneous exchange of molecules takes place in defiance of the law of gravity."

Johnston, who practiced a generation after Callahan, adopted the Callahan method and made several refinements during his early years of research in the 1920's. One of the major refinements was in the canal sealing technique. Callahan used alcohol to displace moisture, followed by heated wires to completely dry or dehydrate the canals. Johnston modified the technique when he discovered that the diffusion action of the chlororesin was enhanced when a trace of alcohol was left; he thus eliminated the use of the hot wires and dehydration of the canals.

Johnston has been credited with being the first dentist to limit his practice to endodontics. He also coined the term "endodontics" and had on his stationery in 1929 "Endodontia Exclusively." Since that time the diffusion technique has been referred to by many as the Johnston-Callahan, or modified Callahan, technique. Johnston made other modifications, such as reducing the strength of the acid solution from 50% to 20% by volume and refining the canal preparation technique.

It seems logical that if it is important to seal the main canal, it is also important to seal every external opening possible. At present I feel the diffusion technique offers a very good opportunity to accomplish this. We naturally should continue our efforts to develop improvements, and I am confident that each generation will do so.

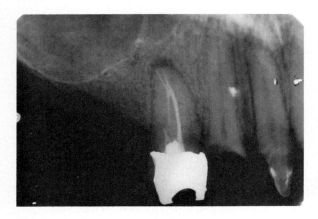

Figure 4–1 Only one canal was located and instrumented in an upper first bicuspid. This unusual canal network is adequately sealed by diffusion, after being adequately debrided by diffusion.

Further modifications have been made by utilizing the many improvements in instruments, materials, and the knowledge gained from the outstanding research during the past few decades. Every effort will be made to explain the technique as it is used in my practice, as well as my philosophy in caring for the endodontic patient.

First, it must be emphasized that the basic principle of thorough debridement and complete sealing of all external canal openings is as sound today as it was when advocated by our predecessors almost a century ago and should be applied to every technique.

Many have modified the diffusion technique to best adapt it to their skills. Basically the technique utilizes the ability of one solution to diffuse into the preceding solution, thus cleansing, debriding, and sealing accessory canals and crevices that could not be reached mechanically, as well as treating the main canal.

Figures 4–1 and 4–2 show the value of the diffusion technique in the treatment of problem cases as well as the so-called routine cases.

The following is a quote from Johnston's presentation read before the Section on Operative Dentistry at the Midwinter Clinic of the Chicago

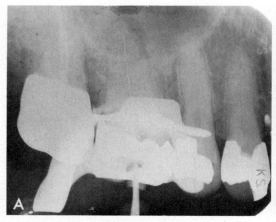
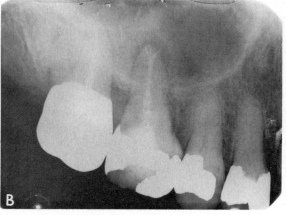

Figure 4–2 An upper first molar with questionable prognosis because of calcified or restriced canals. This main canal and several accessory canals are well sealed, so a favorable prognosis should be expected. *A,* One canal has been located and prepared. *B,* Several apical accessory canals are well filled, demonstrating the value of diffusion.

Dental Society, February 3, 1931. This paper was later published in the Journal of the American Dental Association, October 1931.

This quote pertains to the use of 30% sulfuric acid utilized by Callahan and others:

Dr. Callahan contended that, "It is a practical impossibility to really clean the canal walls of the average tooth except by chemical means." I am convinced that this contention is supported by fact. It is admitted by students of dental anatomy that a canal which is perfectly round throughout its entire length or even any considerable portion of its length, is an anatomic accident. This being the case, even the incisors and cuspids cannot be cleaned with round instruments unless their canals are enlarged sufficiently to render them practically or entirely round. Even when this is done the canal walls cannot be perfectly cleaned of the scrapings, filings or debris from grinding, except by chemical means.

With bicuspids and molars the difficulty of mechanical cleansing becomes even more nearly impossible. The canals become broader and flatter, the roots more curved, rendering reaming out of the question. These canals often are so broad and flat that even if they were straight, they could not be reamed into rounded form without perforating the side.

There is much theoretic objection to the use of sulfuric acid, but this is due either to its abuse or to a lack of accurate knowledge as to its action. Only by the grossest overinstrumentation can any of the acid be carried through the canal. If the instrument is passed entirely through the canal and into the apical tissues, the acid on the instrument will be wiped off by the tissues and retained, but free acid, that is acid not attached to the file, will not be forced through. This is contrary to what seems to be the popular conception, but is perfectly true. Remember, 30% sulphuric acid will not diffuse into tissue, but should it come in contact with tissue, quickly forms a thin coagulum which completely bars its further progress. This applies also to its penetration of dentin, for there it converts the surface calcium into calcium sulphate, which is insoluble, and thereby limits its action to the area being curetted by the operator.

An understanding of the above is important because of certain misconceptions pertaining to the diffusion technique as it is used today. It is important to realize that these outstanding pioneers in the field of endodontics were concerned about the necessity for extreme care and skill in the treatment of all tissues. Even with our continuing efforts to improve technique and avoid periapical irritation, we must recognize that any surgical procedure is traumatic to the tissue cells involved. The simplest cavity preparation requires the skillful use of high speed rotary drills or the careful manipulation of a hand-held excavator. In medicine, the suturing of a laceration or the setting of a fractured bone requires the utmost skill if excess trauma to the involved tissue cells is to be avoided. As trained professionals in the highly skilled and demanding field of dentistry, we should be capable of using both topical and systemic medications, as well as highly sophisticated instruments, with the utmost care. We should not delegate certain procedures to anyone less skilled than our professional training requires. If we, as dentists, feel we are incapable of using certain medicaments or fulfilling the requirements of certain techniques, we should recognize these limitations and refer the patient to someone who is capable or is specially trained.

The philosophy of the diffusion technique, even after three quarters of a century, continues to stress an abundance of care and gentle treatment of the tissues involved.

Much progress has been made in minimizing the use of irritating medicaments, and we must continue our search for improved medications.

We must recognize that removal of diseased tissue cells often requires a certain amount of trauma to adjacent vital tissue cells. The surgeon who removes a cancerous lesion certainly has no hesitancy in extending his surgical procedure into surrounding vital tissue, since the expected favorable results warrant it.

I am convinced that the dental profession is superior to most medical fields in our constant efforts to minimize trauma to the tissues we deal with. However, we should weigh the advantages of certain medications or solutions, even when some temporary tissue irritation is to be expected, against the ultimate result. A certain amount of common sense must accompany our skill. It is sometimes advantageous to use a medication that may cause some temporary irritation to tissues involved. The end result often warrants this. We naturally should be aware of the irritating factor and exert the special care required. It has been shown that the careless application of the most commonly used solution, sodium hypochlorite, will produce more tissue irritation than 20% sulfuric acid if left in contact with tissue too long. The sodium hypochlorite will also cause deterioration of the rubber dam and is more corrosive on the root canal instruments. Both solutions have proved to be valuable aids, and we should be just as capable of using these as we are of using our high speed equipment, x-ray machines, and prescribed medications. Certainly some of the reactions from antibiotics, for example, present more complications than the above solutions do.

We deal with people as a whole, rather than with just their periapical and pulpal tissues. Our efforts, therefore, must be directed toward providing every consideration for our patients' welfare.

PHILOSOPHY

The golden rule should be applied to all aspects of dentistry, meaning "we should treat every patient as we would want our personal dentist to treat us."

First, the patient should understand what is to be done, what results are to be expected, and should generally be put at ease. Understandings avoid misunderstandings. Good communication and an abundance of TLC will make a more satisfactory experience for the doctor and the patient. This basically is our philosophy.

Every effort should be made to eliminate discomfort. The generous use of the improved local anesthetics permits this. With the use of topical anesthetics, sharp needles, slow injections, and an abundance of TLC, the patient's visit to our office can be a pleasant surprise, as opposed to the misconception that it will be an unpleasant ordeal.

TECHNIQUE

Adequate access is essential for every technique. The rubber dam should be used in all cases. It not only provides an aseptic field, but protects against a dropped instrument, which the patient could swallow or aspirate. The dam and the clamp should be carefully applied so that no leakage will occur. If the clamp does not fit snugly or if one wall of the tooth is missing, the clamp can be built up or reinforced with warmed temporary stopping (Fig. 4–3).

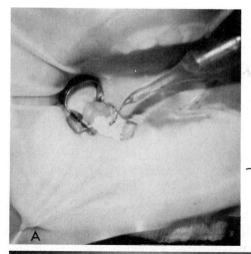

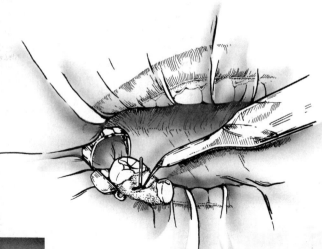

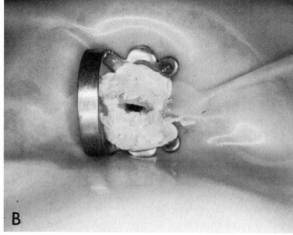

Figure 4–3 *A*, A lower second bicuspid with the crown fractured off, making clamp retention difficult. A clamp is placed on the first molar and the bicuspid is sealed off with temporary stopping. *B*, An upper central incisor with the incisal half and the lingual cusp fractured off below the gingival margin. The warmed temporary stopping stabilizes the clamp and seals against leakage.

The reinforcement with temporary stopping prevents leakage of any saliva into the fields of operation and of any solutions into the patient's mouth, which could be distasteful and irritating to the tissues. The stopping is easily removed before removing the clamp.

Of course, if time and conditions permit, the build-up of the tooth with temporary cement, or whatever method you may choose, would be more desirable. Often a patient is being seen as an emergency, and the condition or time available does not permit the more permanent build-up, which may be accomplished later. In these cases we find the temporary stopping to be very expedient.

Every technique is based on a philosophy. This philosophy affects our thinking and our approach to basic steps, so it is important to alter our thinking as we use different techniques.

In the debridement of canals, some use reamers more than files, or vice versa, but our thinking must be altered with each instrument. The term "reamer" indicates that we should use a reaming or rotating motion with the instrument, whereas the term "file" indicates that an up-and-down filing motion is needed. Any rotation action used with either instrument should be minimal, and extreme care must be taken.

In the filling of canals, we think in terms of condensation, whether this is lateral or vertical or a combination of both. If we think of "packing" the canal space, this denotes pressure.

To establish the proper philosophy when utilizing the diffusion technique, we recommend thinking in terms of "easy-does-it." While debriding and preparing the canal, files and reamers should be used with a gentle touch — *never* with force. These instruments are always used with a lubricant or irrigating solution, starting with the smallest file (or at least a smaller file than the natural lumen of the canal) and gradually working up to the desired size.

Before starting any canal preparation, it is assumed that profound anesthesia has been obtained, the rubber dam is in place, an adequate access opening has been prepared, and all debris has been removed from the pulp chamber so that the canal openings may be located.

If vital or highly inflamed pulp tissue is present and there is any question about profound anesthesia, we inject a few drops of the local anesthetic directly into the pulp tissue and work this into the canal with a small file. Here again "easy-does-it" should be the approach and, with an abundance of TLC, any discomfort is rapidly eliminated. The pulp tissue or any degenerating remnants are removed very carefully with a small barbed broach. In some cases the entire segment is removed intact. If not, the remaining remnants are removed by means of the biomechanical preparation that is to follow.

We flush the pulp chamber with 3% hydrogen peroxide followed by 5.25% sodium hypochlorite. This helps control the bleeding and will minimize the objectionable putrescent odor, when present.

Canal Access, Debridement, and Canal Preparation

Basically, adequate access is essential. The canal opening is located and gradually funneled in the first few millimeters of the coronal portions. In some cases it is necessary to start with a #10 file, then gradually enlarge with a small reamer, an orifice opener, and eventually with Gates-Glidden drills.

Our thinking should always be "easy-does-it"; be patient and avoid the temptation to use force. This will prevent the creation of ledges or perforations, which eventually will require considerable wasted time or even fatal complications to the tooth. "Easy-does-it" and patience are the best ways to prevent broken files. Since the beginning of dentistry, we have all had to worry about the problem of the broken instrument. The ultimate solution is "do not break it." Recommended precautions are to use the best quality instruments available, never force them, and discard the ones that have been bent sharply, show flute distortion, or have been used in a tortuous canal for some time. If in doubt, discard and select a new instrument. Filing in a moist or lubricated canal minimizes stress on the instrument, so frequent flushing of the canal is highly recommended.

Assuming it is necessary to start with a #10 file, a rubber stop is placed on the file to the estimated length that will reach the dentino-cemental junction. An accurate radiograph is essential to make this estimation. Measure from the incisal edge, the tip of the most visible cusp, or the edge of the access opening. This reference point may vary with different teeth but should be the most visible point for constant checking.

Before starting any actual canal preparation, place a few drops of sodium hypochlorite in the pulp chamber or canals; then very carefully work the small file to the estimated dentino-cemental junction. This may be 1 to 2 mm short of the radiographic apex. With experience, this restriction often can be determined by digital feel and interpretation. A radiograph is made and the necessary adjustment is recorded. In some cases, a subsequent film and adjustment may be necessary. The rubber stop placed on the file should correspond to the selected reference point or may need to be adjusted according to feel. Many years ago one of my colleagues stated during a presentation — ''I would never proceed past the dentino-cemental junction in debriding or filling the canal *if* I were clever enough to always be able to determine this junction.''

We certainly subscribe to this objective and strive to accomplish it, recognizing our inability to always succeed. Our thinking should be in terms of debriding the entire canal network and not just enlargement of the main canal. While debriding and preparing the main canal, every effort should be made to maintain the integrity of the constriction at the dentino-cemental junction. This constriction can usually be determined by digital feel if a certain amount of concentration is used. Once this terminal point is determined and this measurement is recorded, carefully position rubber stops on subsequent files so that the periapical tissues are not unduly traumatized. We rarely use reamers to this point, because there is some curvature in most canals before this point is reached, and reamers are more likely to create a ledge. The files are used in an up-and-down motion, attempting to remove all debris that may be attached to the walls of the canal and eventually establishing a smooth, polished surface to the entire lumen. The flushing action of the irrigating solutions is constantly removing tissue fragments and filings.

After the initial use of the sodium hypochlorite and peroxide, the canals are dried with suction or paper absorbent points. A small portion of ethylenediamine tetra-acetic acid (EDTA) and urea peroxide in a water-soluble glycol base is placed at the mouth of the coronal opening and then worked into the canal or canals with a gentle filing motion. This preparation was developed by Stewart and associates[3] and is marketed under the trade name R-C Prep.* R-C Prep works as an excellent lubricant as the canal is gradually shaped to the desired size. In small canals we start with a #10 file and gradually work up to a #20 or #25, allowing only the tip of the file to slightly penetrate the dentino-cemental junction. Of course, some apical foramina will be larger to begin with, in which case we strive to cleanse or debride the foramen but not to enlarge it. The larger the foramen, the more difficult it is to obtain a tight seal and at the same time avoid overextension of the filling material. As the filing and preparation of the canal progress, we should strive to establish a *mental picture* of the size and shape of the main canal. This helps in the selection of our master filling point as well as providing a better idea as to how many additional points may be needed.

Every few minutes we irrigate the canal with a concentrated solution of sodium bicarbonate. We find that the effervescent action of the R-C Prep and sodium bicarbonate is more active, or explosive, than the mild effervescence of the sodium hypochlorite and peroxide. To enhance the effervescent action, 1 or 2 drops of 20% sulfuric acid (by volume) may be added to

---

*Premier Dental Supply Co., Philadelphia, Pa.

the R-C Prep. This, of course, increases the diffusion action in accessory canals, crevices, and dentinal tubules. The coronal half of the canal should be enlarged or funneled so as to enhance the entry and positioning of the gutta percha points. In this part of the canal we use the reamers very carefully, as well as the orifice openers and Gates-Glidden drills.

With the exception of the normally larger canals, we strive to keep the apical opening to a size #25 or smaller. Beyond the size #20 file there is practically no flexibility in the tip of the file, even when the tip is curved or flexed. The danger of creating a ledge or perforation increases rapidly as the size of the file increases.

Once the canals are debrided and shaped to the desired size, the last solution used is removed with absorbent points. In our case this would be sodium bicarbonate or sodium hypochlorite.

The canal medication of choice is placed and sealed with temporary cement until the next appointment, or if the canal is ready for filling, we proceed accordingly.

A loose pellet of cotton is moistened, but not saturated, with the medication of choice and is then placed in the pulp chamber. We use Cresanol,* which has proved to be very effective clinically. The coronal opening is sealed with Cavit,* which is ready mixed and provides an adequate seal in most cases.

The condition of the tooth, the comfort of the patient, and the time involved dictate the number of appointments required.

If a tooth has been prepared during a previous appointment and a treatment has been sealed, we proceed at the filling appointment as follows: adequate anesthesia is obtained, the rubber dam is placed, and the cement and cotton dressing are removed. The canals are dried with paper points and again cleansed with R-C Prep, using a carefully measured file one size smaller than the largest file used in the preparation. After a few seconds the preparation is flushed with the sodium bicarbonate solution; then the canals are dried with paper points. If there is any question, the procedure is repeated until the canals are clean and dry. We then proceed with the sealing of the canal network.

Canal Sealing

All solutions used in the debridement up to this point have been aqueous. It is essential to remove this moisture before placing the chlororesin, which is the solvent used to assist in the adaptation of the gutta percha cones or points. Chlororesin and moisture are like oil and water — they will not mix or diffuse.

To accomplish this, several drops of pure 95% grain alcohol are placed in the pulp chamber, and with gentle agitation of a small file, the alcohol will diffuse into all crevices, absorbing any trace of moisture that may be present. The solvent used to assist in adapting the gutta percha is a mixture of chloroform and rosin. Chloroform will not diffuse into any trace of moisture, but will diffuse into alcohol. The alcohol absorbs the moisture, thus acting as a very important link in the diffusion process. The alcohol is

---

*Premier Dental Supply Co., Philadelphia, Pa.

allowed to remain for several minutes. During this period the master gutta percha point is selected and in some cases may be tried in. Ideally the tip of the point should meet resistance 1 or 2 mm short of the dentino-cemental junction, provided the constriction at this junction has not been destroyed by overenlargement. The majority of canals may be prepared to the dentino-cemental junction with a #25 file. If more than a slight curvature is present in the apical third, it is necessary to prepare this opening with a curved or flexed #20 file or, in extreme cases, a #15 file. As these flexed files work back and forth through this curved area, they actually make the opening larger than the size of the file. During this time it is important to establish a clear mental picture of the opening you plan to adapt the gutta percha to. This mental picture is very valuable in selecting the proper-sized master gutta percha point.

If the apical opening is larger than the #25 file, the standard gutta percha points are used, selecting one size larger than the largest file used. Example: If #25 was the largest file used to open the apical stricture, we select a #30 gutta percha point. If a #30 file was used, we probably would select a #40 gutta percha point, provided it does not bind in the main body of the canal. The larger the apical opening, the more demanding the selection of the proper point will be. This step requires practice and experience and never allows you to become complacent. For some unusually large canals, it may be necessary to roll a special point (Fig. 4–4).

To minimize inventory of gutta percha points, the great majority of canals could be sealed by using the regular-sized points, fine-fine, fine, and fine-medium. Experience helps in determining how much of the tapered tip should be cut off, so that the tip of the point will correspond to the standardized points of #30, #40, #50, and so on.

Utilizing the standardized points #30, #40, #50, and so forth does make it possible for the auxiliaries to be of more help in selecting and premeasuring the points to be used for each canal. It is important for the dentist to make the final decision and adjustment of the master point because he is the only one who has a mental picture of the shape and size of the canal.

A minimum selection of the standardized points #60 through #120 should be available.

When the canals are smaller than #25, such as the mesial canals of lower molars, upper first bicuspids, buccal canals of upper molars, lower anteriors, and partially calcified canals that may be encountered in any tooth, we usually select a size fine-fine regular gutta percha point and trim off the fine tapered tip to be slightly larger than the tip of the #20 or #15 file, which has been used because of its flexibility. This flexibility of the file allows you to maneuver the curves and avoid perforations. Even in these small canals, we are able to enlarge the coronal portion of the canal, which allows us to position these small flexible gutta percha points. Of course it requires a more gentle touch and a little more practice. It may also require the use of a plugger, usually a finger plugger, to vertically condense and encourage the diffusion in these more restricted areas.

Here again we must adjust our thinking compared with our thinking in other techniques. For instance, if you were to use a sealer and expect to seat the master point to the end of the canal, you should select a point that corresponds to the same size as the largest file used.

With the diffusion method we are using a solvent of chlororesin (a

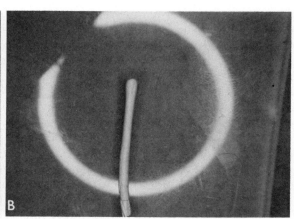

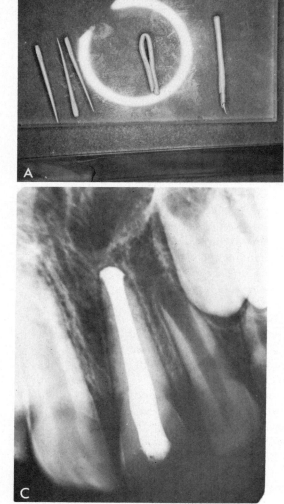

Figure 4–4 *A, B,* and *C,* Several large gutta percha points are placed on a warm agate slab and with a warm agate spatula are rolled into a 30 to 40 mm rope. This is doubled over and rolled to the special size needed. Some gentle lateral condensation and additional points to fill the coronal portion of the canal should provide an adequate solution to one of endodontics' more difficult problems.

mixture of chloroform and rosin). Chlororesin is mixed by adding enough rosin to a small amount of chloroform to give a very light golden color. We use a 30 ml bottle with a ground-glass stopper. This tapered ground-glass dropper seals the bottle each time you replace it. Even so, a certain amount of chloroform evaporates, so it may be necessary to add additional chloroform occasionally to maintain the very light color and thin consistency. If it is too sticky (thick), it will not soften the periphery of the gutta percha point enough to adapt to the irregularity of the canal or diffuse into the accessory canals.

Chlororesin, when thin (as it should be), has very little surface tension, so extra care must be used in carrying it from the dispensing bottle to the tooth. We recommend using a 3 ml Luer-Lok type syringe with a 5/8 inch 25 gauge needle. More than 1 ml of solution will rarely be needed, and usually less will be required, since only a few drops are needed to fill the canal network.

Since the chlororesin has so little surface tension, it is recommended that a 2 × 2 gauze sponge be held at the tip of the syringe, so that it cannot accidentally spill on the patient's clothing or face. We recommend this precaution when carrying all solutions from the working area to the tooth.

This solvent combines with the periphery of the firm gutta percha point, making a sticky mixture of chloroform, rosin, and gutta percha. By this softening action of the periphery of the point, the mixture will adapt to the irregular shape of the canal. The inner core of the gutta percha point remains firm, which allows it to move past the point of resistance. The coronal end of the point is crimped or cut off to correspond with the established measurement. When this crimped mark is even with the point of reference on the incisal edge or cusp tips, the apical end of the point should be seated at the dentino-cemental junction. During this gentle agitation and seating of the master point, a thin mixture of chloroform-rosin and gutta percha is formed. This diffuses into the dentinal tubules, crevices, and lateral canals.

Robert P. Bethea,[4] in his research project as a graduate student, under the direction of Herbert Schilder,[5] demonstrated that dentinal tubules and minute accessory canals were sealed with rosin as well as chloropercha (Fig. 4–5).

Bethea made a detailed study of the history of the diffusion technique and quoted John R. Callahan's contention that

> Chlororesin was superior to chloropercha as a solvent for adaptation of the master gutta percha point in three ways:
>
> 1. The rosin penetrates deeply into the tubuli and foramina, leaving a solid, inert, insoluble substance when the chloroform evaporates — that seals the tubuli and foramina.
> 2. The rosin and chloroform cause the gutta percha to adhere closely to the walls of the root canal.
> 3. The incorporation of rosin makes an unshrinkable and impervious mass about the gutta percha cone.

Bethea also quoted Harry B. Johnston, Sr., who claimed that "his modification of the Callahan method, later referred to as the Johnston-Callahan Diffusion Technique, made it not only possible, but easy to fill and hermetically seal canals that were before considered impossible."

This filling stage in the procedure calls for "easy-does-it" as much as any other step. We are striving to *adapt* the filling material rather than *pack* the filling material, so through the years revisions have been made in this step. Originally the point was carefully selected, gently pumped or agitated to place as described, and then condensed vertically with appropriate

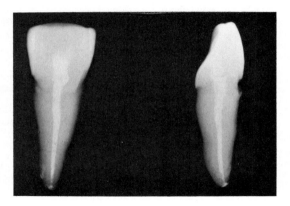

Figure 4–5 Mesio-distal and bucco-lingual view of central incisor filled by diffusion. The photomicrograph (× 100) shows excellent adaptation of the gutta percha to the main canal as well as a minute accessory canal filled with rosin.

pluggers. We then altered this procedure by using lateral condensation after the first point with a #3 spreader and adding the necessary extra points to fill the coronal portion of the canal.

To minimize pressure even more, as well as to minimize the occasional overextention, we have altered the procedure further by *not* using the plugger or spreader immediately after placing the master point. I refer to the way we used to do it because there has been very little published in the last decade or so about diffusion. Many were hesitant to try the diffusion technique because numerous misconceptions and lack of a clear understanding of its principles discouraged its use. Many also felt it was a difficult procedure to learn and had difficulty working with the filling material in its tacky or sticky form because they were thinking in terms of "packing" or "condensing" rather than adaptation.

Any technique requires a thorough understanding, followed by a certain amount of practice to develop the skill. An accomplished musician or a star athlete is certainly not the result of a few lessons or an all-day course. Many do not have the talent or temperament to be an athlete or a musician but could be a fine surgeon or attorney. There are many fine endodontists who would not excel as general practitioners and vice versa. Therefore, many may find a different technique more adaptable to their skills. We feel that this technique offers another choice and are presenting it as a modality that has proved to be very successful for many years. This is the way we have refined the diffusion technique, having had a very sound foundation to build on.

With the above explanation and a *mental picture* of how the point is adapted to the irregular-shaped canal, we will recapitulate by starting at the step at which the canal has been flooded with 95% alcohol and proceed

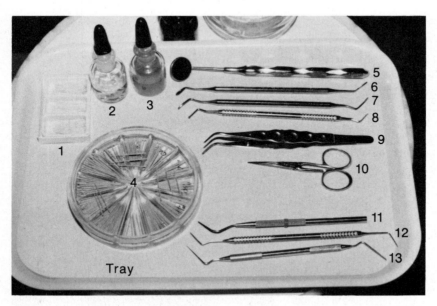

Figure 4–6 Tray set-up for canal sealing. *1*, Absorbent points; *2*, Alcohol (95%); *3*, Chlororesin; *4*, Gutta percha dish (points have been selected, measured, and positioned to fill a lower molar); *5*, Mouth mirror; *6*, Glick #1 (Starlight); *7*, Glick #2 (Starlight); *8*, Double end excavator (Starlight #32); *9*, Cotton tweezers (151 G., Emil Huber); *10*, Buttonhole scissors; *11*, Shortened plugger (made by cutting off a bent or used #3 spreader); *12*, Double end explorer (sometimes used as a spreader when access is difficult); *13*, Sherard #1 (Premierlite) (has a short #3 spreader on one end and a plugger, approximate size #6 or #7, on the other).

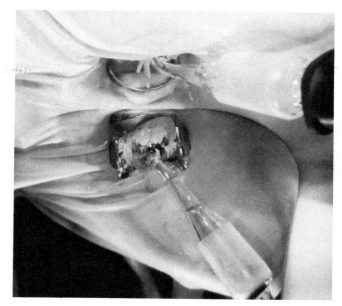

Figure 4–7 Upper first molar with extensive distal cavity. This has been built up with temporary stopping, which also surrounds the tooth at the junction of the clamp. This insures a good seal and prevents any leakage of the solutions into the patient's mouth. Paper points have been placed in each canal and serve as a wick in carrying the thin chlororesin into each canal.

through each step of sealing the canal, as we currently utilize the power of diffusion. The tray set-up is shown in Figure 4–6.

While the canal, or canal network, is flooded with alcohol, we use these few minutes to select and accurately measure the master gutta percha point. We actually select and measure two, and sometimes three, points for each canal. The points are then placed on an appropriate part of the treatment tray for ready access. Having the extra points already measured saves time in case the first point is inadvertently bent or dropped. The extra points can then be used as supplementary points.

The excess alcohol is now removed with absorbent points but not to the degree of dehydration. After the excess alcohol is removed, an extra fine paper point is placed in each canal. The pulp chamber is then filled with chlororesin. The paper points become saturated, serving as a wick and thus carrying the chlororesin to the apical opening of the canal. Of course, capillary attraction and the power of diffusion play a major role in this step. Using the paper points as a wick is particularly helpful in upper molars because the chlororesin has very little surface tension, and care must be used not to flood the pulp chamber to overflowing, since the chloroform softens the rubber dam and could result in leakage. Care and skill are required here, as with the use of so many of the materials and medicaments that we work with. A few additional drops of chlororesin are added as the paper points are removed. This fills the canals with the solvent (Fig. 4–7).

The master point is then selected and gently placed in the canal, accompanied by a gentle pumping motion. This gentle agitation of the point should start before the tip of the point encounters any resistance from the canal wall. Once this gentle motion is started, it should not stop, because the sticky periphery will bind against the wall. With only a few pumping movements, you should be able to seat the point according to the exact measurement. If measured and selected accurately, the crimp mark on the coronal end of the point should correspond to the reference point on the tooth, such as the incisal edge, cusp tip, and so on. The tip of the point should be seated at the dentino-cemental junction.

There is no way to describe how much pressure to use in positioning the master point. It must be gentle, yet steady. If too much apical pressure is used, the point may bend or buckle in the midsection. The gentle up and down motion is not rapid but is steady, keeping in mind that you are gently softening the periphery of the gutta percha point in the chlororesin solvent so that the firm inner core of the point can assist you in adapting the entire gutta percha–chlororesin mass as near to the dentino-cemental junction as possible.

If the canal is large, the amount of pumping action may require only one or two strokes to position the point at the apical opening. If the canal is curved or narrow, a smaller point is used, and this may require a more gentle "easy-does-it" approach. If the point has been selected properly for size and measured accurately, the gentle pumping stroke will allow you to work it to place with a minimum of pressure. Here too, you must adjust your thinking, because when the term "pumping motion" is used, most of us naturally think of a vigorous forward and backward movement. Actually the forward and backward stroke should be as minimal in each direction as possible. If you try to seat the point with force, there is the chance of bending the point or not allowing the periphery of the terminal millimeter or so to soften sufficiently to adapt to the irregular shape of the dentino-cemental junction. Think in terms of adapting a pliable material to a mold, similar to developing an inlay pattern. Pliable is defined in the dictionary as "easily influenced," thus "easy-does-it." By using this gentle motion combined with the tacky surface tension of the chloropercha-rosin combination, we are not forcing the solvent of chlororesin through the apical opening nor are we exerting undue pressure on the periapical area.

Once the master point is adapted, we now add the necessary supplementary points as needed. Here again it is necessary to adjust our thinking and utilize our *mental picture* as to what we are trying to accomplish. A certain amount of finesse is required. Using our mental picture, we determine that a tapered size *fine* gutta percha point will gently wedge beside the master point to approximately 3 to 4 mm short of the measured apical opening. This *fine* point may enter easily; therefore you determine another point is needed. You then enter gently alongside this point, using the small #15 or #20 file and a few more drops of chlororesin, to approximately 5 to 6 mm short of the overall measurement; then you may place a medium gutta percha point in this space. Of course, each case is different, but the mental picture that you have established helps you select the proper-sized points. It is *very important* to remember that these supplementary points are placed with a firm apical insertion, and *not* with the pumping motion used with the master point. If a pumping motion is used, it may pull the master point backward, thus disturbing the apical seal. As additional points are added, they exert a gentle lateral and vertical pressure that enhances the diffusion action of the filling material into any accessory canals that may be present.

With multiple canals the most distal canal is filled first, then the next most distal, and finally the canal nearest to the point of entry. For example, on a lower right first molar, fill the distal, then the mesio-lingual, and finally the mesio-buccal. Exceptions are often necessary, such as first filling the canal that is most difficult to locate or gain access to. For example, the most difficult canal may be the mesio-buccal canal of an upper second molar in a small mouth. Every technique should be flexible enough to allow for the necessary alteration in the treatment plan to accommodate each individual case. Using the lower first molar as an example, I would proceed as follows: Flood all three canals with chlororesin, adapt the master point to the distal canal, and add a supplementary-sized fine point. If my mental picture indicates a third point, or possibly that this distal root has two canals, an additional supplementary point may be added. This usually requires only a minute or so. If more time has been required, I might add another drop or two of chlororesin to the two mesial canals and then proceed by adapting the master point to the mesio-lingual canal, followed by a supplementary-sized fine-fine or fine point. The excess gutta percha may be removed with a heated plastic instrument or excavator so as to eliminate any interference in adapting the master points in the mesio-buccal canal. An extra drop of chlororesin may be added if indicated; then the master point is adapted, followed by an auxiliary point.

At this stage a radiograph is made to determine how well the filling is adapted. If all has gone well, remove the excess gutta percha in the pulp chamber and gently condense the filling material in the coronal portion of the canal with a root canal plugger only slightly smaller than the coronal opening. The type of case will determine whether to use a long handle or a finger plugger. This condensing pressure should be gentle, so that undue pressure is not exerted on the apical seal. By allowing the apical filling material a few minutes to "set" while making and developing the radiographic film, the chance of overfilling is minimized. The larger the apical opening, the more care in vertical and/or lateral condensation is required. The apical opening is considered large if it has been prepared large enough to accommodate a size #40 or greater master cone.

If measurements have been accurate, if correct judgment was used in the selection of the master point, and if execution was correct in positioning the points with a reasonable amount of skill, the radiograph will reveal a well-sealed root canal network, as shown in Figures 4–8 and 4–9. This should result in a very favorable prognosis.

On occasion the radiograph will indicate that the body of the canal needs additional condensation. To correct this we first insert the #3 spreader either mesial or distal to the main body of the filling. As the spreader is inserted, it should be rotated back and forth while exerting gentle pressure on the back of the spreader with the middle finger of the free hand. We try to keep the spreader point in contact with one wall of the canal, rather than going through the middle of the filling. If the apical end is sealed now, this lateral condensation should not disturb this seal, because it has had several minutes to set while the film is being developed and checked. A few drops of chlororesin are gently worked into this space made by the spreader. This is done with a #15 or #20 file. The appropriate-sized gutta percha point is then inserted. The excess gutta percha is removed, followed by gentle condensation with a plugger. *If this lateral condensation with the spreader is done before the apical portion of the filling has had a few minutes to harden, there is more chance of overextention.*

If by chance the filling is short of the estimated apical opening, the measurement is double checked and corrected if necessary. This usually indicates an error in measurement, selection of too large a point, or too much pressure exerted in adapting the master point, causing it to buckle or bend rather than soften and adapt. In any event it indicates that additional softening and condensation are needed. The measurement stop is adjusted on a small file, size #15 or #20, and a few drops of chlororesin are worked

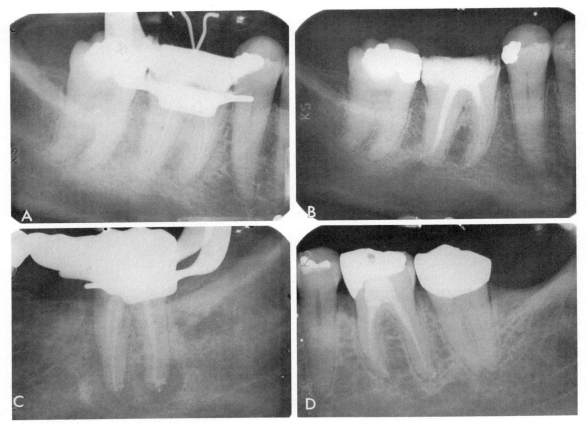

Figure 4–8 *A*, Mandibular molar well sealed by adaptation only. Mesial canals were filled with a standardized #30, one fine-fine, and one fine gutta percha point. At this stage no spreader or plugger has been used. *B*, Mandibular molar canals, being very fine and curved, were shaped and enlarged up to size #20 file in the mesial canals and a #25 file in the distal canals. Working with the curved flexible file actually enlarges the opening by one or two sizes. The master gutta percha point must be selected accordingly. *C*, #30 gutta percha points were used as master points in the mesial canals. A #40 point, plus the necessary supplementary points, was used in the distal canals. Minimal vertical condensation was used. *D*, Note filled accessory canal opening to mesial canal slightly apical to mid-root. No lateral condensation was necessary other than that obtained by the insertion of supplementary points.

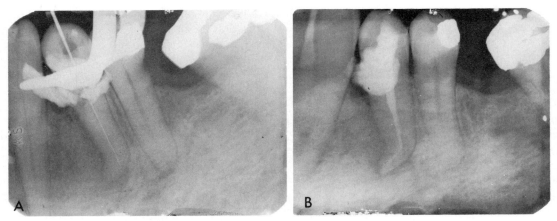

Figure 4–9 *A*, Mandibular bicuspid with sharply curved, fine canal. Maneuvering curvature with file was not possible; therefore, stopped at this point rather than risk a perforation. *B*, Diffusion plus gentle lateral and vertical condensation provided a very good seal.

into the space made by the spreader. This time, however, the file must be worked all the way to the apical opening, thus creating a pliable mixture of chlororesin and gutta percha. A supplementary gutta percha point is inserted into this space. Usually the tapered size fine gutta percha point is the point of choice, but the size of the canal may dictate that one size smaller or larger would be better. Each time the spreader is used, a certain amount of vertical as well as lateral condensation is exerted, so that the "easy-does-it" approach is very important during this stage (Fig. 4–10).

When this resoftening is necessary, there is more likelihood of developing some overextention, but we prefer this to an underfilled (more specifically an undersealed) canal in the majority of cases. The escaped material is thin chloropercha, most of which will be resorbed in time. It, of course, is not as cosmetically acceptable as we would like, but we have found that our success is far greater with a well-sealed canal, even with some overextention, than with the poorly sealed canal that may result with underfilling.

Figure 4–11 shows a variety of teeth in which the excess assured a complete seal of the irregularly shaped apical openings, but did not prevent excellent healing of the periapically involved area.

Accessory canals rarely can be seen on preoperative radiographs. Areas of periodontal ligament involvement often suggest the presence of an accessory canal and the final filling will confirm this when such canals are present (Figs. 4–12 and 4–13).

Many canals are properly cleansed, medicated, and rendered sterile; however, if they are not completely sealed, a high percentage of success cannot be expected.

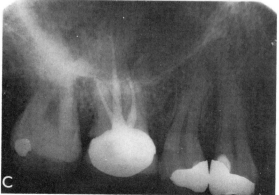
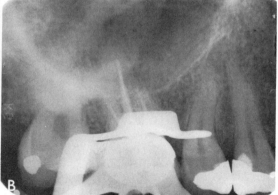
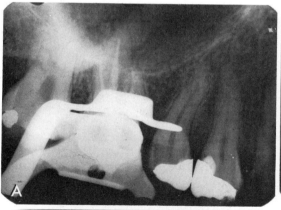

Figure 4–10 *A*, The check radiography of an upper first molar shows the lingual root to be incompletely filled. *B*, A #3 spreader is worked into the canal to make room for softening of the gutta percha and refilling. A #20 file is used for this, after carefully double checking the measurement. A few drops of chlororesin are worked into the canal with the file, then the carefully selected point is positioned as if it were the first point. In this case a size fine point with the apical 2 mm cut off was used, followed by a fine-medium supplementary point. *C*, Final radiograph showing all three canals well sealed.

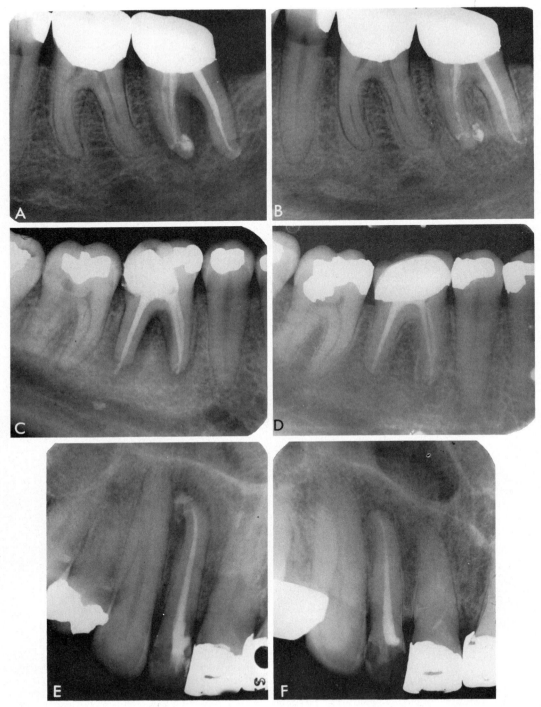

Figure 4–11 *A*, Lower second molar showing extensive periapical breakdown involving the entire bifurcation. The irregular apical foramen is well sealed, although there is some thin overfill. *B*, Two year follow-up radiograph shows excellent repair and some resorption of the overfill, which is well tolerated. *C*, Lower first molar showing overextension of distal filling point, but well sealed. *D*, Six year follow-up radiograph shows perfect repair and complete resorption of the overfill. *E*, Upper lateral incisor showing accessory canal and some thin overfill. *F*, Fourteen year follow-up radiograph shows perfect repair and complete resorption of overfill.

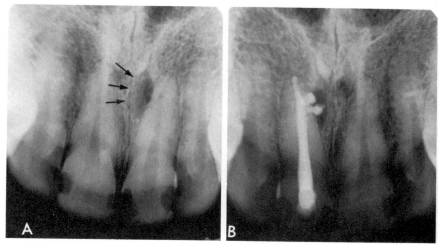

Figure 4–12 *A*, Preoperative radiograph of upper right central incisor suggests an accessory canal on mesial at junction of apical third. The location of the area of breakdown indicates this to be the main site of trouble. Arrows point to the bone lesion caused by the endodontic problem and indicate a probable accessory canal. *B*, Two large accessory canals confirm that this is the main site. It also emphasizes that all accessory canals are not small.

Figure 4–13 Accessory canals opening in the coronal half of the root often account for the perioendodontic problems. Sealing the accessory canal on the distal of this lower molar should enhance the prognosis.

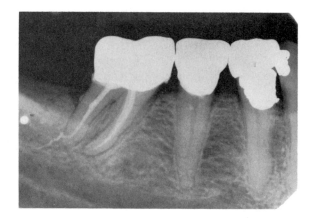

Figure 4–14 *A*, Incompletely filled upper central incisor. Apparently the point was measured accurately but lacks adaptation and did not seal the canal, which resulted in failure. The patient was referred to us for retreatment and the canal was completely sealed. *B*, Two year follow-up radiograph shows excellent healing.

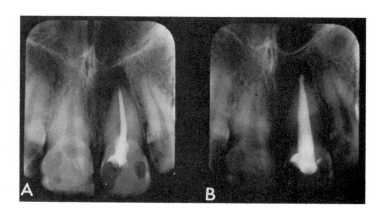

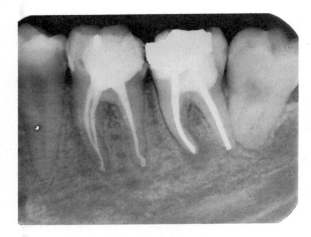

Figure 4–15 A lower first molar filled by diffusion, showing the adaptation of the gutta percha to the irregularly shaped canals. The second molar is filled with silver points after the canals were considerably enlarged.

Figure 4–14 shows a tooth that, according to the patient, was thoroughly debrided and rendered sterile after several appointments, which resulted in a negative culture. A year later periapical trouble recurred. Apparently the master point had been selected reasonably well as to size and length, but had not been properly adapted, thus failing to seal the canal. Obviously, supplementary points were needed but not used.

To expect the highest percentage of success, certain basic principles must be fulfilled, no matter which technique is used.

Figure 4–15 shows a second molar treated by another endodontist and a first molar treated by this author, using the diffusion technique. Both teeth should have a very favorable prognosis. Note the difference in canal preparation to accommodate the different filling techniques.

We make every effort to prepare and seal all canals to the dentino-cemental junction and feel slight overseal provides a higher percentage of success compared with underseal.

In the majority of cases, if the canals have been debrided and prepared properly and measured accurately and if the gutta percha points have been selected accurately and adapted with care, the canals will be well sealed without the worry of overfill or underfill, as shown in Figure 4–16. Practice is necessary to develop any skill or technique. This certainly is true with any endodontic procedure.

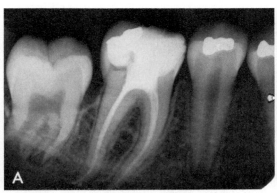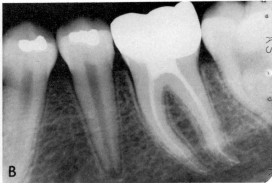

Figure 4–16 *A*, Lower first molar with long, curved, fine canals. *B*, Excellent adaptation and complete seal resulted in a very favorable prognosis, as shown on the 2 year follow-up radiograph.

PRACTICE FOR TECHNIQUE DEVELOPMENT

Debriding and filling extracted teeth allow you to observe the difference in the effervescent action of different combinations of solutions. Compare the gentle effervescence of sodium hypochlorite and peroxide, then R-C Prep and sodium hypochlorite, and then R-C Prep and sodium bicarbonate. Next you might add a drop or two of 20% sulfuric acid to the small portion of R-C Prep placed in the pulp chamber, use the file for 30 to 60 seconds, and then flush with sodium bicarbonate. This will allow you to observe the action more closely, and you may choose the combination that suits your needs best. The purpose of the effervescent action (which is the liberation of nascent oxygen) is to flush out filings, debris and so forth. The stronger the affinity of one solution for the preceding solution, the stronger the diffusion action will be.

Constant efforts are made to standardize many of our endodontic procedures, and we should continue to do so, but it will never be completely possible. Therefore, we must recognize the importance of perfecting our individual talents. One particular technique is certainly not the best choice for everyone. Most of us have found very valuable steps in other techniques, such as the warm gutta percha and the lateral condensation methods, which are adaptable to the procedure we may find most successful.

Many who utilize the diffusion technique may use a different combination of irrigating solutions in the debridement step and a different method for adapting the gutta percha, but the basic principles of thorough debridement and complete sealing of the entire root canal network are the same.

While practicing filling of canals by using extracted teeth, it wil help to understand how the chlororesin softens the periphery of the gutta percha cone by making a few in-and-out strokes with the cone and then removing it. This allows you to observe how the cone conforms to the irregular shape of the canal. Working with extracted teeth does not give the same feel, but does allow you to establish a better mental picture of what is taking place and what you are striving to accomplish.

POSTOPERATIVE CARE

Preparing the patient for the postoperative healing period is very important. Experience allows us to estimate healing time and the degree of postoperative discomfort to be expected.

Of course, some cases are unpredictable and errors will be made in judgment. If the effort has been made to explain this to patients, they will be prepared and much more understanding when unpredicted events arise.

We explain to all patients that endodontic treatment is a surgical procedure and as such some postoperative discomfort is to be expected during the 3 to 4 day to 1 week initial healing period. In some cases we explain how the repair process progresses during the 6 to 24 month period following treatment.

In most cases the discomfort will be controlled by one or two aspirin tablets, or the equivalent, at 3 to 4 hour intervals. If the history or condition indicates that a stronger analgesic is needed, we explain this in detail and prescribe accordingly. Usually one of the codeine preparations, ½ to 1 grain, or the equivalent, will be sufficient.

Antibiotics are not prescribed routinely but should be used in selected cases when indicated.

When in doubt, we prescribe for the greater need. If the need does not arise, both the patient and the doctor will be very happy.

If it is suspected that the patient may experience more than the minor discomfort or possibly some swelling, a follow-up phone call during the next 24 to 48 hours will pay tremendous dividends. Even though an explanation has been given, it will be reassuring to patients to know that we have a continuing interest in their welfare.

The patient is encouraged to have the crown portion restored as soon after the initial healing period as possible (1 or 2 weeks), so that this area may be returned to normal use.

Naturally, proper protection against crown fracture and careful adjustment of occlusion are essential for the comfort and longevity of any tooth, particularly an endodontically treated tooth.

Usually these teeth have not been used normally for several weeks, so that the supporting tissues have lost some of the tissue tone and toughness stimulated by use. When returned to the stress of mastication, they will naturally be tender. Hard, tough foods should be avoided at first. Even though some limping may be necessary, the patient should be encouraged to use this area to chew soft or semi-hard foods, which will stimulate the supporting tissues and re-establish the healthy tone and toughness needed for comfortable use.

We compare this return to use of the tooth to a sprained ankle or a broken limb that has been immobilized in a cast for some time. Once the ankle or limb is returned to use, it is tender or sore, but it must be used and exercised to work this soreness out. Limping, light use, and exercise are essential, but overuse should be avoided. This approach is recommended for a "lame" tooth as well.

Fulfilling the following basic principles is very important:

1. An aseptic technique.
2. Complete debridement.
3. Careful shaping of the canals.
4. Complete sealing of the entire root canal network.
5. An abundance of TLC in the treatment of the disease process and the individual patient's anxieties.
6. Careful explanation and patient communication.

Accomplishing the above, no matter what technique is used, should render a very high percentage of success.

Acknowledgments

I am very much indebted to Dr. Harold Gerstein and his staff for editing and assistance with the slides and art work, to Dr. Robert P. Bethea for his assistance in compiling the section on the history of endodontics in general and diffusion specifically, and to Mrs. Robin Morris for help with typing and editing.

REFERENCES

1. Callahan, J. R.: Rosin solution for the sealing of dentinal tubuli and as an adjuvant in the filling of root canals. J. Allied Dent. Soc. 9:53, 1914.

2. Johnston, H. B.: A method for the filling of the pulp canaliculi by diffusion. J. Dent. Res. 4:117, 1922.
3. Stewart, G. G., Kapsimales P., and Rappaport, H.: EDTA and urea peroxide for root canal preparation. J. Am. Dent. Ass. 78:335, 1969.
4. Bethea, R. P., and Schilder, H.: Comparison of warm gutta percha and diffusion with gutta percha. Thesis, Boston University School of Dentistry, 1973.
5. Schilder, H., Professor and Chairman, Department of Endodontics, Assistant Dean, Continuing Education, Boston University School of Graduate Dentistry.

SOFTENED GUTTA PERCHA TECHNIQUE

LEO GRUDIN, D.D.S.

A three-dimensional filling technique for the complete obliteration of the canal system apically and laterally with gutta percha is outlined in this section.

For a number of years, I have been using various methods of filling root canals, e.g., lateral condensation,[1a,b, 2] Johnston's diffusion technique,[3] and Ostby's Kloroperka N-O techniques.[4] A far greater degree of successful results has been obtained by adapting some modifications and additions to Johnston's diffusion technique. This alteration justified my continuing this method of filling canals.

OBJECTIVES

The objectives of endodontic therapy are:

1. Elimination of pain and/or infection from the tooth and surrounding periapical tissue.
2. Obliteration of the canals.
3. Restoration of the crown for the completed endodontically treated tooth.

The obturation of the canal is a mechanical procedure that includes the following aspects: (1) access, (2) length of tooth, (3) cleaning and shaping, (4) filling material, and (5) actual obturation.

ANATOMY AND MORPHOLOGY

Knowledge of the anatomy and morphology of the involved tooth is extremely important before beginning any endodontic therapy; this includes information about the crown, the root, the canal system, and the apical third of the root, including accessory canals and the apical foramen (Fig. 4–17). The apical foramen (dentino-cemental junction) may be located within a radius of 0.05 mm of the end of the root. The radiograph should disclose the crown, direction of the root, and size of the pulp chamber and canal, as well as the surrounding periapical tissue. With improved local anesthetics, perfected instruments, and controlled procedures, successful endodontic treatment can be achieved on virtually any tooth with the exception of those exhibiting extreme metaplastic changes.

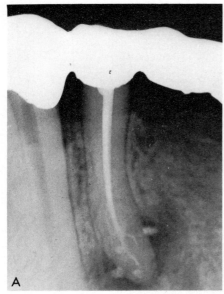

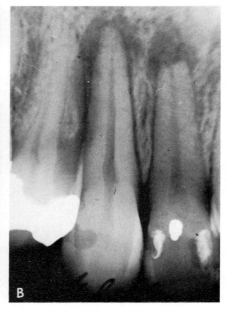

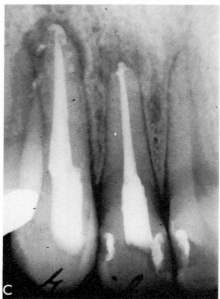

Figure 4–17 *A*, Mandibular first premolar showing the canal arborization in the apical third. *B*, Maxillary lateral and cuspid showing the lateral with a craterlike apex due to resorption and the cuspid with normal anatomy. *C*, Lateral and cuspid filled. Lateral filled by lateral condensation and the cuspid with softened gutta percha.

ACCESS

All pre-endodontic treatment should be completed before proceeding with the endodontic therapy. Openings into the pulp chamber, as a rule, are normally made through the middle third of the lingual surface of anterior teeth and through the central groove, slightly mesial to the center of the occlusal surfaces of posterior teeth. The size and shape of the internal anatomy of the pulp chamber and the direction of the individual canals will develop the outline form. Additional modifications are necessary to gain direct access through the pulpal orifice to the apical foramen. A visual examination of the involved tooth is important before applying the rubber dam, in order to determine rotation or inclination of the crown.

LENGTH OF TOOTH

In order to avoid over- or under-instrumentation, it is necessary to establish the length of the tooth. Using the radiograph as a guide, a rubber stop is placed on the shaft of a #10 style B file approximately 2 mm short of the measured length of the tooth.[5] The file is carefully inserted into the canal to a point of resistance or until the rubber stop reaches a reference point on either the incisal or the occlusal surface. If the file is too loose, change to a size larger or one that holds at the reference point. A radiograph is now made, and an adjustment is made to the rubber stop position so the file will be 0.05 mm short of the radiograph apex. The recorded length now becomes the working length.

COMMANDMENTS OF CLEANING AND SHAPING

1. Never proceed until an exact measurement of the canal length has been established.
2. Be sure the working lengths of all instruments have been accurately calibrated by means of a rubber stop.*
3. Pre-moisten the canal with sodium hypochlorite[6] (NaClO)† or a similar solution before filing. Never file a dry canal.
4. Irrigate copiously with sodium hypochlorite after the use of each file before proceeding to the next size.
5. Always use a curved instrument in a curved canal. Restore the curve to the instrument when re-entering the canal.
6. At no time should a file with debris be allowed to re-enter the canal. Constantly clean the instruments as they are being used.
7. Use instruments in sequence — never omit any sizes while advancing to instruments of a larger diameter.
8. Never force an instrument if it binds. The file should be given only a quarter turn and withdrawn.
9. Re-establish and taper the apical constriction by returning with #10, 15, and 20 files to working length following the use of each size instrument. In larger canals, return to the size that approximates the initial size of the apical structure.
10. Debris and drugs must not be forced through the apical foramen.

CLEANING AND SHAPING

Cleaning and shaping has been considered to be the most important single phase of endodontic therapy.

Technique

The canals should be prepared, keeping in mind the indicated filling material and method for filling the canal.

---

*A 32 gauge rubber band cut in squares.
†NaClO — one part Clorox to three parts distilled water by volume = 1.3% NaClO.

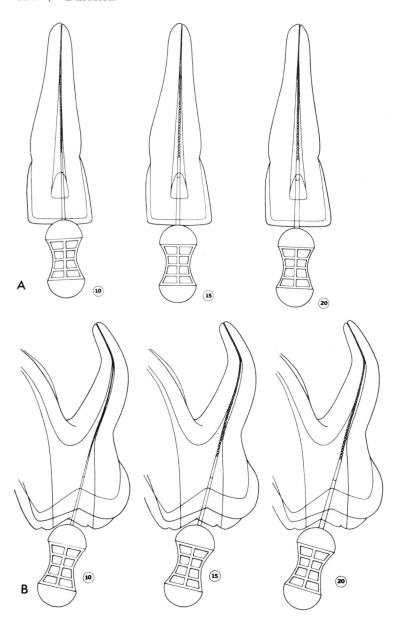

Figure 4–18 *A*, Anterior tooth. Files #10, #15, and #20 sequentially used to the working length. *B*, Posterior tooth. Files #10, #15, and #20 sequentially used to the working length.

    1. The working length is established from the last radiograph, 0.05 mm from the radiographic apex. Using the small flexible style B files with rubber stops, #10, 15, and 20 in sequence, enlarge the canal to its working length. Each time a file is removed from the canal or increased in size, the canal is irrigated with a solution of sodium hypochlorite. Mandibular teeth are irrigated first with sodium hypochlorite, then with peroxide followed by sodium hypochlorite. This causes an effervescent action, which helps to float debris to the surface. With the # 20 file placed in the canal, a radiograph is again made for the verification of the working length (Fig. 4–18). In larger canals, return to the size file that approximates the initial size of the apical structure.

    2. With the larger, more rigid files, style B #25, 30, 35, 40, and so on, again in sequence, enlarge the canal only to the point of resistance until the

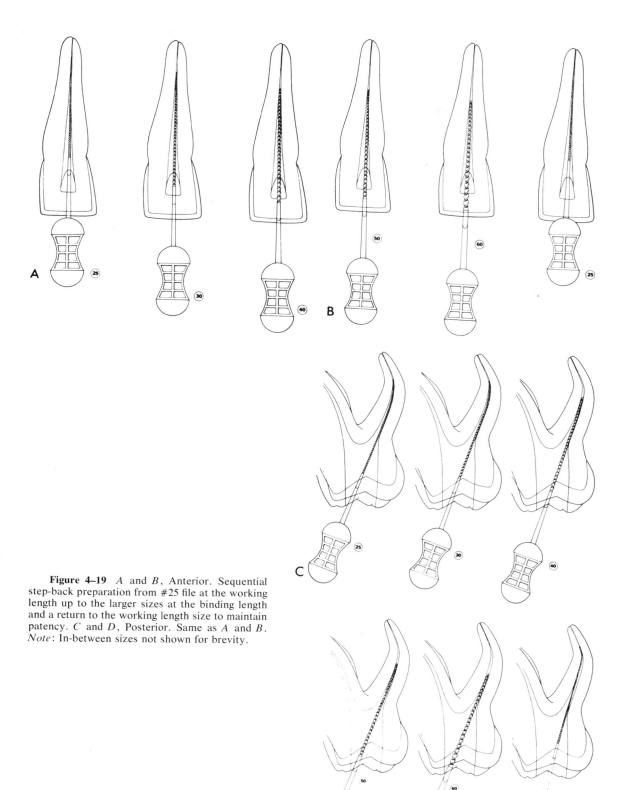

Figure 4–19 *A* and *B*, Anterior. Sequential step-back preparation from #25 file at the working length up to the larger sizes at the binding length and a return to the working length size to maintain patency. *C* and *D*, Posterior. Same as *A* and *B*. *Note*: In-between sizes not shown for brevity.

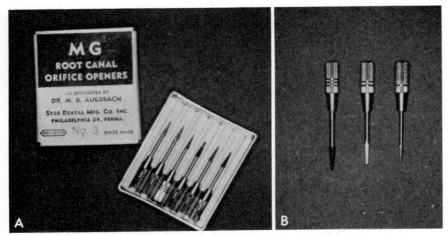

Figure 4–20 *A*, Orifice openers as packaged, and *B*, orifice openers sizes 1, 2, 3, (Auerbach openers, Star Dental Mfg. Co.).

desired enlargement is obtained. *Never force a file if it binds.* As each file is increased in size, the apex is refiled with the #20 or 25 file to the original working length (Fig. 4–19).

3. To avoid any ledges in the canal and to insure a smooth taper to the apex, a reverse procedure is followed; first filing with the #50 file, then using the #40, 30, and 20 files at the working length.

4. The orifice wideners (Auerbach) #1 and 2 (Fig. 4–20) are now used in the pulpal floor opening of the canal, each size about ten turns, by hand, to enlarge and funnel-shape the orifice, so that a gutta percha cone may be inserted with ease for lateral condensation and apical packing.

INSTRUMENTATION

All canal preparations for cleaning and shaping are made with the style B files #8 to 60. The taper varies with each canal according to the size of the canal and the age of the patient. At the completion of cleaning and shaping a canal, the size of the file at the working length would be #20 or 25. The initial size varies in larger apices; however, the largest file used in a canal is always #60.

FILLING MATERIAL

Gutta percha is the most universally used and accepted root canal filling material available for endodontic therapy. It is classified as a solid and, in solvent form, as a plastic. When softened with chloroform and used as a root canal filling, it is considered a combination filling.[7]

OBTURATION OF THE CANAL

Assuming that the tooth has been comfortable since the last appointment and the canal is dry, it is ready to be filled.

A. A gutta percha cone (Mynol, regular style) is fitted in the canal at least 5

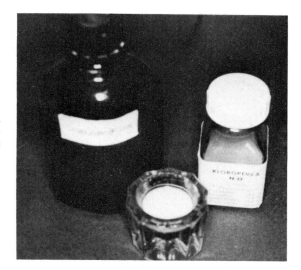

Figure 4–21 Chloroform, Kloroperka N-O and a dappen dish with the mixture. Kloropercha powder is composed of Canada balsam, rosin, gutta percha, and zinc oxide. (Kloroperka N-O, Union Broach Co.)

mm short of the working length with tug-back. The fitted cone and accessory cones are now immersed in 99% isopropyl alcohol until ready to be used. When ready to be used, they are placed on a 2 × 2 sterile gauze square and allowed to dry.

B. The canal(s) are now thoroughly flushed with 99% isopropyl alcohol and dried with absorbent paper points. Each point is measured to the working length before being inserted into the canal to avoid perforating the apex.

C. A solution of Kloroperka N-O and chloroform is made (consistency of milk) in a dappen dish and covered (Fig. 4–21).

    1. The apical one third of the fitted gutta percha cone is now immersed in this solution for 5 to 10 seconds and then inserted into the canal with a slight pumping action apically until seated. It will now move 2 to 3 mm.

    2. Following the same procedure as in lateral condensation, additional accessory cones are added *dry* until the canal is filled (Fig. 4–22).

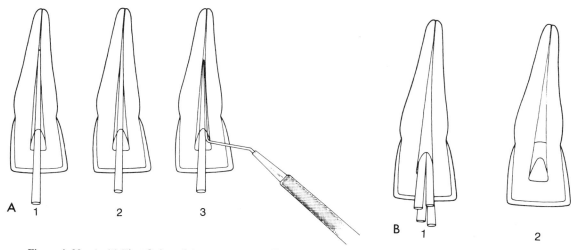

A
1   2   3

B 1   2

Figure 4–22 *A*, (1) First fitting of the master cone, (2) cone softened with Kloroperka and inserted, and (3) spreader in place, starting the lateral condensation. *B* (1) Completed obturation, and (2) apical condensation completed and excess gutta percha removed.

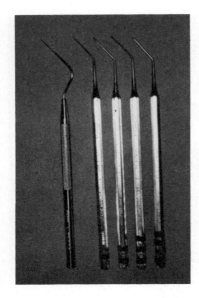

Figure 4–23 Kerr spreader #3 (left) and Luks pluggers #1, 2, 3, and 4 (right).

3. The excess gutta percha is removed from the pulp chamber with a heated plastic instrument. Luks hand pluggers, #1, 2, and 3, are used for additional apical condensation (Fig. 4–23).
D. A radiograph is now made to check the filling in the canal.
   1. When there are several canals to be filled in the same tooth, the other orifice(s) are blocked with sterile or flamed silver cones (Fig. 4–24). Each canal is filled separately and radiographed.
E. When the canal(s) are completely filled, a thin layer of gutta percha is softened and packed in the floor of the pulp chamber and covered with crown and bridge cement.
   1. The rubber dam is now removed. The occlusion is checked and all interferences are relieved or removed. A final radiograph is made for the completion of the root canal treatment.

CORRECTION TECHNIQUE

If the root canal filling is not completely satisfactory, correction can be made at the time of filling or at the next appointment. A rubber dam is again placed on the tooth involved, the chamber is opened, and the gutta percha is removed from the floor of the chamber and the top of the canal with a heated instrument.

Figure 4–24 Filling procedure of a lower first molar, radiographs only. *A*, Gutta percha cone fitted in distal canal. *B*, Cone softened with Kloroperka and inserted into canal. *C*, Lateral condensation. *D*, After apical condensation and removal of excess gutta percha, cone is fitted in mesial-lingual canal. *E*, Silver cone placed in mesial-buccal canal to keep canal patent. *F*, Softened cone is inserted into canal. *G*, Lateral condensation. *H*, After apical condensation, excess gutta percha is removed. *I*, Silver cone is removed from mesial-buccal canal; gutta percha fitted in canal. *J*, Softened cone inserted into canal. *K*, Lateral condensation. *L*, After apical condensation, a layer of gutta percha is softened and packed on the floor.

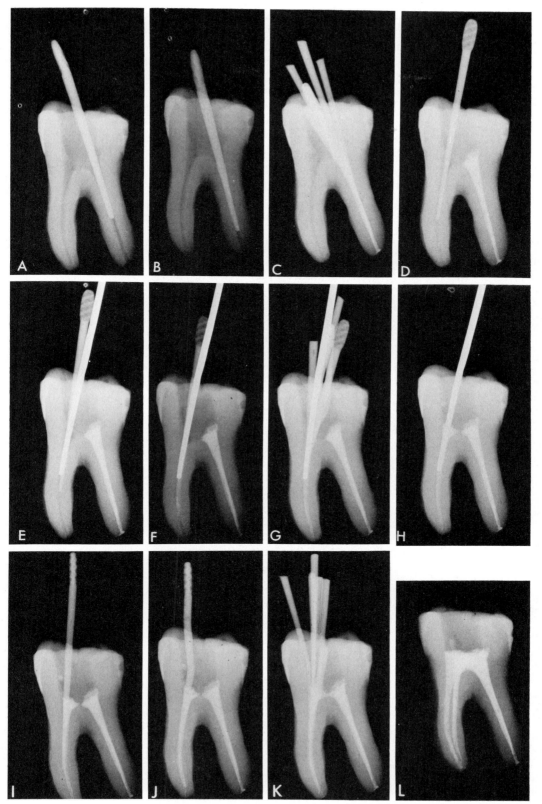

Figure 4–24 *See legend on opposite page*

1. A sterile #20 file with a rubber stop 1 mm short of the working length is inserted into the canal with a few drops of chloroform. Using a pumping action, the gutta percha is made plastic within the canal.[4]

2. The root canal is now repacked, using the lateral condensation technique, with additional dry accessory gutta percha cones. The excess is removed and packed apically.

3. A radiograph is now made, and if satisfactory, a thin layer of gutta percha is now packed on the floor of the pulp chamber and covered with crown and bridge cement. The rubber dam is now removed, the occlusion adjusted, and another radiograph made.

4. This technique can also be used in very fine and curved canals, as well as in canals with internal resorption.

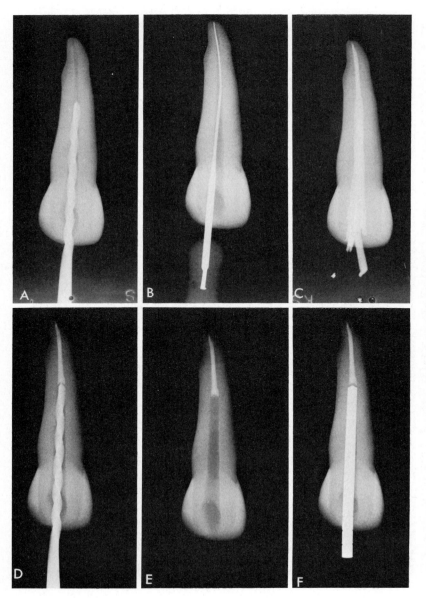

Figure 4–25 A, After cleaning and shaping the canal, reamers, sizes #70 to #100 in sequence, enlarge canal to the desired length. Last reamer used in making post space. B, A #25 file smoothes and tapers walls to working length. C, Lateral condensation. D, Gutta percha is removed from canal with a heated instrument, packed apically and sized with the last reamer used in preparing the post space. E, Post space cleared to the proposed desired length. Fitted endo post in place. F, Post space fitted with endo post, same size as the last reamer used.

POST SPACE

If post space is required, it should be prepared at the time of cleaning and shaping. Post space should be at least equal to the length of the crown. Allow no less than 5 mm of gutta percha at the apex. Post space is prepared with large style B reamers #70 through 100 with stops. In sequence, the canal is sized with #70, 80, 90, and 100 instruments to the depth desired, using a reaming and filling action. The canal is filled with gutta percha, as described in the filling technique. The excess gutta percha is removed from the canal space with a heated instrument, and the last reamer is used to create the post space (Fig. 4–25). The space can now be used with either an endo post or an endowel post or can be easily enlarged for those wishing to make a cast post. *No motor-driven drills should be used in canal(s) — only hand reamers.*

RADIOGRAPHIC CONTROL

Cleaning and Shaping

To maintain a controlled method for establishing the length of canals, the following procedure has been used for identification of canals in bicuspids and molars:

1. Bicuspids with two canals — the file in the canal nearest to the root of the mesial tooth would be the lingual canal.
2. Maxillary molars — use two films. The first radiograph would be of the lingual canal, the second of the mesial and distal buccal canals.
3. Mandibular molars — the first radiograph would be of the distal and mesial-lingual canals, the second of the mesial-buccal canal.

Obturation of Canals

It is desirable to have your instruments organized so the filling technique becomes habitual (Fig. 4–26). A radiograph of each canal is made

Figure 4–26 A set-up preferred by the author, with heat source, dappen dish containing Kloropercha with a glass cover to prevent evaporation, paper points, storage and sterilizing facility, scissors, ruler, mouth mirror, cotton pliers, endodontic explorers, Luks pluggers, Kerr #3 spreader, plastic instrument, glass syringe for 99% isopropyl alcohol and a tray with gutta percha or paper points.

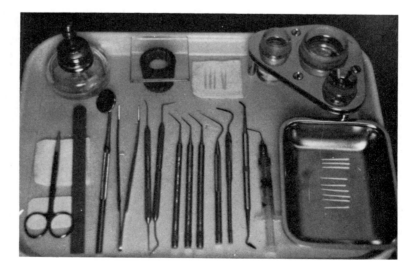

at the time the canal is filled. The following procedure is employed in filling anterior and posterior teeth with multiple canals:

1. Anteriors and pre-molars with two canals — the labial or buccal canal is blocked with a silver cone to keep the canal patent. The lingual canal is filled first, then the labial or buccal canal.

2. Maxillary molars — the mesial-buccal canal is blocked with a silver cone and the distal-buccal canal is filled first, the mesial-buccal canal next, and, finally, the lingual canal.

3. Mandibular molars — the first canal to be filled is the distal canal, the mesial-buccal canal is blocked with a silver cone, and the mesial-lingual canal is filled next. The final canal to be filled is the mesial-buccal canal.

In using this method of obturation, each canal can be observed without any obstruction before proceeding to the next canal.

SUMMARY

The advantages of the softened gutta percha technique are as follows:[8]

1. Since it is impossible to prepare a round root canal,[9] the softened gutta percha most nearly conforms to the root canal system.

2. Since no sealer is used, any material visable on the radiograph is gutta percha and is not resorbable.

3. Fitting a gutta percha cone short and using the minimum of Kloroperka N-O on the apical third of the cone keeps shrinkage to a minimum.

4. No trial cone radiograph is necessary.

5. The technique is efficient and lends itself to office procedure.

REFERENCES

1a. Grossman, L. I.: Root Canal Therapy, 3rd ed. Philadelphia, Lea and Febiger, 1950, p. 289.
1b. Grossman, L. I.: Post Graduate Course, University of California, 1952.
2. Ingle, J. I.: Practical Root Canal Therapy. Post Graduate Course, University of Southern California, 1956.
3. Johnston, H. B.: Endodontics. Post Graduate Course, University of California, 1950.
4. Nygaard-Ostby, B.: Endodontics. Post Graduate Course, University of Southern California, 1957.
5. Ingle, J. I.: Endodontics. Philadelphia, Lea and Febiger, 1965, p. 181.
6. Witaker, D., and Miller, R.: Personal correspondence.
7. Grossman, L. I.: Endodontic Practice, 6th ed. Philadelphia, Lea and Febiger, 1965, p. 338.
8. Wantulok, J. C.: Graduate Student Presentation.
9. Davis, S. R., Brayton, S. M., and Goldman, M.: Morphology of the prepared root canal: A study utilizing injectable silicone. Oral Surg. (accepted for publication).

5

Pulp Therapy for Children and Adolescents

RONALD J. PRUHS, D.D.S., M.S.

PULP THERAPY PROCEDURES FOR PRIMARY TEETH

Criteria for Successful Pulp Therapy

In order to select and perform successful pulp therapy for primary teeth, the clinician must be knowledgeable in three important areas. First, he must be aware of histologic changes that occur in response to an advancing carious lesion. Second, he must be able to interpret signs and symptoms of histologic changes and relate them to the extent of pulpal damage. Third, he must be familiar with the various pulp therapy procedures and use them in the appropriate situation.

Knowledge of Histologic Changes

As a carious lesion approaches the pulp, the pulp defends itself with an inflammatory reaction. When the defense mechanisms are overcome, the pulp can no longer survive. Cohen and Massler[1] showed that, although a deep carious lesion may be very close to the pulp, damage to the pulp is usually reversible until bacteria actually enter the pulp. Reeves and Stanley[2] showed, and Shovelton[3] confirmed, that irreversible degeneration of the pulp occurs at a late stage of the carious process and that the thickness of remaining dentin can be very small, 0.5 mm in many cases.

The point at which bacteria enter the pulp, although difficult to determine, is diagnostically critical. Prior to bacterial colonization, carious teeth can be successfully treated with conservative techniques, including indirect and direct pulp capping. Teeth with pulps that have been invaded by bacteria are irreversibly damaged. Because of the extent of pulpal involvement, they can be treated successfully only with pulpotomy or pulpectomy.

A dental clinician does not have the advantage of the histologist; he cannot remove the diseased tooth and study it microscopically. Consequently, it must be determined whether the inflammatory changes of the pulp are reversible or irreversible, based on symptoms and clinical and radiographic signs, and treatment must be planned accordingly.

Interpretation of Symptoms and Signs of Pulpal Degeneration

History of Pain. One of the most important factors in determining the condition of the pulp in carious primary teeth is a history of pain. The clinician is interested in two types, elicited and spontaneous.

Elicited pain was described by Massler[4] as "characterized by its sharp lancinating quality and is evoked by mechanical, thermal or chemical agents." It disappears after the stimulus is removed. In shallow carious lesions involving the dentinal-enamel junction, pain is frequently initiated by sugar. In deep carious lesions, it may be the result of toxic by-products of the carious process affecting the dentin or pulp. It can also result from food impaction occurring between primary molars with compromised interproximal surfaces. *Elicited pain indicates a reversible pulpal condition; the pulp has the capacity to heal if the process is stopped.*

Spontaneous pain is characterized by a dull throbbing ache that is increased by temperature change or lying down. It occurs in the absence of stimuli and tends to alter the normal behavior of the child. *It is related to a severe inflammatory reaction in part or all of the pulp and indicates irreversible pulpal damage.*

Because of the subjective nature of pain and the problem of interpreting information given by children, it is often difficult to obtain a reliable history of pain. A question relating to pain should be included in the office history form. It is best phrased in general terms; for example, "Has your child ever had a toothache or complained about tooth discomfort?" If the answer is yes, the parents should be asked more specific questions in order to differentiate between spontaneous and elicited pain. Specific questions might be "Was your child ever awakened during the night by pain or did it ever keep him/her from sleeping at bedtime?" or "Did a toothache ever keep your child from playing or doing his/her schoolwork?" A positive response to any of these questions indicates a history of spontaneous pain.

In addition to a history of pain, clinical and radiographic signs are used to determine pulpal degeneration.

Clinical Signs. Local inflammation may be present in the tissues adjacent to an infected tooth. The tissues exhibit a brighter than normal red color and swelling. The degree of change may be determined by comparing affected tissue with adjacent normal tissue or with normal tissue on the opposite side of the arch.

Mobility due to inflammation may be present and is detected by tactile examination. It must be differentiated from the mobility occurring in the exfoliation process of primary teeth. Comparing the amount of movement of an affected tooth with the movement of its antimere may help in making this judgment.

In children, a frequent sign of an infected tooth is the presence of a fistula. Because of the soft consistency of the jaw bones of children, liquefied waste products are often able to form an opening and drain. The fistula is usually found in the buccal or facial mucous membrane about midway between the gingival and vestibular tissues or in the gingival sulcus.

Radiographic Signs. Calcified bodies in the pulp or internal resorption of the pulp chamber or canal(s) may be found. They reflect defense reactions of tissue that is still vital despite the intensity of the carious insult. However, they indicate irreversible damage to the pulp.

Once the process of pulpal degeneration has extended into the perio-

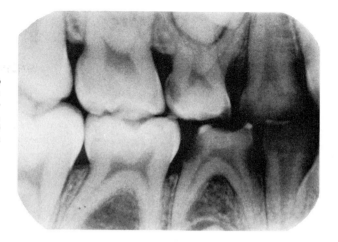

Figure 5–1 Careful scrutiny is necessary to detect the subtle pulpal pathosis evident in the mandibular first primary molar. The pathologic findings include internal resorption in the distal canal, diffuse calcification in the distal half of the pulp chamber, and pathologic bone loss in the bifurcation area.

dontal tissues, bone loss may occur. In primary molars it usually occurs initially in the furcation area and extends to the apical region. These areas appear radiolucent on the radiograph. Spouge[5] reported that 30 to 60 per cent of the hard structures of bone must be demineralized before it can be detected radiographically and that this takes about 10 days to occur.

Tissue degeneration may also be associated with premature root resorption of the primary molar roots. This must be differentiated from root resorption occurring normally during the process of exfoliation.

In many cases radiographic signs of pathosis are obvious. However, they are easily overlooked; therefore, careful scrutiny is frequently necessary to make a diagnostic interpretation (Fig. 5–1).

When pathologic changes are radiographically apparent, irreversible pulpal damage has occurred.

Procedure Selection

It is poor judgment to excavate caries in order to determine what therapy is necessary. A careful diagnostician can utilize available information to determine the treatment of choice prior to the removal of caries.

Conservative treatment is indicated in primary teeth with large carious lesions approximating the pulp in the absence of clinical and radiographic signs of pulpal involvement and when there is no history of spontaneous pain. A history of elicited pain indicates a vital pulp in which the inflammatory changes are reversible. Conservative techniques can also be used successfully in these cases.

Primary teeth with a history of spontaneous pain or with clinical or radiographic signs of pulpal involvement indicate an irreversible inflammatory reaction and should be treated by the removal of the infected pulpal tissue and the application of an appropriate medication.

Some clinicians feel that the pulps of primary teeth with deep carious lesions are frequently irreversibly involved, even in the absence of a history of spontaneous pain and clinical and radiographic signs. Consequently, they feel uneasy about using conservative techniques and tend to enter the pulp more often than necessary. However, this has not proved true in the experience of the author and is not supported by dental research.[4, 6]

After a diagnosis has been made, a clinician can choose one of the following four therapy procedures: direct pulp capping, indirect pulp capping, pulpotomy, or pulpectomy.

Direct Pulp Capping

Direct pulp capping is the covering of an exposed pulp with a material that provides protection against external stimuli and promotes healing. It is indicated for mechanical exposures in primary and permanent teeth or small carious exposures in permanent teeth in which the exposure is surrounded by sound dentin. It is not indicated for teeth with a history of spontaneous pain or for those teeth exhibiting clinical or radiographic signs of irreversible pulpal inflammation.

Direct pulp capping has been traditionally considered the least desirable pulp therapy technique because of its unpredictable prognosis. Many clinicians do not use it for exposures in primary teeth but prefer to perform a pulpotomy, especially when exposure occurs while excavating caries. However, if it is reserved for carefully selected cases of obvious mechanical exposures and if carefully performed, direct pulp capping can be a satisfactory treatment.

Haskell et al.[7] substantiated the value of the direct pulp capping procedure on permanent teeth over a long period of time. They were 87.3 per cent successful over an average interval of 11.7 years. The authors concluded that pulp capping procedures can be used effectively.

Research has shown that the presence or absence of bacteria is the most important factor in the determination of pulpal healing after exposure. Kakehashi et al.[8] compared healing of exposed pulps in germ-free and conventional laboratory rats. No evidence of pulpal degeneration was found in the germ-free rats even in the presence of gross food impactions; however, granulomas and abscess formation occurred in all the conventional rats.

The medication of choice for direct pulp capping procedures is calcium hydroxide. It stimulates the formation of new reparative dentin, which covers the site of the exposure with a dentin bridge. The quality and quantity of the new dentin are unpredictable. However, in cases in which complete bridging has occurred, the hard tissue provides a satisfactory protection for the pulp.[9]

Early studies have shown that isobutyl cyanoacrylate,[10] mixtures of calcium hydroxide and vancomycin,[11] or calcium hydroxide and creasatin[12] are equal to or superior to calcium hydroxide alone as pulp capping agents. Continued research is indicated.

Calcium hydroxide has been introduced into various vehicles that improve the clinical handling of the material. One of the most successful combinations is Pulpdent* paste, which contains 52.5 per cent calcium hydroxide in an aqueous methyl cellulose solution.[13]

The following procedure is utilized after a pulp has been accidentally exposed (Fig. 5–2):

1. All instruments are sterile and available on a pulp therapy set-up at the chairside.

---

*Pulpdent Corp. of America, 75 Boylston Street, Brookline, Mass.

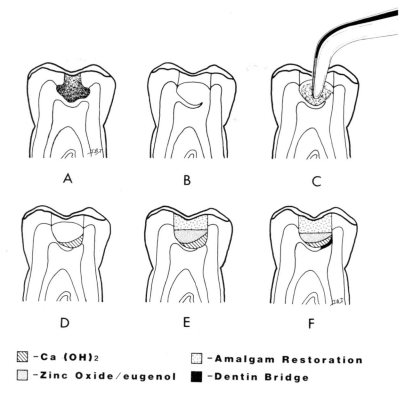

Figure 5–2 Direct pulp capping procedure. *A*, A moderately deep carious lesion is present but is not affecting the pulp. *B*, Caries removal resulted in an inadvertent pulpal exposure. *C*, Cleanse the cavity with sterile cotton pellets and sterile water and dry with sterile cotton pellets. *D*, Place calcium hydroxide over the exposure site. *E*, Carefully seal the cavity with zinc oxide–eugenol, cavity varnish, and an amalgam restoration. *F*, Six weeks later a dentin bridge has formed at the exposure site.

2. The cavity is washed with a sterile cotton pellet and sterile water.

3. The area is dried with sterile cotton pellets, and one pellet is left in place until the bleeding stops.

4. A thin layer of calcium hydroxide paste (Pulpdent) is carefully placed over the exposure site.

5. The calcium hydroxide is covered with a fast-setting, creamy mixture of zinc oxide and eugenol.

6. A thin layer of cavity varnish is applied to the walls of the cavity. These materials prevent microleakage of the final restoration.

7. The cavity is restored with an amalgam or stainless steel crown restoration.

Indirect Pulp Capping

Indirect pulp capping is the removal of all peripheral caries along the dentinal-enamel junction and all soft caries over the pulp except for a thin layer of residual dentin directly over the pulp, which, if removed, would result in pulpal exposure. A medication that promotes healing of the pulp is placed over the residual dentin; it reduces inflammation and stimulates the formation of reparative dentin. The medication also promotes remineralization of the residual dentin. The procedure is indicated for teeth with deep carious lesions in the absence of spontaneous pain or clinical and radiographic signs of irreversible pulpal inflammation (Fig. 5–3).

Since G. V. Black recommended in 1908 that it was safer to remove all decay in carious permanent teeth,[14] it has been difficult for many dentists to

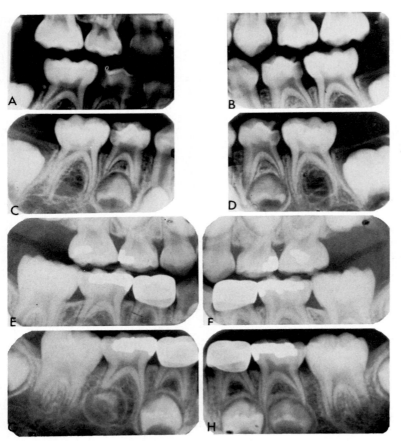

Figure 5–3 A radiographic examination of the right and left first primary molars in this 4-year-old patient revealed deep carious lesions approximating the pulp (*A* to *D*). However, there was no sign of pulpal pathosis. The patient complained of minor discomfort while eating but there was no history of spontaneous pain. The discomfort was attributed to tissue irritation caused by food impaction in the interproximal areas. One-visit indirect pulp capping procedures were performed on both teeth. Two and one half years later the teeth were asymptomatic and there was no radiographic evidence of pulpal pathosis (*E* to *H*).

adopt the use of the indirect pulp capping procedure. The traditional method of excavating deep caries in an asymptomatic primary tooth was to remove all traces of caries, to feel for a possible pulpal exposure with a sharp explorer, and to render appropriate pulp therapy when the pulp was exposed. This approach has been strengthened by the clinical success rates reported for the formocresol pulpotomy technique in primary teeth. Clinicians argue that it is better to perform a pulpotomy to "be sure" of the results. *However, because of the high rate of success possible with indirect pulp capping, in a large number of cases pulpotomy constitutes overtreatment.*

Dimmaggio and Hawes[15] reported a study in which complete caries removal in 244 primary and permanent teeth with deep carious lesions but with no signs or symptoms suggestive of irreversible pulpitis resulted in an exposure rate of 75 per cent. They also showed in subsequent study[16] that 99 per cent of primary teeth selected on the same basis could be successfully treated with indirect pulp capping.

Medications used in indirect pulp capping are selected according to their ability to inactivate bacteria, promote healing of the pulp, stimulate the formation of reparative dentin, and remineralize residual dentin. Either calcium hydroxide or zinc oxide–eugenol can be used as a base in indirect pulp capping. Both cause remaining bacteria to become inactive or die, thereby arresting the carious process.[17] The differences between the two medications are not clinically significant. It is thought that zinc oxide–eugenol is a better sedative and prevents microleakage and that calcium hydroxide is better for stimulation of reparative dentin and the remineralization of residual dentin. Leung et al.[18] suggested the placement of calcium hydroxide (Dycal*) over the residual dentin and sealing it with zinc oxide–eugenol.

The application of stannous fluoride prior to the placement of the base has been shown to improve the remineralization of residual dentin. Nordstrum et al.[19] applied a 10% solution to the residual dentin for 5 minutes before placing a zinc oxide–eugenol base. After 12 weeks the remineralized dentin was harder, and it showed greater radiodensity than dentin treated with calcium hydroxide. The application of stannous fluoride to deep carious lesions does not cause significant pulpal reaction.[20, 21] However, when the remaining dentin layer is extremely thin, the application time should be reduced.[22]

The clinical application of the indirect pulp capping technique may take one of three forms: caries control, a two-visit technique, and a one-visit technique.

Caries control in primary teeth is indicated for children with large carious lesions that cannot be treated immediately. It makes use of the general principles of indirect pulp capping in order to stop the carious process and prevent further pulpal involvement until permanent treatment can be provided. All lesions are treated at one visit. A large round bur and spoon excavators are used to peel away the bulk of caries. Care should be taken to remove caries adjacent to the cavo surface margins. A thick mix of polymethyl methacrylate–reinforced zinc oxide–eugenol cement (IRM)* should then be placed. It has good marginal sealing properties and is able to withstand normal stresses for long periods of time.[23] During subsequent visits the teeth can be treated and restored.

The two-visit technique involves an initial visit during which an indirect pulp capping procedure is performed and a second visit, at least 6 weeks later, at which time a permanent restoration is placed.

Indirect Pulp Capping Procedure (Fig. 5–4)

1. *Obtain profound anesthesia* using the appropriate infiltration or block method. In the maxillary molar region the needle should be inserted high enough to include the long lingual root of the primary molars. In the mandible a mandibular block injection should be given that includes the inferior alveolar, lingual, and long buccal nerves. The area should be checked for profound anesthesia before placing the rubber dam, in order to eliminate the need to reanesthetize a painful tooth once the procedure has been started.

2. *Isolate the tooth* with a rubber dam to prevent contamination and to help the patient cope with the various instruments, washes, debris, and medications. A tooth mesial and distal to the treated tooth should be included in the rubber dam in order to facilitate placement of the restoration.

3. Remove all undermined or unsupported enamel so that the carious dentin can be easily visualized and excavated. Use a large bur running at a slow speed to remove caries completely. Remove the caries from the dentinal-enamel junction first. Then remove all soft caries over the pulp

---

*L. D. Caulk Co., Division of Densply International Inc., Milford, Del.

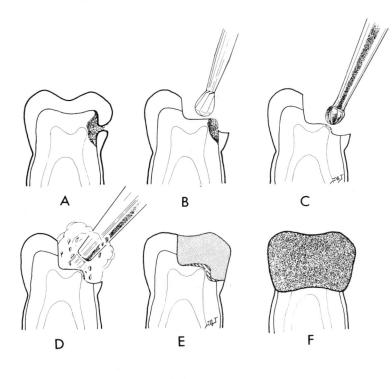

A B C

D E F

Figure 5-4 Indirect pulp capping procedure. *A,* A deep carious lesion is approximating the pulp. *B,* Using a high speed bur, remove all undermined or unsupported enamel so that the entire periphery of the carious lesion can be visualized. *C,* Completely remove caries from the dentinal-enamel junction using a large round bur and remove all soft caries over the pulp except for a thin layer of residual dentin. *D,* Cleanse the area with a water spray and dry with cotton pellets. *E,* Place a calcium hydroxide base over the residual dentin and a polymethyl methacrylate reinforced zinc oxide–eugenol temporary restoration. (An experienced clinician may place a permanent restoration at this time.) *F,* After a minimal period of 6 weeks, remove any remaining soft material, place a zinc oxide–eugenol base, and place a permanent restoration. A stainless steel crown is usually the restoration of choice for primary teeth.

▦ –Residual Dentin   ▤ –Reinforced ZOE

▨ –Ca (OH)₂   ▦ –Stainless Steel Crown

except for a thin layer of residual dentin that, if removed, might result in a pulpal exposure.

4. Cleanse the area with a water spray and dry with cotton pellets.

5. Place a calcium hydroxide base and a polymethyl methacrylate–reinforced zinc oxide–eugenol temporary restoration. If a zinc oxide–eugenol base is preferred, it can be used as both base and temporary restorative material. The placement of a cotton pellet saturated with a 10% solution of stannous fluoride for 5 minutes over the residual dentin prior to the placement of a base is optional.

6. After a minimal period of 6 weeks the tooth is reanesthetized, isolated, and re-excavated. The residual dentin should be darker in color and harder. Any soft material should be removed, a zinc oxide–eugenol base placed, and the tooth permanently restored.

During the interval between the two visits the pulp forms reparative dentin adjacent to the lesion and some remineralization of the residual dentin occurs. This procedure is especially indicated for asymptomatic young permanent teeth with deep carious lesions when the dentist is unsure if all infected dentin has been removed.

In the one-visit technique an indirect pulp capping is done, but because of the experience of the clinician in performing the procedure, no follow-up visit is necessary. A permanent restoration is placed immediately. Paul Starkey explained this when he stated:

As dentists become experienced in the use of the indirect pulp-capping procedure they more and more question the need to reenter the tooth. They see no reason not to restore the tooth permanently at the first sitting. I believe the question is justified when one considers the high percentage of success in using the procedure. In addition, when one refines his approach and finds at the second sitting that the residual dentin is now dehydrated and can only be "dusted" away, it does seem like an unnecessary step. Perhaps one should consider his prognosis of the individual case when deciding if a two-sitting procedure should be used. In other words, if from experience in using the technique he questions the prognosis and feels it may not be successful, then he should reenter the cavity and determine if the treatment has enabled him to avoid an exposure. If, however, from experience, he feels there is little doubt but the prognosis is excellent, he might well justify a one-sitting procedure.[24]

The indirect pulp capping procedure depends on (1) the ability of the dentist to excavate a deep carious lesion without exposing the pulp and (2) the ability to distinguish between dentin that should be removed and dentin that can be allowed to remain.

In excavating a large carious lesion the tendency of the operator is to use burs that are too small, to focus attention on the caries over the pulp, and to remove the caries first in order to determine how close the lesion is to the pulp. Pulpal exposure is a too frequent result. Using this approach, once it is determined how deep the lesion is, the operator must still remove the peripheral caries before initiating the appropriate pulp therapy. The technique of choice is to use the largest round bur possible and to work from the outside or periphery of the lesion toward the pulp. This provides good access and visualization of the lesion and helps the operator to develop a sense of touch for the caries.

Some research has been published relative to the problem of distinguishing between dentin that should be removed and dentin that can be allowed to remain. Fusayama and Terashima[25] and Ohgushi and Fusayama[26] found two distinct layers in the carious soft dentin of human teeth. The first, or infected, layer consisted of deteriorated collagen fibers, lacked odontoblastic processes, and contained invading bacteria. The second layer showed sound collagen fibers, swollen odontoblastic processes, and no bacterial invasion. This layer was recalcifiable. In another study it was found that the first layer, but not the second, could be stained red with 0.5% basic fuchsin–propylene glycol solution and that this provided a practical clinical aid for the removal of infected dentin.[27] An experienced dentist can accomplish this procedure with regularity.

Formocresol Pulpotomy

A pulpotomy is the removal of the coronal portion of the pulp and the placement of a medication at the amputation site over the tissue remaining in the pulp canals. The medication widely used for pulpotomy is formocresol.

Formocresol is a strong germicidal medication that causes "fixation" of living tissue. When placed on the amputation site, formocresol causes coagulation necrosis of the tissue in direct contact with it. As it diffuses into the pulpal canals, it causes a wide range of tissue reactions, including a reduction in the number of cells and changes in pulpal morphology as a result of calcific deposits and resorption. Closer to the apex there may be an attempt at healing, including an accumulation of inflammatory cells and fibrosis.[28, 29] These reactions occur within 4 days of the pulpotomy procedure.[30] After longer periods of time, even though pulpotomy with formocresol is clinically successful, inflammatory reactions and necrosis frequently occur, along with dentinal resorption followed by apposition of hard tissue.[31]

The indications for pulpotomy are:

1. When pulpal exposure inadvertently occurs while removing decay during an indirect pulp capping procedure. The condition of the pulp is considered reversible. There is no history of spontaneous pain and no evidence of clinical or radiographic pathosis.

2. For teeth with early clinical or radiographic signs of pulpal degeneration or a history of spontaneous pain. In these cases pulpotomy can be used to retain teeth that, if extracted, would create a difficult situation for space management.

There are two pulpotomy procedures: a one-visit and a two-visit procedure. The one-visit procedure is used for teeth inadvertently exposed while attempting an indirect pulp capping. The two-visit procedure is used for teeth with irreversibly involved pulps.

One-Visit Formocresol Pulpotomy Procedure (Fig. 5–5)

1. Profound anesthesia, isolation of the tooth, and caries removal have been accomplished, as described for the indirect pulp capping procedure.

2. Using a 702R bur and high speed, remove the roof of the pulp chamber. Extend the opening laterally with a 702R safe-end bur, eliminating any overhanging ledges (see Chapter 1 for technique). Remove the entire coronal pulp with slow speed and a large round bur. Complete removal of any residual tissue tags makes it easier to control hemorrhage at the amputation sites. Care should be taken not to perforate the floor of the chamber walls.

3. Cleanse the chamber of blood and debris by flushing with air and water. Locate the canals that should be exposed and check to see that the floor of the pulp chamber has not been perforated.

4. Control bleeding from the amputation site by: (a) Gently absorbing the excess blood from the area with a damp cotton pellet, being careful not to touch the amputation site. This is preferable to packing the site with cotton because the cotton pellets may tear away the clot when they are removed. (b) After 3 to 4 minutes, if the bleeding has not stopped, place a moistened cotton pellet saturated with Thrombin Topical* over the amputation site for 1 minute.[32] If the bleeding does not stop at this point, the tissue in the canal is considered irreversibly involved and a two-visit procedure is indicated.

5. Place a cotton pellet moistened with formocresol over the amputation site for 5 minutes. The pellet should not be saturated but rather should be blotted on a gauze sponge. After 5 minutes, the stumps will appear darker in color because of "fixation" of the surface layer. The formocresol mixture commonly used is Buckley's solution† (cresol 35 per cent and formaledhyde 19 per cent in aqueous glycerin solution). However, Morawa et al.[33] obtained equal, if not better, clinical results using Buckley's solution diluted

---

*Parke Davis & Co., Detroit, Michigan.
†King's Specialty Co., Fort Wayne, Indiana.

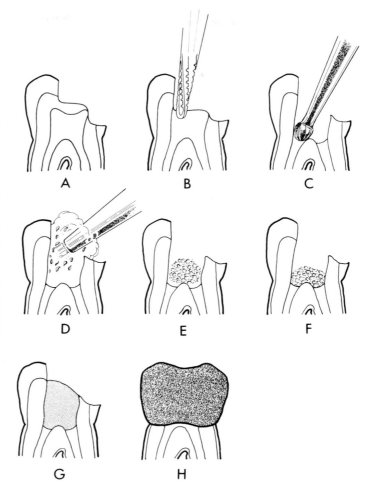

Figure 5–5 Formocresol pulpotomy — one-visit procedure. *A*, Complete caries removal has resulted in a pulpal exposure. *B*, Use a 702R bur to gain access to the chamber and a 702R safe-end bur to create the chamber outline form (see Chapter 1 for technique). *C*, Completely remove the coronal portion of the pulp using a large round bur. *D*, Flush the chamber of blood and debris using a stream of air and water. *E*, Gently place a dry cotton pellet in the chamber, being careful not to touch the amputation sites. Remove the pellet after 3 to 4 minutes. If bleeding has not stopped, place a cotton pellet saturated with thrombin over the amputation site for 1 minute. If the bleeding does not stop at this point, a two-visit pulpotomy procedure is indicated (see text). *F*, Place a cotton pellet moistened with formocresol over the amputation site for 5 minutes. *G*, Fill the chamber with a "putty-like" mixture of zinc oxide–eugenol. *H*, Restore the tooth with a stainless steel crown.

to a 1/5 concentration with a mixture of one part water and three parts glycerin.

6. Fill the chamber with a "putty-like" mixture of zinc oxide–eugenol containing an accelerator and restore the tooth with a stainless steel crown. A zinc oxide–eugenol combination is used because of its excellent sealing quality. Many clinicians prefer to add formocresol to the eugenol in a 1:1 ratio in order to prolong the effects of the drug. This may be desirable if a dilute solution is used. However, Beaver et al.[28] showed that when using undiluted Buckley's solution, incorporating the formocresol into the subbase prior to placing the final restoration did not basically alter the histologic changes of the pulp.

7. A stainless steel restoration is generally necessary because of the amount of tooth structure removed in the process of excavating caries and preparing the pulp chamber.

When a pulp with no irreversible damage is inadvertently exposed, a direct pulp capping procedure, rather than a one-visit pulpotomy, may be considered. However, in this situation the prognosis following a pulpotomy is better than a direct pulp capping procedure; there is a better chance of maintaining the tooth until the permanent tooth erupts.

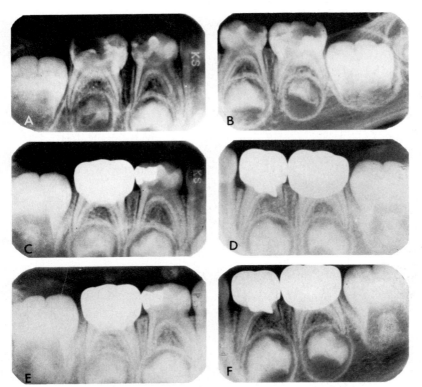

Figure 5–6 Radiographs (*A*) and (*B*) were taken prior to treatment of a 4-year-old child. A one-visit pulpotomy was performed on the mandibular left second primary molar. In the mandibular right first primary molar, hemorrhage from the amputation site was difficult to control. Consequently, a two-visit pulpotomy procedure was performed. Radiographs (*C*) and (*D*), taken 6 months after treatment, showed a common abnormal response to pulpotomy, i.e., pathologic resorption of the distal root of the mandibular right first primary molar. The tooth was asymptomatic. Radiographs (*E*) and (*F*), taken 1 year after the procedure, showed that treatment of the mandibular left second primary molar was apparently successful. The mandibular right first primary molar was unchanged. It was decided to leave this tooth without further treatment and to reevaluate it periodically. (Courtesy of Dr. Mahmoud H. Ashrafi.)

Various studies showed a clinical and radiographic success rate of 70 to 97 per cent.[30, 34, 35] A comprehensive study of 98 teeth by Rolling and Thylstrup[36] over a period of 3 years reported a survival rate of 90 per cent, 83 per cent, 78 per cent, and 70 per cent at intervals of 3, 12, 24, and 36 months after treatment, respectively. Failures were observed to have inter-radicular bone destruction combined with pathologic root resorption.

Although the survival rate following the one-visit pulpotomy procedure is considered clinically and radiographically successful, it must be noted that, because of the unpredictable tissue reactions to the procedure, "the formocresol method should be regarded only as a means to keep primary teeth functioning for a limited period of time"[31] (Fig. 5–6).

Two-Visit Formocresol Pulpotomy Procedure (Fig. 5–7)

1. Profound anesthesia, isolation of the tooth, caries removal, and cleansing of the chamber have been accomplished, as indicated for the one-visit procedure.

2. Seal a cotton pellet moistened with formocresol and blotted with gauze into the chamber with a zinc oxide–eugenol temporary restoration.

3. After 4 to 7 days, administer a local anesthetic, isolate the tooth with a rubber dam, and remove the temporary restoration and the cotton pellet.

4. Fill the chamber with a putty-like mixture of zinc oxide–eugenol in which formocresol has been added to the eugenol in a 1:1 ratio.

5. Restore the tooth with a stainless steel crown.

The results of the two-visit pulpotomy are usually limited to clinical successes. The teeth remain asymptomatic, although they may continue to show bone loss. Success is probably due to the strong germicidal properties of formocresol and its ability to diffuse into the periodontal tissues rather than its fixation properties.

The decision as to whether or not to use the procedure in a questionable situation depends on the value of the tooth to the oral health of the patient and the feasibility of alternative treatments.

Full[37] established some requirements for treating abscessed primary teeth with the two-visit pulpotomy procedure. He recommended the use of formocresol because it: "(1) renders devitalized tissue sterile, (2) maintains the sterility of the root canals for an unlimited time and, (3) diffuses and permeates easily throughout the root canals without disturbing the biological reactions of normal tissue beyond the apices." In a study of 20 primary molars with draining fistulas, showing radiographic demonstration of inter-radicular radiolucency and no evidence of root resorption, clinical success was obtained in all cases after a period of 18 months. Each of the fistulas had resolved, with no evidence of pathosis in the vestibule adjacent to the treated tooth. The teeth were free of pain during the treatment period. The size of the radiolucency tended to increase or remain the same. In only one case did it appear to be replaced with normal bone. Full concluded the treatment "offers some degree of success dependent on the operator's objectives."

Adverse Effects of Formocresol Pulpotomy Procedures

Recent research has shown certain side effects to the use of formocresol for pulpotomy procedures in primary teeth. Myers et al.[38] showed that during a 5 minute application of formocresol to the pulp, 1 per cent was absorbed into the system and extensive concentrations could be found in the pulp, dentin, periodontal ligament, and bone. Even in successful treatments, the pulpal tissue at the apex may remain chronically inflamed.

An increased rate of root resorption,[35] early exfoliation of pulpotomized teeth,[39] and enamel defects in the permanent successors[40] have been

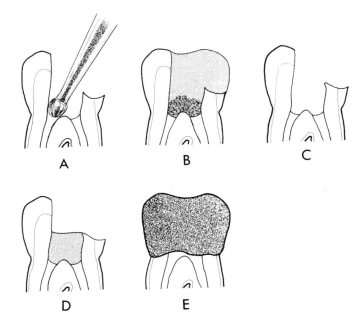

Figure 5–7 Formocresol pulpotomy — two-visit procedure. *A,* Caries removal and amputation of the coronal portion of the pulp have been accomplished, as indicated for the one-visit procedure. *B,* Seal a cotton pellet moistened with formocresol and blotted with gauze into the chamber with a zinc oxide–eugenol temporary restoration. *C,* After 4 to 7 days remove the temporary restoration and the cotton pellet. *D,* Fill the chamber with a putty-like mixture of zinc oxide–eugenol to which formocresol has been added to the eugenol in a 1:1 ratio. *E,* Place a stainless steel crown restoration.

reported. Messer et al.[41] found an increased prevalence of rotation of the succedaneous premolar teeth and enamel surface defects. The defects were more common when a pulpotomy was performed early in the coronal development of the premolar (two thirds formed or earlier) and when the pulpotomy became unsuccessful. The prevalence of caries and restorations on the premolars was unaffected and there was no change in morphology. However, these authors recommended that pulpotomized teeth should be monitored postoperatively, that teeth with unsuccessful pulpotomies should be removed, and that careful case selection should be used before treating teeth with nonvital pulps.

Pulpectomy

Pulpectomy is the complete removal of pulpal tissue and replacement with an appropriate medication.

Pulpectomy in primary teeth, especially molars, is complicated because of the bizarre morphology of the canals and the root resorption associated with exfoliation. There are differences in the number of canals, lateral branching, connecting fibrils, and apical ramifications.[42] Despite the difficulties, Rabinowitch,[43] in an extensive clinical study, demonstrated the effec-

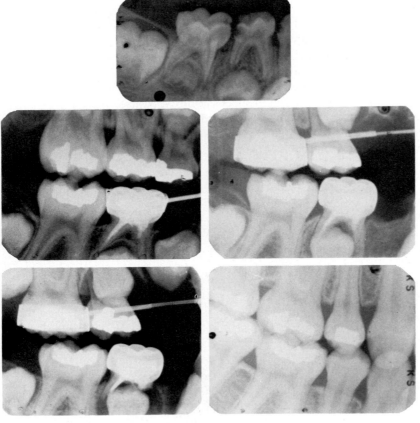

Figure 5–8 A pulpectomy was performed on the abscessed pulp of the mandibular second primary molar of this 4-year-old child. Radiographs taken at various intervals show that the tooth was successfully maintained for 8 years until its successor erupted. (Courtesy of Dr. William Sievert.)

tiveness of the pulpectomy on infected primary molars. In 1363 patients treated, he had only seven known failures. The average number of patient visits necessary to complete treatment was 7.7 for infected nonvital primary molars (periapically involved) and 5.5 for infected vital primary molars (no periapical involvement).

Routine use of the pulpectomy procedure for primary molars remains controversial because of the time and expense involved and the guarded prognosis. However, good clinical success can be achieved using a two-visit procedure and rational endodontic principles (Fig. 5–8).

Indications and Contraindications

Based on an extensive review of the literature, Frankl[44] outlined a comprehensive list of factors that should be evaluated before considering endodontic procedures for primary teeth:

1. The clinician needs to consider the value of the tooth in the arch relative to occlusal function, the length of time the tooth will remain before exfoliation, and its importance in maintaining arch length stability. A common indication for pulpectomy is a case in which the second primary molar is abscessed prior to the eruption of the first permanent molar. Endodontic therapy is more desirable than removal of the tooth and the placement of a distal shoe space maintainer.

2. Enough tooth structure must be present for it to be isolated with a rubber dam and ultimately restored with a stainless steel crown.

3. The periodontal tissues should provide adequate support, and at least two thirds of the root structure should still be present. A fistula and/or furcation radiolucency should not represent a contraindication to treatment.

4. Endodontic therapy is not indicated for teeth in which the floor of the pulp chamber has been perforated by caries or overinstrumentation. It is also contraindicated in the presence of extensive internal resorption, a dentigerous cyst, or pathologic resorption of bone over the permanent tooth.

In most situations primary molars with infected pulps should be extracted and the occlusion analyzed for space maintenance procedures. In recent years clinicians have obtained clinical success treating infected primary teeth with either pulpotomy or pulpectomy procedures. There has been no definitive research comparing the effectiveness of the two procedures. However, it is reasonable to assume that the probability of success would be increased using pulpectomy, as more of the infected pulp tissue is mechanically removed and replaced with an appropriate medication (Fig. 5–9).

Pulpectomy Procedure for Primary Molars (Fig. 5–10)

1. After giving an appropriate local anesthetic and placing a rubber dam, remove all undermined or unsupported enamel and completely remove all caries.

2. Use a 702R bur to gain access to the chamber and a 702R safe-end bur to create a chamber outline form (see Chapter 1 for technique).

3. Remove the contents of the pulp chamber with a large round bur using light pressure. Care should be taken not to perforate the floor of the

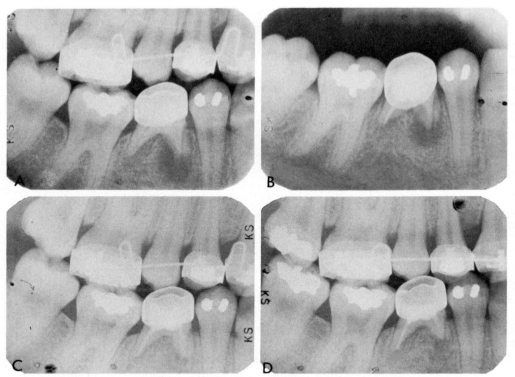

Figure 5–9 Radiograph *(A)* shows a mandibular first primary molar previously treated with a pulpotomy. Treatment was not successful and a periapical lesion developed *(B)*. The tooth was subsequently treated with a pulpectomy. Radiographs taken 6 months *(C)* and 1 year *(D)* post-treatment indicate that the periapical lesion is healing. (Courtesy of Dr. William Sievert.)

chamber. The operator should be able to visualize and probe the orifice of each canal.

4. Radiographically determine the lengths of the files necessary to instrument the canals approximately 2 mm from the apex and mark them with a rubber stop. It is important that infected tissue is not pushed beyond the apex with instruments that are too long.

5. Hedstrom files are recommended for preparing the canals of primary molars. They are sharp cutting instruments and are especially effective in teeth with irregular walls that may contain considerable debris. These instruments should be used with a filing action only, in order to prevent breakage. Using 21 mm files, start with a No. 8 or 10 and file circumferentially, progressing to the largest size that can be conveniently inserted and removed without binding. Frequent irrigation with sodium hypochlorite is recommended. A 610 Proxabrush* (Fig. 5–11) is useful as a handle to file the mesial canals of molar teeth.[45]

6. Irrigate the canals with a 5 ml syringe, flushing first with a 3% solution of hydrogen peroxide followed by sodium hypochlorite, and dry with paper points. A 70% isopropyl alcohol solution can be used as an aid to drying because of the difficulty of negotiating the small canals.

7. Seal a cotton pellet dampened with formocresol in the chamber with a zinc oxide–eugenol temporary restoration for approximately 1 week.

8. At the second visit remove the temporary restoration and the cotton

*John O. Butler Co., 540 N. Lake Shore Drive, Chicago, Ill.

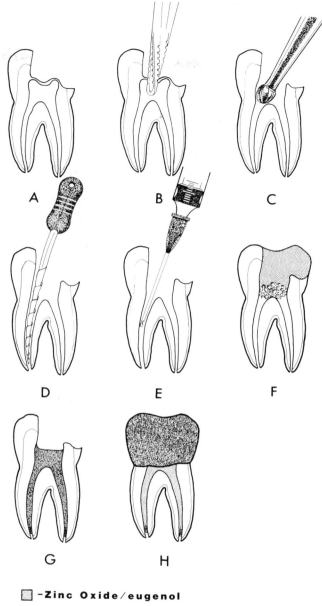

Figure 5–10 Pulpectomy procedure for primary molars. *A,* Remove all undermined or unsupported enamel and complete caries removal. *B,* Use a 702R bur to gain access to the chamber and a 702R safe-end bur to create chamber outline form (see Chapter 1 for technique). *C,* Remove the contents of the pulp chamber with a large round bur. *D,* Prepare the canals with flexible Hedstrom files using circumferential filing to within 2 mm of the apices. The action is purely filing or rasping of the walls without an attempt to create a specific size. *E,* Irrigate the canals with a 3% solution of hydrogen peroxide followed by sodium hypochlorite. Dry with paper points. *F,* Seal a cotton pellet dampened with formocresol in the pulp chamber with a zinc oxide–eugenol temporary restoration for approximately 1 week. *G,* At the second visit complete any necessary filing. Irrigate, dry, and fill the canals with zinc oxide–eugenol to which formocresol has been added to the eugenol in a 1:1 ratio. *H,* Restore the tooth with a stainless steel crown.

☐ –Zinc Oxide/eugenol

▨ –Zinc Oxide/eugenol and formocresol

pellet. Finish any additional necessary filing and irrigate the canals, as in the first appointment. Fill the canals with a mixture of generic zinc oxide–eugenol. Zinc oxide–eugenol is the filling material of choice because of its superior sealing quality, its hygroscopic property, and the fact that it resorbs along with the roots of the primary teeth. Force a creamy mix into the canals as far as possible using a C-R Syringe* (Fig. 5–11) with a disposable plastic tip. Cover the creamy mix with a thick doughy mix (Cavit† works well) and plunge the medication into the canals with finger pressure. Generic zinc

---

*Cavitron Corp., 15400 Commerce Park Drive, Brook Park, Ohio.
†Premier Dental Products Co., Norristown, Pa.

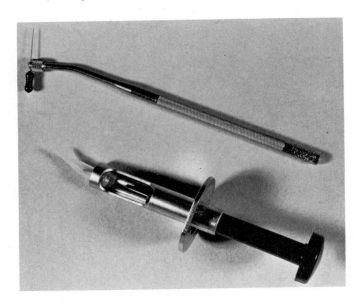

Figure 5–11 A 610 Proxabrush is useful as a file handle to file the mesial canals of primary molars A C-R syringe is useful for placing creamy zinc oxide–eugenol in the pulp chamber.

oxide–eugenol does not contain an accelerator and sets very slowly. A postoperative radiograph can be taken to evaluate the fill. If necessary, the filling material can be forced further into the canals. A Root Canal Pressure Syringe* may be used to place zinc oxide–eugenol into the canals. However, one must be careful not to extrude the materials beyond the apical foramen. In any case, if a small amount of filling material is forced beyond the apex, it can be expected to be absorbed without complication.

9. Take a postoperative radiograph to evaluate the fill. Ideally, it should be within 2 mm of the apex. It is better to be short than to extrude the filling material beyond the apex. However, if the fill is too short, the zinc oxide–eugenol may be forced further into the canals before it sets. If a fistula is present, filling material may extrude through the tract and it can be removed with a large spoon excavator.

10. The tooth should be restored with a stainless steel crown in order to prevent complications occurring as a result of the failure of a large amalgam restoration.

11. Occasionally a pulpectomy is indicated for a primary incisor. The procedure is discussed in the following section.

Pulp Therapy Procedures for Traumatized Primary Incisors

Treatment of a child who has sustained a traumatic injury of the primary incisors presents a special challenge in clinical decision-making and treatment planning. Emergency treatment is complicated by the distress associated with a blow to the mouth and the young age of the child. The assessment of pulpal degeneration is complicated by the fact that the customary clinical examinations of electric pulp testing and the application of heat and cold are generally unsatisfactory. Radiographic interpretation is difficult because of root resorption of the primary incisors and the superimposition of the permanent incisors over their roots. In addition, the time and expense associated with the treatment of a primary incisor that will soon exfoliate must be justified.

---

*Pulpdent Corp. of America, 75 Boylston Street, Brookline, Mass.

Because of the soft cancellous bone surrounding the primary incisors, traumatic forces most often result in luxation type injuries — loosening or displacement. Teeth with a moderate degree of mobility that have not been displaced do not need emergency treatment. They should be periodically evaluated for pulpal degeneration for at least 1 year. Teeth displaced to the lingual or extruded can be brought back into their correct position by applying slow, firm pressure. A local anesthetic is usually not necessary. Some cases do not require stabilization. However, if the tooth is quite mobile or if it tends to move into a position in which it would interfere with centric occlusion, it should be stabilized with a flat wire secured to the adjacent teeth with an acid-etched resin.

Intruded teeth can be expected to erupt spontaneously within 6 months.[46] They should be watched closely for infection and removed if this occurs. After re-eruption it is likely that the pulp will degenerate. The teeth should be closely watched for signs of pathosis.

In rare cases, the crown of a primary incisor may be fractured and the pulp exposed. In these cases a pulpotomy is indicated.

After a period of time, pulpal degeneration of an injured primary incisor may become radiographically evident by the presence of pathologic root resorption, pathologic bone loss, internal resorption, or diffuse calcifications

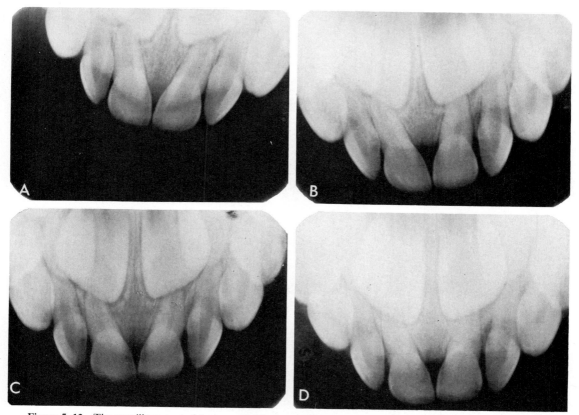

Figure 5–12 The maxillary central incisors of this 2-year-old child were injured in a fall. The teeth were slightly mobile but did not require emergency treatment. Radiograph *(A)* was taken on the day of the injury. Radiograph *(B)* was taken 1 year later. The canals were undergoing calcific metamorphosis. Radiograph *(C)*, taken 18 months after the injury, and radiograph *(D)*, taken 2½ years later, showed continued progress of the calcific metamorphosis. No additional pathosis was evident. Consequently, no treatment was recommended. (Courtesy of Dr. Clifford Hartmann.)

in the pulp. However, the first sign quite often is the failure of secondary dentin to form along the canals. This can be determined radiographically by comparing the size of the canal of the injured tooth with its antimere. The injured tooth will appear to have a larger canal because of its failure to form new dentin.

Occasionally, diffuse calcification of the pulp will cause complete obliteration of the chamber (calcific metamorphosis). The situation should be considered pathologic. However, many of these teeth progress through a normal process of exfoliation and can be allowed to remain untreated. The teeth should be evaluated periodically and extracted if any additional pathologic changes occur (Fig. 5–12).

In addition to radiographic changes, tooth discoloration shortly after an injury is an indication of blood congestion in the pulp chamber with possible pigment formation in the dentinal tubules. The tooth may still be vital and may even lighten after a few weeks. The prognosis is poor, however, and the tooth should be regularly evaluated for radiographic signs of degeneration. Teeth that become dark in color months after the injury have necrotic pulps and should be treated with root canal therapy or extraction.[47] Primary

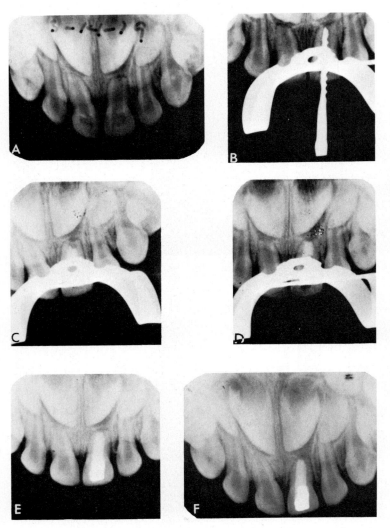

Figure 5–13 The right central incisor of this 3½-year-old child darkened several months after a luxation injury. A radiographic examination (A) revealed a pulp canal wider than its antimere, accelerated resorption of the apex, and a small amount of periapical pathosis. A pulpectomy was indicated. The pulp was removed to a point just short of the apex (B) and the canal was prepared to a #80 file. Zinc oxide–eugenol filling material was placed just short of the apex (C) with a Glick-placing instrument. The material was pushed further apically before filling the remainder of the canal (D). The rest of the canal was filled and a restoration placed (E). One year later the situation was unchanged and stable (F). (Courtesy of Dr. Clifford Hartmann.)

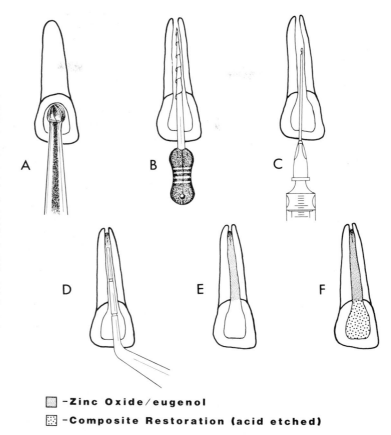

Figure 5–14 Pulpectomy for primary anterior teeth. *A*, Obtain access to the pulp chamber with a high speed bur and completely remove the pulpal tissue from the crown of the tooth. *B*, File 1 to 2 mm short of the apex to at least #80 file. *C*, Irrigate the canal with hydrogen peroxide followed by sodium hypochlorite and dry with paper points. The needle should not bind in the canal. It is best to use an endodontic irrigating needle. *D*, Place a small ball of zinc oxide–eugenol just short of the apex using a Glick calibrated placing instrument. If it is difficult to seat the Glick instrument, check to see if it is binding at the coronal opening and enlarge it if necessary. *E*, Fill the rest of the canal with a thick mixture of zinc oxide–eugenol. *F*, Restore the tooth with an acid-etched composite restoration.

▨ –**Zinc Oxide/eugenol**

▨ –**Composite Restoration (acid etched)**

incisors with necrotic pulps should not be left untreated because of the possibility of infection. The tendency is to extract them, because complicated pulpal procedures are difficult to perform on young children. However, preservation of healthy tissue is the goal of dentistry, and these teeth may provide additional years of good service.

Teeth with little or no periapical bone loss can be successfully treated with a one-visit pulpectomy procedure (Fig. 5–13). The following technique, especially appropriate for primary maxillary central incisors, is recommended by Hartmann and Post of Milwaukee (Fig. 5–14):

1. Local anesthesia. After the application of a topical anesthetic inject 4 to 5 drops of anesthetic solution just beneath the gingiva at the approximate level of the root apex. Inject the rest of the Carpule cartridge after 5 minutes, making sure the needle is superior to the apex. This two-step technique creates little discomfort for the child in a sensitive area and provides profound anesthesia.

2. Isolation is best attained with the placement of a rubber dam. A No. 6 S.S. White* dam clamp will hold the dam snugly in place on most primary maxillary incisors.

3. Access to the chamber should be made from the lingual with a small pear-shaped bur. The openings should be kept in the gingival two thirds of the crown in order to maintain incisal strength in the likelihood of incisal wear. Enlarge the access opening with a No. 4 round bur running at slow

---

*S.S. White Dental Products International, Three Parkway, Philadelphia, Pa.

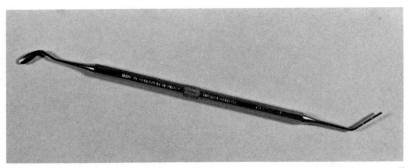

Figure 5–15 A Glick 1 calibrated placing instrument can be used to place a small amount of zinc oxide–eugenol just short of the apex in primary central incisors.

speed. Make sure all the pulpal tissue has been removed from the crown of the tooth in order to decrease the probability of future tooth discoloration. Mack and Halterman[48] have proposed a labial opening followed by a composite restoration in an effort to improve access for instrumentation and esthetic appearance of the tooth.

4. Start with a No. 30 file. Confirm the working length with a radiograph and file 1 to 2 mm short of the apex. Care should be taken not to force necrotic tissue through the apical opening into the periapical tissue.

5. File to a No. 80 file. At this size insert a Glick 1 calibrated placing instrument* (Fig. 5–15) to check that it can be used to place the apical medication.

6. After each increase in file size, rinse the canal with hydrogen peroxide and sodium hypochlorite in a 5 ml syringe. The needle should not bind, so that the solution is not expressed past the apex. Dry with paper points after the last irrigation.

7. Prepare a heavy, doughlike mixture of zinc oxide–eugenol without an accelerator. It should be able to be rolled into a small ball about 1 mm in diameter. A thick mixture prevents the ball from sticking to the walls of the canal. Place the ball just short of the apex, using a Glick 1 calibrated placing instrument. The length of the placing instrument should be 1 mm less than the working length of the files in order to compensate for the thickness of the ball.

8. Take another radiograph in order to ensure proper placement of the filling material. If necessary, the material can be moved further apically.

9. Fill the rest of the canal with a thick mixture of zinc oxide–eugenol.

10. Restore the access preparation with an acid-etched composite restoration. The restoration should help prevent microleakage and crown discoloration. The pulpectomy lightens dark teeth. However, treated teeth frequently turn a light yellow color after a period of time.

PULP THERAPY FOR IMMATURE PERMANENT TEETH AFFECTED BY DEEP CARIOUS LESIONS OR TRAUMA

A special problem in providing pulp therapy for young people is the treatment of permanent teeth with pulpal involvement and incompletely

---

*Star Dental, P.O. Box 896, Valley Forge Corporate Center, Valley Forge, Pa.

formed roots. Newly erupted first permanent molars and permanent incisors are affected most often. Because they erupt at an early age (6 years), parents often mistake the first permanent molars for primary teeth and do not seek dental treatment, even in the presence of obvious caries. Occlusal caries may begin shortly after eruption and progress toward the pulp at a rapid rate. The incisor teeth erupt at an age when the child engages in rough play and activity and are frequently injured before they have time to mature.

The root apices of permanent teeth close approximately 1½ to 2 years after the teeth erupt. Pulpal involvement prior to this time is complicated and requires treatment that promotes further formation of the roots, so that if complete root canal therapy is indicated, it can be accomplished with standard endodontic procedures.

Asymptomatic permanent teeth with deep carious lesions but no clinical or radiographic evidence of pulpal degeneration should be treated with a two-visit indirect pulp capping procedure (see page 137). All caries involving the dentino-enamel junction should be removed. However, in removing the caries directly over the pulp, extreme care and a light touch with a large round bur running at slow speed should be used. Because of the high activity and rapid penetration of these lesions, reparative dentin is usually thin, of poor quality, and easily perforated. Spoon excavators should not be used because they cut into the floor too quickly or may lift remaining dentin off the pulp, thereby causing an exposure. The probability of success is high, and the need for further pulpal treatment is usually unnecessary.

If an inadvertent pulpal exposure should occur during an indirect pulp capping procedure in an otherwise asymptomatic permanent tooth with incomplete root formation, the clinician has two alternatives of treatment. First, if the exposure is small and surrounded by sound dentin, a direct pulp capping procedure should be performed (see page 136). If the exposure is large or if it is surrounded by soft carious dentin, a calcium hydroxide pulpotomy should be performed.

Posterior teeth can be prepared using the one-visit pulpotomy technique discussed on page 142. However, an aqueous methylcellulose mixture of calcium hydroxide (Pulpdent) is placed over the amputation site rather than formocresol. The tooth should be restored with a zinc oxide–eugenol temporary restoration or an amalgam restoration with a zinc oxide–eugenol base in order to prevent microleakage. The tissues in the canals retain their vitality, and a calcific bridge forms below the amputation site. The bridge may be visible radiographically at a 3 month recall visit. Root formation should progress normally (Fig. 5–16).

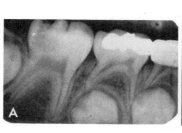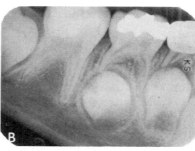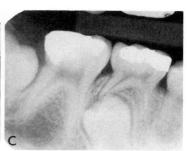

Figure 5–16 Indirect pulp capping is the treatment of choice for young permanent teeth with deep carious lesions in the absence of pathologic symptoms. A preoperative radiograph *(A)*, a 6-month postoperative radiograph *(B)*, and a 1-year follow-up radiograph *(C)* show a successful indirect pulp capping procedure that allowed continued root maturation of a cariously involved young permanent molar.

The calcium hydroxide pulpotomy is also indicated for traumatized immature permanent incisors with incomplete root formation. Teeth with large pulpal exposures in which the injury has occurred several hours prior to treatment are candidates for pulpotomy. However, if the apex has developed to a point where a conventional root canal filling can be accomplished, this procedure should be done. The procedure includes the following steps:

1. Administer a local anesthetic.
2. Isolate the tooth with cotton rolls or a rubber dam. A rubber dam is not indicated if the tooth is mobile, because a taut rubber dam may extrude a mobile luxated tooth from its socket. A rubber dam may sometimes be used if retention is provided by placing the rubber dam clamp on teeth other than the injured one.
3. Obtain access to the pulp chamber in order to amputate the coronal portion of the pulp. Because the objective of this procedure is to maintain vital pulp tissue, it should be carried out in a meticulous manner that avoids contamination with bacteria or debris. A modified version of a technique described by Krakow et al.[49] can be used:
   a. With a small pear-shaped bur running at high speed, cut a preparation that extends to the periphery of the pulp chamber but does not penetrate it.
   b. Circumscribe the dentin over the pulp chamber, just barely penetrating it with the same pear-shaped bur. This operation will leave a thin island of dentin overlying the pulp.
   c. Thoroughly wash the preparation with a stream of air and water in order to ensure a clean cavity. Bacteria, dentin dust, or other debris produces inflammation and retards healing.
   d. Remove the island of dentin with a spoon excavator.
4. Amputate the coronal portion of the pulp 1 to 2 mm below the cemento-enamel junction, using a long, sharp spoon excavator.
5. Control bleeding from the amputation site by gently absorbing excess blood from the area with a dry cotton pellet, being careful not to touch the amputation site.
6. Carefully cover the amputation site with an aqueous methylcellulose calcium hydroxide paste (Pulpdent).
7. Seal the cavity with a hard-setting zinc oxide–eugenol temporary cement.

The reparative dentin bridge forms in approximately 6 weeks. It is relatively impermeable and isolates the remaining pulpal tissue in the canals from further irritation.[9] The procedure is considered successful if root formation continues to completion. At this point, because of the possibility of calcific pulpal degeneration, Patterson[50] recommended perforating the dentin bridge and completing a root canal filling. However, Krakow et al.[49] suggested that calcification of the canals was an infrequent occurrence and that it would be better to evaluate the teeth periodically and to perform a root canal filling only when the need became apparent (Fig. 5–17).

Pulpotomy using formocresol has also been suggested in these cases.[51] However, there is a strong tendency for calcified tissue to form in the canals.[52] The tissue may be difficult to remove and complicate future endodontic therapy. If the technique is used, it should be followed by root canal treatment as soon as the root apex has closed (Fig. 5–18).

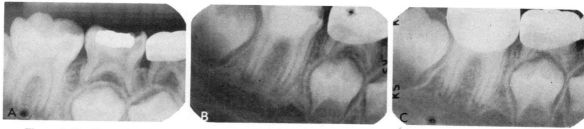

Figure 5–17 The pulp of this cariously involved young first permanent molar was inadvertently exposed during caries removal. There were no preoperative signs or symptoms of pulpal pathosis (A). A calcium hydroxide pulpotomy was performed (B) to permit continued maturation of the roots. (Six months later (C) the roots were continuing to mature. However, condensing osteitis was evident at the apex of the mesial root.) The tooth will be observed periodically for continued maturation and signs of pulpal degeneration, at which time root canal therapy would be indicated.

If pulpotomy treatment is not successful and root formation does not proceed to completion or if an immature tooth has already undergone pulpal degeneration, additional treatment is indicated. The tooth may be treated with a periapical surgical procedure in which the root apex is filled through a surgical flap and an alveolar window. However, this procedure should be avoided whenever possible because of the following reasons: it is not a pleasant experience for a child; there may be postoperative discomfort; and the thin dentin walls present in the apical region of an incompletely developed root may complicate the procedure. A more desirable method of treatment involves the induction of a calcific closure at the apex and the

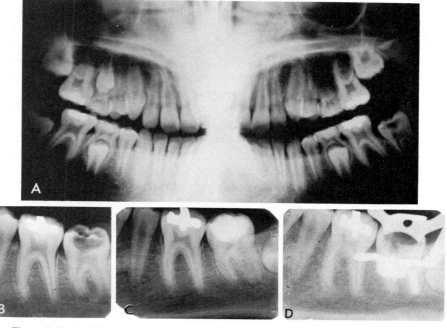

Figure 5–18 In this unusual case a panoramic radiograph (A) revealed an unerupted second permanent molar with a large carious lesion. Fourteen months later (B), just prior to eruption, the patient complained of pain in the area of the cariously involved tooth. The soft tissue over the crown of the tooth was surgically removed and a formocresol pulpotomy was performed. Eight months later (C), after further root maturation had taken place, a root canal procedure was completed (D).

subsequent filling of the root canal with a conventional technique. The procedure is described in Chapters 6 and 7.

Once a young permanent tooth has undergone complete root formation, infection of the pulp should be treated with root canal therapy. Initially this may appear to be a relatively easy procedure because the canals have not matured, they are relatively large, and internal calcifications have not occurred, as they might in an older person. However, successful endodontic treatment may be more complicated owing to the large number of furcal and lateral canals in younger teeth and the fact that the apical constriction, although appearing closed on a radiograph, may still be slightly open.

Kerkes et al.[53] studied the results of endodontic treatment on 166 traumatized incisors occurring in 9- to 18-year-old patients. They found that the standardized technique of circular canal preparation was acceptable for patients older than 13 years of age. However, in younger patients the apical seal was frequently defective. They confirmed the limitations of the radiographic technique to assess the anatomy of the apex of an immature tooth, the difficulty of tissue removal in wide oval canals, and the difficulty of achieving an apical seal in these teeth. These authors concluded that the treatment of 9- to 12-year-old patients should include apexification treatment and a modified obturation technique.

Furcal involvement is a frequent finding in pulpally involved young permanent teeth. However, the gingival attachment is usually unaffected. Furcal involvement should not be flapped and curetted; conventional root canal therapy is indicated. In most instances the affected area will regenerate over a period of time.

Some keys to success in root canal therapy in young permanent teeth include:

1. Step back 1.5 to 2 mm from the apex instead of the recommended 1 mm for more mature teeth. This provides a better apical seal for canals that may have a slightly open apical constriction.
2. Use Hedstrom files — never below size 25 and never above size 40 — to plane the walls. This is the most efficient flexible instrument that can be used with circumferential filing to plane and smooth the walls of the canals. No attempt should be made to use larger files to create a standard-sized preparation.
3. Customize a master cone in large canals in young teeth in order to ensure better adaptation to the irregular walls of the canals. Bence[54] described a practical technique for customizing cones:
   a. Fit a premeasured master cone approximately 2 mm from the apex.
   b. Hold the cone with a locking type plier, dip the tip of it in chloroform, and place it into the canal with slight pressure. The softened tips will take the shape of an irregular canal and provide a superior apical seal. The procedure may have to be repeated in order to achieve a good imprint of the canal. The locking type plier allows the operator to reseat the cone in the same position.
   c. When the master cone has been made, cover the tip with sealer and position it in the canal. A lateral condensation technique can be used to complete the fill.
   d. If a canal is too large for conventional-sized gutta percha cones, three of them can be wrapped together, heated, and rolled between two glass slabs to obtain an approximate fit.

SUMMARY

The histologic response of the pulp to caries is virtually the same in primary and permanent teeth. The criteria for success, however, are different. In permanent teeth it is necessary to obtain histologic success, whereas in primary teeth, under certain circumstances, radiographic or clinical success is acceptable. In addition, in primary teeth there is a tendency to accept the histologic presence of chronic inflammation or slow degenerative changes, knowing that the tooth will be replaced in due time. For this reason pulpotomy is an acceptable procedure for primary teeth but is considered as an interim procedure for permanent teeth.

Direct pulp capping is the least predictable of the pulp therapy procedures in primary teeth and should be used only in carefully selected cases. Indirect pulp capping is highly predictable when used on teeth with large carious lesions that have no apparent clinical or radiographic pathosis and no history of spontaneous pain. The clinical procedure, especially when accomplished in one visit, requires minimal manipulation and is the least expensive pulp therapy procedure for deep carious lesions. The one-visit pulpotomy procedure has limited indications — primary teeth with pulpal involvement of the coronal portion of the pulp and normal tissue in the canals. This occurs as a result of an inadvertent pulpal exposure while excavating caries during an indirect pulp capping procedure. The two-visit pulpotomy procedure and pulpectomy can be effective in the treatment of infected primary teeth. However, the result is unpredictable, so that these procedures should be used only after careful consideration of the prognosis and alternative treatment procedures.

Acknowledgments

Special thanks to John B. Jones, Jr., Department of Learning Resources, Marquette University School of Dentistry, for the illustrations and Jeffrey F. Seipel, Department of Learning Resources, Marquette University School of Dentistry, for the photographs.

REFERENCES

1. Cohen, S., and Massler, M.: Pulpal response to dental caries in human primary teeth. J. Dent. Child. *34*:130, 1967.
2. Reeves, R., and Stanley, H. R.: The relationship of bacterial penetration and pulpal pathosis in carious teeth. Oral Surg. *22*:59, 1966.
3. Shovelton, D. S.: A study of deep carious dentin. Int. Dent. J. *18*:392, 1968.
4. Massler, M.: Preventive endodontics: vital pulp therapy. Dent. Clin. North Am. *11*:663, 1967.
5. Spouge, J. D.: Oral Pathology. St. Louis, The C. V. Mosby Co., 1973.
6. Shovelton, D. S.: Studies of dentin and pulp in deep caries. Int. Dent. J. *20*:283, 1970.
7. Haskell, E. W., Stanley, H. R., Chellemi, J., and Stringfellow, H.: Direct pulp capping treatment: a long-term follow up. J. Am. Dent. Ass. *97*:607, 1978.
8. Kakehashi, S., Stanley, H. R., and Fitzgerald, R. J.: The effects of surgical exposures of dental pulps in germ-free and conventional laboratory rats. Oral Surg. Oral Med. Oral Path. *20*:340, 1965.
9. Holland, R., de Souza, V., de Mello, W., Nery, M. J., Berabe, P. F. E., and Otoboni Filko, J. A.: Permeability of the hard tissue bridge formed after pulpotomy with calcium hydroxide: a histologic study. J. Am. Dent. Ass. *99*:472, 1979.
10. Bhaskar, S. N., Beasley, J. D., Ward, J. P., and Cutright, D. E.: Human pulp capping with

isobutyl cyanoacrylate. J. Dent. Res. *51*:58, 1972.

11. Gardner, D. E., Mitchell, D. F., and McDonald, R. E.: Treatment of pulps of monkeys with vancomycin and calcium hydroxide. J. Dent. Res. *50*:1273, 1971.

12. Citron, C. I.: The clinical and histological evaluation of creasatin with calcium hydroxide on the human dental pulp. J. Dent. Child. *44*:294, 1977.

13. Phaneuf, R. A., Frankl, S. N., and Ruben, M. P.: A comparative histological evaluation of three calcium hydroxide preparations on the human primary dental pulp. J. Dent. Child. *35*:61, 1968.

14. Black, G. V.: Operative Dentistry, Vol. 2. Chicago, Medico-Dental Publishing Co., 1908.

15. Dimmaggio, J. J., and Hawes, R. R.: Evaluation of direct and indirect pulp capping. Int. Ass. Dent. Res., Program and Abstracts of Papers. Vol. 40, No. 86, 1962 (Abst.).

16. Dimmaggio, J. J., and Hawes, R. R.: Continued evaluation of direct and indirect pulp capping. Int. Ass. Dent. Res., Program and Abstracts of Papers. Vol. 41, No. 22, 1963 (Abst.).

17. Fairbourn, D. R., Charbeneau, G. T., and Loesche, W. J.: Effect of improved Dycal and IRM on bacteria in deep carious lesions. J. Am. Dent. Ass. *100*:547, 1980.

18. Leung, R. J., Loesche, W. J., and Charbeneau, G. T.: Effect of Dycal on bacteria in deep carious lesions. J. Am. Dent. Ass. *100*:193, 1980.

19. Nordstrum, D. O., Wei, S. H. Y., and Johnson, R.: Use of stannous fluoride for indirect pulp capping. J. Am. Dent. Ass. *88*:997, 1974.

20. Weiss, M. B., and Massler, M.: Pulp reactions to fluorides. Int. Ass. Dent. Res., Program and Abstracts of Papers. Vol. 47, No. 663, 1969 (Abst.).

21. Langeland, L. K., Tobon, G., Eda, S., and Langeland, K.: Histological response of the dental pulp to fluorides applied to freshly cut dentin. Int. Ass. Dent. Res., Program and Abstracts of Papers. Vol. 46, No. 348, 1968 (Abst.).

22. Brannstrom, M., and Nyborg, H.: Pulp reaction to fluoride solution applied to deep cavities: an experimental histological study. J. Dent. Res. *50*:1548, 1971.

23. Hutchins, D. W., and Parker, W. A.: Indirect pulp capping: clinical evaluation using polymethyl methacrylate reinforced zinc oxide–eugenol cement. J. Dent. Child. *39*:55, 1972.

24. Starkey, P. E.: Management of deep caries and pulpally involved teeth in children. Current Therapy in Dentistry, Vol. 3. St. Louis, The C. V. Mosby Co., 1968.

25. Fusayama, T., and Terashima, S.: Differentiation of two layers of carious dentin by staining. Bull. Tokyo Med. Dent. Univ. *19*:83, 1972.

26. Ohgushi, K., and Fusayama, T.: Electron microscopic structure of the two layers of carious dentin. J. Dent. Res. *54*:1019, 1975.

27. Sato, Y., and Fusayama, T.: Removal of dentin by fuchsin staining. J. Dent. Res. *55*:678, 1976.

28. Beaver, H. A., Kopel, H. M., and Sabes, W. R.: The effect of zinc oxide–eugenol cement on a formocresolized pulp. J. Dent. Child. *33*:381, 1966.

29. Massler, M., and Mansukhani, N.: Effects of formocresol on the dental pulp. J. Dent. Child. *26*:277, 1959.

30. Doyle, W. A., McDonald, R. E., and Mitchell, D. F.: Formocresol versus calcium hydroxide in pulpotomy. J. Dent. Child. *29*:86, 1962.

31. Rolling, I., and Lambjerg-Hansen, H.: Pulp condition of successfully formocresol-treated primary molars. Scand. J. Dent. Res. *86*:267, 1978.

32. Shoaf, H. K., Pashley, E. L., Myers, D. R., and Pashley, D. H.: Quantitation and control of pulpal bleeding. Pediatr. Dent. *1*:177, 1979.

33. Morawa, A. P., Straffon, L. H., Han, S. S., and Corpron, R. E.: Clinical evaluation of pulpotomies using dilute formocresol. J. Dent. Child. *42*:360, 1975.

34. Law, D. B., and Lewis, T. M.: Formocresol pulpotomy in deciduous teeth. J. Am. Dent. Ass. *69*:601, 1964.

35. Wright, F. A. C., and Widmer, R. P.: Pulp therapy in primary molar teeth: a retrospective study. J. Pedodontics *3*:195, 1979.

36. Rolling, I., and Thylstrup, A.: A 3-year clinical follow-up study of pulpotomized primary molars treated with the formocresol technique. Scand. J. Dent. Res. *83*:47, 1975.

37. Full, C. A.: Pulpotomy treatment of fistulated primary molars. Quintessence Int. *10*:73, 1979.

38. Myers, D. R., Shoaf, H. K., Dirksen, T. R., Pashley, D. H., Whitford, G. M., and Reynolds, K. E.: Distribution of 14C-formaldehyde after pulpotomy with formocresol. J. Am. Dent. Ass. *96*:805, 1978.

39. Lauterstein, A. M., Pruzansky, S., and Barber, T. K.: Effect of deciduous mandibular molar pulpotomy on the eruption of the succedaneous premolar. J. Dent. Res. *41*:1367, 1962.

40. Pruhs, R. J., Olen, G. A., and Sharma, P. S.: Relationship between formocresol pulpotomies on primary teeth and enamel defects on their permanent successors. J. Am. Dent. Ass. *94*:698, 1977.

41. Messer, L. B., Cline, J. T., and Korf, N. W.: Long-term effects of primary molar pulpotomies on succedaneous bicuspids. J. Dent. Res. *59*:116, 1980.

42. Hibbard, E. D., and Ireland, R. L.: Morphology of the root canals of the primary molar teeth. J. Dent. Child. *24*:250, 1957.
43. Rabinowitch, B. Z.: Pulp management in primary teeth. Oral Surg. *6*:542, 671, 1953.
44. Frankl, S. N.: Pulp therapy in pedodontics. *In* Siskin, M. (ed.): The Biology of the Human Dental Pulp. St. Louis, The C. V. Mosby Co., 1973.
45. Rifkin, A.: A simple, effective, safe technique for the root canal treatment of abscessed primary teeth. J. Dent. Child. *47*:435, 1980.
46. Ravn, J. J.: Sequelae of acute mechanical traumata in the primary dentition — a clinical study. J. Dent. Child. *35*:281, 1968.
47. McDonald, R. E.: Dentistry for the Child and Adolescent, 3rd Ed. St. Louis, The C. V. Mosby Co., 1978.
48. Mack, R. B., and Halterman, C. W.: Labial pulpectomy access followed by esthetic composite resin restoration for nonvital maxillary deciduous incisors. J. Am. Dent. Ass. *100*:374, 1980.
49. Krakow, A. A., Berk, H., and Gran, P.: Therapeutic induction of root formation in the exposed incompletely formed tooth with vital pulp. Oral Surg. Oral Med. Oral Path. *43*:755, 1977.
50. Patterson, S. S.: Pulp calcification due to operative procedures — pulpotomy. Int. Dent. J. *17*:490, 1967.
51. Weine, F. S.: Endodontic Therapy. St. Louis, The C. V. Mosby Co., 1972.
52. Willard, R. M.: Radiographic changes following formocresol pulpotomy in primary molars. J. Dent. Child. *43*:414, 1976.
53. Kerkes, K., Synnove, H., and Jacobson, I.: Follow-up examination of endodontic treatment in traumatized juvenile incisors. J. Endo. *6*:744, 1980.
54. Bence, R. B.: Handbook of Clinical Endodontics, 2nd Ed. St. Louis, The C. V. Mosby Co., 1980.

6

Calcium Hydroxide Root Closure

ROBERT J. OSWALD, D.D.S.
HENRY J. VAN HASSEL, D.D.S., M.S.D., Ph.D.

INTRODUCTION

Therapy for incompletely developed teeth with pulpal involvement in young patients can be a troublesome part of dental care. Whenever vital pulp tissue can be demonstrated in the canal, either a pulp capping or a pulpotomy technique is the treatment of choice. If vital pulp tissue can be maintained, tooth development can be expected to continue and result in normal length and thickness of the root with commensurate narrowing of the apical canal.

Vital pulp can generally be found in the following situations:

1. When the pulp has been exposed to saliva for no more than 24 hours.

2. When clinical signs of irreversible pulpitis do not exist.

3. When the pulp tissue is pink or red and bleeds freely when manipulated with an explorer.

When endodontic treatment is necessary, it is difficult to employ conventional root canal debridement and obturating techniques because of the divergent or "blunderbuss" form of the apical canal. Frequently the apical canal divergence is greater in the labio-lingual dimension than in the mesio-distal plane seen in clinical radiographs (Fig. 6–1).

In immature teeth in which the pulps are necrotic or are unlikely to survive, other forms of therapy must be instituted. Although surgical treatment of these patients is possible, it is undesirable both from a patient management standpoint (since most of the patients are quite young) and because surgical intervention will eliminate any potential that additional root length may be achieved. Root lengthening is known to occur in some instances in which pulpless teeth are treated in the nonsurgical manner described below (Fig. 6–2). Alternatives to surgical treatment have been available for some time. These techniques are known as "apexification" or "root end induction" procedures. The principal therapeutic agent that is common to these procedures is calcium hydroxide.

Although the use of calcium hydroxide in dental treatment can be traced at least as far back as 1838 when Nygren[1] reported on this technique, the incorporation of the material into a regimen for conservative endodontic

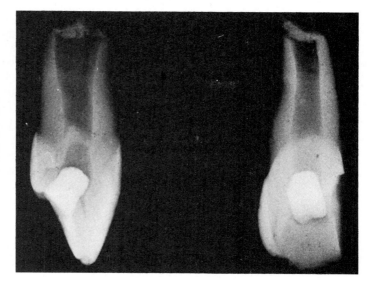

Figure 6-1 Proximal and clinical view radiographs of an incisor that has undergone calcium hydroxide root closure. The problems of instrumentation and obturation are obvious, particularly in consideration of the extreme labio-lingual width of the apical canal. (Courtesy of Dr. Gerald W. Harrington.)

treatment of teeth with incompletely formed roots was not reported until about 1959 when Granath[2] described such an application. Ingle and Beveridge[3] later credit Kaiser, in 1964, with the radiographic and histologic demonstration of root end closure subsequent to induction with calcium hydroxide. Since that time, Frank,[4] Steiner and Van Hassel,[5] and others have aided in establishing root induction as a widely accepted and reasonably predictable technique.

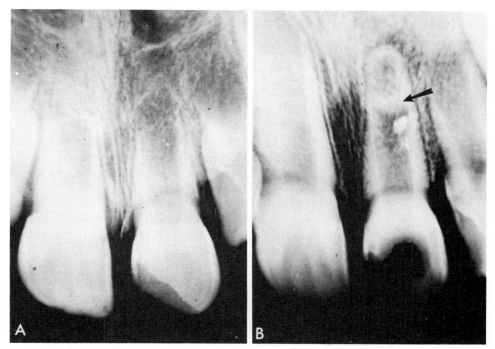

Figure 6-2 Calcium hydroxide root closure in a pulpless tooth. *A*, Clinical preoperative appearance. *B*, Clinical postoperative appearance demonstrates additional root formation apical to the calcium hydroxide–induced bridge (*arrow*). (From Steiner, J. C., Dow, P. R., and Cathey, G. M.: J. Dent. Child. *35*:47, 1968. Used with permission.)

In spite of the widespread use of root induction procedures, there are certain controversies regarding such techniques. For example, the exact mechanism by which root induction occurs is not well understood. It appears, however, that calcium hydroxide may not play an active role in calcification. Pisanti and Sciaky,[6] for example, showed that calcium hydroxide does not contribute calcium ions but that the calcium is derived from the circulation.

Since closure of immature roots by a calcified tissue barrier has been reported with a myriad of techniques, it is only reasonable to suppose that some common element must be associated with all the techniques. At this point, it appears that thorough biomechanical preparation of the root canal is that common factor and that the calcium hydroxide, in whatever form it is used, merely aids in providing the appropriate microenvironment in which calcification can occur. Nevertheless, the calcium hydroxide technique is predictable and accepted and thus is the treatment of choice for nonvital open-apex cases at present. The following procedure for calcium hydroxide use is representative of the calcium hydroxide techniques presently utilized in the United States.

PROCEDURE FOR ROOT END INDUCTION IN IMMATURE TEETH WITH NECROTIC PULPS

In all patients in whom acute clinical symptoms are present, emergency endodontic procedures should be carried out before starting root induction. Once the patient is asymptomatic, the following treatment sequence can be used:

First Appointment

1. Anesthetize the patient when appropriate, place a rubber dam, and establish conventional access.
2. Debride the coronal two thirds of the canal with broaches and large Hedstrom files.
3. Irrigate the canal thoroughly with an acceptable endodontic irrigant such as 2.5% sodium hypochlorite.
4. Dry the canal to the level that you approached with your files, using large sterile paper points.
5. Medicate the canal with camphorated monochlorophenol (CMCP). The medicament should be placed on a sterile cotton pellet; the pellet is then squeezed dry in a sterile gauze sponge.
6. Temporarily seal the chamber with Cavit.

Second Appointment

1. Place a rubber dam and remove the temporary filling. (Anesthesia is generally not used at this visit.)
2. Irrigate the canal thoroughly.
3. Establish a working length. Because of the irregular shape of many incompletely formed teeth, it may not be possible to make the length

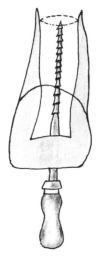

Figure 6–3 Diagram of a reasonable level at which working length is established.

determination with the same degree of precision that is possible in fully formed teeth. Since the canal walls in the apical region may be paper thin, there is probably some advantage to establishing working length approximately 2 mm coronal to the most apical root edge (Fig. 6–3). By working at this slightly coronal level, there is less likelihood that the thin apical root structure will be torn by files. By restricting filing to within the root canal, there is also less likelihood that periapical tissue that may still have the potential to participate in further root development will be damaged; hence, additional root structure may form apical to the level to which you ultimately place calcium hydroxide.

4. Instrument the canal. Large sized (#70 to #90 Hedstrom) files are recommended. Instrumentation in these instances should be thought of as planing of all walls of the canal without an attempt to increase the size of the canal. In order to contact all surfaces of the canal, it is necessary to place a curvature on the file. In particular, it is difficult to adequately debride the labial and lingual portions of the canal, since, as noted above, the pulp chambers in the apical portion of these roots are frequently much wider labio-lingually than they are in a mesio-distal dimension (see Fig. 6–1).

5. Dry the canal. Coarse sterile paper points should be used for drying. The paper points should be grasped with cotton pliers held at the working length so that the point does not go beyond the canal. Once the canal is dry, a medicament (CMCP) should be placed in the manner previously described.

6. The access cavity is then sealed with Cavit.

Third Appointment

1. Place the rubber dam and remove the Cavit and the medicated pellet.

2. Freshen the canal walls with the same size file used at the second appointment, then thoroughly irrigate the canal again to remove debris.

3. Dry the canal as you did at the second visit. In some instances, you may find some bleeding due to ingrowth of periapical inflammatory tissue. The bleeding can generally be controlled by irrigation and by measuring the

paper points so that they do not go beyond working length. Slight bleeding that continues to dampen the apical canal should not, however, be of concern.

4. Prepare the calcium hydroxide paste. On a sterile glass slab, mix U.S.P. calcium hydroxide powder with camphorated monochlorophenol. When mixed to proper consistency, the mass should have a putty-like thickness and should hold its shape when mounded on the slab. The paste can be carried into the canal with a sterile amalgam carrier (one that is small enough to fit into the access cavity is most effective.) Alternatively, special syringes can be used to introduce the calcium hydroxide paste into the canal.

5. Next, begin moving the paste into the apical canal with a long plugger that can be introduced to within 2 to 3 mm of working length without binding on any of the canal walls. The first plugger insertion should be slow, and the patient should be warned that he may experience slight pain. Although material that is forced beyond the canal into periapical tissue will generally resorb, it is desirable to attempt to confine the calcium hydroxide paste to the root canal. It is generally helpful to place a rubber stop on the plugger and set it so that you insert the instrument only to within 2 to 3 mm of your working length. Once the first mass of the paste has been moved apically, additional paste can be placed in the canal with the amalgam carrier, and the condensation procedure repeated. As the canal begins to fill, it may be helpful to use a larger size plugger than you used for the initial condensation. Although pluggers work well, some operators prefer to tamp the paste in place with the butt ends of large sized paper points.

6. A radiograph should be taken to assess the quality of the obturation. If voids are evident, particularly in the apical segment of the canal, it may be necessary to reinsert the smaller plugger and then add additional paste.

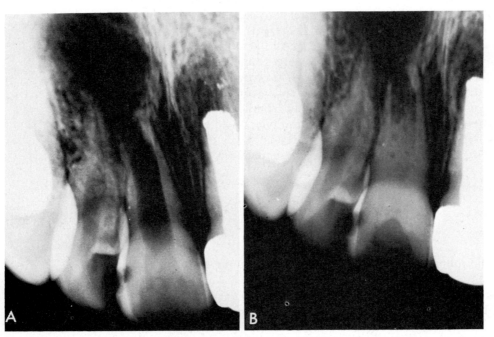

Figure 6–4 *A*, Preoperative appearance of the canal. *B*, Calcium hydroxide paste has been placed; note the relatively more opaque appearance and loss of the canal outline, particularly in the coronal portion of the canal.

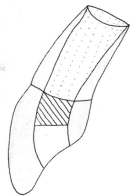

Figure 6–5 Diagram of temporary restoration of a tooth undergoing calcium hydroxide root closure. Dotted area = calcium hydroxide, diagonal lines = cavit or zinc oxide and eugenol, and the clear area = zinc phosphate or silicate.

Although the calcium hydroxide paste does not have the radiodensity of conventional root canal filling materials, you should begin to lose the clarity of the canal outline when the material has been properly condensed (Fig. 6–4).

7. Excess paste should be removed from the chamber with a spoon excavator and moist cotton pellets. A large, dry cotton pellet is then placed over the canal orifice, and additional condensation with a large plugger is performed. In some instances you may find that the entire paste mass will move apically.

8. A durable temporary filling should be placed in the access cavity. If the pulp chamber is large, a double seal composed of a layer of Cavit or thick mix of zinc oxide and eugenol followed by a final layer of zinc phosphate cement or silicate is recommended (Fig. 6–5). In instances in which the access size is limited, a single layer of either zinc phosphate cement or silicate is generally acceptable. Cavit alone is not recommended at this stage of the procedure, since the temporary filling must function for at least six months and in some instances for as long as 1½ years. Coronal leakage may prevent root induction from occurring and will necessitate that the canal be reinstrumented and resealed before a satisfactory result can occur.

RECALL SEQUENCE

Generally patients remain comfortable after the placement of the calcium hydroxide–CMCP. In the event that pain occurs during the first few days after the procedure, appropriate analgesics can be prescribed.

As long as the patient remains asymptomatic, the first scheduled recall should be at approximately 6 months. At that time a radiograph is taken, in addition to making a clinical evaluation of mobility, palpation and percussion tenderness, and the status of the temporary filling. The radiograph should be examined to determine: (1) if any calcification has occurred in the apical region (Fig. 6–6), and (2) if paste can still be seen in the root canal.

If root end closure is occurring but is not complete, the paste can be seen in the canal, and the temporary filling is intact, the paste should not be disturbed. In the event that you cannot see signs of apical closure, the paste is not evident in the canal, or the temporary filling is breaking down, the tooth should be reopened and the instrumentation procedure and calcium hydroxide placement should be repeated in the manner previously described.

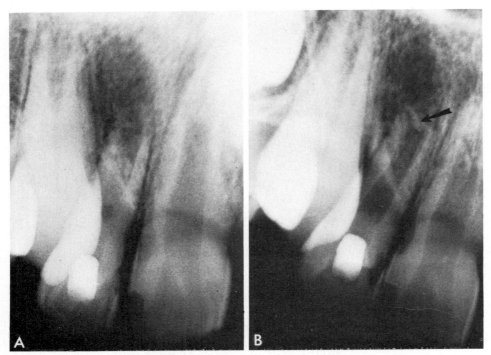

Figure 6–6 *A*, Appearance of the apical canal immediately after placement of the calcium hydroxide. *B*, A recall radiograph after several months demonstrating the initial formation of a calcified apical bridge (*arrow*). (Courtesy of Dr. Gerald W. Harrington.)

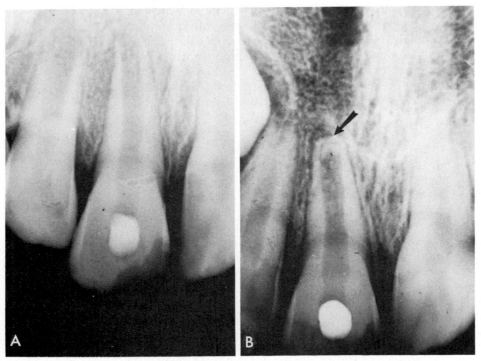

Figure 6–7 *A*, Initial radiographs at the time the calcium hydroxide paste was placed. *B*, Subsequent recall radiograph demonstrating good radiographic evidence of root closure (*arrow*). The bridge should be tested with instruments at this stage to determine if the barrier is complete. (From Steiner, J. C., Dow, P. R., and Cathey, G. M. J. Dent. Child. *35*:47, 1968. Used with permission.)

Recall visits should be continued at 6 month intervals. The examination and/or treatment procedures just described should be repeated until there is good radiographic evidence that the root end has closed (Fig. 6–7).

Although in some patients closure may occur within 6 months, you should routinely advise the patient, and particularly the patient's parents, that the treatment may take as long as 18 months or more.

Final Appointment

When you have radiographic evidence of root end closure, the tooth should be isolated and reopened. The final test that the root end has in fact calcified is made with a #25 file, since in some cases the bridge will be incomplete regardless of the radiographic appearance. The files should be used to probe the entire surface of the calcified bridge. If the clinical test demonstrates a "dead stop" in all areas, obturation with gutta percha can be performed. If, on the other hand, voids are found in the bridge, consideration should be given to replacing the calcium hydroxide paste for another 6 months or until the bridge is complete.

Procedure for Final Obturation

After probing the bridge, a radiograph is taken to confirm the final working length, the canal is flooded with an irrigant, and all the walls of the canal are filed gently. A final irrigation is then completed and the canal is dried with large sterile paper points.

Although the apical barrier will prevent overfilling, the canals of teeth that have undergone root end induction still do not lend themselves to routine gutta percha obturation techniques, primarily because of the extensive labio-lingual dimension of the canals.

In order to completely obturate such teeth, it is necessary to soften large gutta percha cones with a solvent such as chloroform and then use vertical condensation as well as lateral condensation to distort the gutta percha into the irregularities. Vertical condensation of gutta percha that is first softened with a hot plugger is another method of filling these irregular canals.

Once obturation is complete, a final restoration such as silicate can be placed.

ROOT END INDUCTION IN ADULT PATIENTS

Occasionally it may be desirable to use the root end induction procedure just described in an adult patient in whom pulp injury at a young age prevented complete root formation. Root end induction is particularly desirable in those adult patients in whom surgical intervention would be difficult, as for example, with a palatal root of a maxillary molar or a distal canal of a mandibular second molar.

Although successful results have been obtained in adults (Fig. 6–8), there is not good evidence available on the comparative success rates in adults and children.

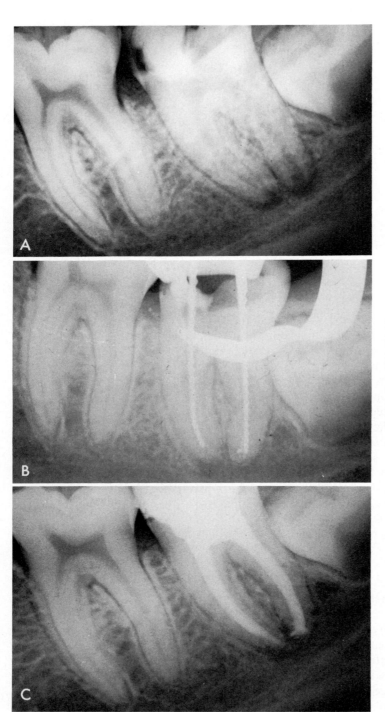

Figure 6–8 Root end closure in the distal canal of an 18-year-old patient. *A*, Preoperative appearance (the tooth had been left open for approximately 2 years). *B*, Seven months after calcium hydroxide placement a bridge was present at the level shown in the radiograph. *C*, Final filling radiograph demonstrating some extrusion of sealer through porosity in the bridge but control of the primary filling material.

REFERENCES

1. Nygren, J. A.: Rådgivare angående bästa sättet att värda och bevara tändernas friskhet. Stockholm, 1838.
2. Granath, L. E.: Några synpunkter på behandlingen av traumatiserade incisiver på barn. Odont. Revy 10:272, 1959.
3. Ingle, J. I., and Beveridge, E. E. Endodontics, 2nd ed. Philadelphia, Lea & Febiger, 1976, p. 689.
4. Frank, A. L.: Endodontic endosseous implants and treatment of the wide open apex. Dent. Clin. North Am. 11:675, 1967.
5. Steiner, J. C., and Van Hassel, H. J.: Experimental root apexification in primates. Oral Surg. 31:409, 1971.
6. Pisanti, S., and Sciaky, I.: Localization of calcium placed over amputated pulps in dogs' teeth. J. Dent. Res. 39:1128, 1960.

7

Traumatic Injuries and the Expanded Endodontic Role of Calcium Hydroxide

RAYMOND T. WEBBER, D.D.S., M.S.

INTRODUCTION

Resorptive or iatrogenic perforations, root fractures, and root loss from external resorption can create special endodontic difficulties and an unfavorable prognosis. In this chapter, the calcium hydroxide technique employed in various clinical situations is discussed, along with a suggested course of therapy that will aid in the treatment of these endodontic difficulties. The basic endodontic principle, i.e., complete obturation of the root canal system, is especially applicable to obturation with calcium hydroxide. Scientific articles describing failure of the calcium hydroxide technique may not take into account the necessity of introducing the paste completely into the apex and ensuring that the mixture is placed without voids. Canal obturation is essential, as are thorough cleaning and shaping of the root canal system to achieve predictable healing.

The added benefits of calcium hydroxide treatment (or its alkaline pH) are biologic stimulation of hard tissue deposition at the defect, stimulation of the repair process, and bactericidal effects. Further advantages include easy preparation and a favorable influence on the local environment of resorptive defects by raising the acid pH to an alkaline pH (thus stimulating the healing process). Also resorption of the calcium hydroxide occurs if it is extruded out of the canal system. The calcium hydroxide therapy advocated in this chapter is not intended to be a panacea for all endodontic treatment, but if a proper diagnosis is made, the prognosis is much brighter in many situations.

Immunologic Response. Spangburg's studies showed that calcium hydroxide was extremely toxic to HeLa cells. Kawahara et al. showed that dispersed calcium hydroxide was extremely toxic to tissue culture cellular growth. Jones et al. used radioisotope determination to measure the carbon dioxide release resulting from pulp respiration in rat incisors and demonstrated that Dycal is quite cytotoxoid. Stuart et al., using in vivo skin tests on rabbits, showed that USP Calcium Hydroxide (Eli Lilly and Co.) is inflammatory. However, in vitro assessments for antibody detection against the calcium hydroxide were negative. Their conclusion was that calcium hydroxide is a nonspecific irritant. Campbell et al., in an earlier study, arrived at the same conclusion as the later investigators: specifically, they were unable to show antigenicity by migratory inhibiting factor (MIF) assay in guinea pigs. Calcium hydroxide does cause an initial inflammatory response when it contacts viable tissue. Patients often have some initial inflammation comparable to that of root canal sealer contacting a viable periodontium. On the average, discomfort lasts 1 or 2 days after each proper placement of the paste and can be relieved by aspirin or its equivalent. In some rarer instances, the patient does have discomfort 3 to 10 days after $Ca(OH)_2$ placement. This correlates with Campbell et al.'s study, which showed the inflammatory response to manifest itself 2 to 3 days after placement of the paste in guinea pigs. However, Goldberg and Gurfinkel reported that, when employing Dycal as their root canal sealer, they observed less postoperative pain than after using conventional root canal filling cements.

Commercial Preparations. Multi-Cal is a preparation that has been premixed in a water-soluble base that softens or melts at body temperature. It is composed of 34 per cent calcium hydroxide, 15 per cent barium sulfate, and 51 per cent Chloro-Thymonol. The active ingredients of Chloro-Thymonol are 1 per cent phenacaine hypochloride, 5 per cent thymol, and 6 per cent camphorated parachlorophenol. Pulpdent is composed of calcium hydroxide mixed with a methyl cellulose vehicle. Hypo-Cal contains 45 per cent calcium hydroxide, 5 per cent barium sulfate, 2 per cent hydroxyethyl cellulose, and 48 per cent water. The commercial preparations are in soft paste form, which makes vertical condensation difficult. Burke describes mixing Pulpdent with calcium hydroxide powder to obtain a thicker mix to aid in condensation. Multi-Cal can be condensed more easily if it is kept refrigerated until time of use.

Calcium Hydroxide Preparation. Calcium hydroxide is very slightly soluble in water and insoluble in alcohol. USP (Lilly #40) or chemically pure powder of calcium hydroxide is desired, since contaminants in the powder may adversely affect healing. The author prefers the powder rather than the commercial preparations because the powder can be mixed with a vehicle to variable consistencies for ease of condensation in the root canal system. The fewer noncontributory materials, the better the preparation. Because of the antibacterial effect of calcium hydroxide, a germicide is not needed as a vehicle. Therefore, a desirable liquid vehicle is one that is tissue compatible and nonirritating to the surrounding tissue if the vehicle is extruded. *Suggested vehicles* are sterile water, isotonic saline, or dental anesthetic (preferably without a vasoconstrictor).

A clean, sterile glass slab and spatula with no residual cement are necessary to avoid contamination of the medicament. Barium sulfate powder is added to the paste to provide opacity and thus aid in radiographic interpretation of the extent of the calcium hydroxide paste in the root canal system. A ratio of one part barium sulfate to eight to ten parts calcium

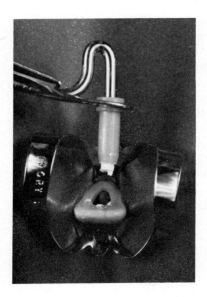

Figure 7–1   Amalgam carrier with Teflon sleeve.

hydroxide is recommended. To obtain an even distribution of the opacity through the paste, add the barium sulfate to the liquid vehicle first and then add small increments of calcium hydroxide. The powders and liquid are mixed to a very dry, thick consistency comparable to that of a dry resin. It is important that the mix possesses enough body to allow vertical condensation while minimizing occlusal reverse flow.

Introduction to Paste.   An amalgam carrier is suggested for introducing the calcium hydroxide paste into the canal. A clean carrier with a plastic or Teflon sleeve (Fig. 7–1) is recommended, because the calcium hydroxide can corrode metals and contaminate the paste.

Condensation.   The canal system is usually packed with the calcium hydroxide at the instrumentation appointment. In cases of acute apical abscess, the canal should not be packed with the calcium hydroxide medication until drainage of the purulent exudate from the periapical lesion has occurred. This can be aided by direct aspiration of the canal through the access opening.

Various diameters of blunted endodontic pluggers are needed for vertical condensation to ensure a dense filling. The pluggers are prefitted for the correct size and length. First, a plugger is selected that nearly occludes the canal at a distance of 2 to 3 mm short of the radiographic apex and yet does not bind against the dentinal walls. The mix is introduced in small increments, using the small barrel only half full. The pluggers should be firmly pressed against the mix in a vertical direction, and the sizes should be gradually increased as the canal is filled. Introduction of small increments of the paste will provide a denser filling. In order to prevent root fracture, the pluggers should not bind against the canal walls, but a technique employing depth control is preferable. A thickness of 4 mm of temporary filling (IRM or ZOE) is required to create an adequate seal.

Refilling Procedures.   For a more predictable result, the calcium hydroxide should be changed routinely at the *first* 6 week observation visit. In some instances, the paste may need to be changed earlier. Holland and associates demonstrated better results with a paste change.

The placement of calcium hydroxide is not limited to the first and second appointments; rather, it should be replaced as often as necessary. If the paste is found to be dry *to* the apex at the first recall visit, the patient can be placed on a 2 to 3 month recall. If the paste is found to be wet in the apical half or (in instances of root perforations) wet in the vicinity of the perforation, the paste should be changed at the second 6 week recall. A radiographic observation of the status of the paste in the canal system assists in determining when the paste needs changing at the recall appointments. If there appears to be a dilution of the paste in the canal (i.e., it becomes more radiolucent), the calcium hydroxide should be changed. The final determination for a calcium hydroxide change is made at the time of removal of the temporary filling by probing the paste with an endodontic explorer, file, or reamer to ascertain if the paste is still dry. If a patient redevelops a sinus tract and/or develops symptoms in the early months of treatment, this is an indication that the paste needs changing. Remedial results can be obtained with persistent calcium hydroxide treatment, provided that the apex or the odontogenic defect is completely *within osseous tissue* or osseous-forming tissue (e.g., below the crestal bone level and within the architecture of the cortical plate). A lateral perforation of the tooth less than 2 or 3 mm below the crestal bone height has a guarded prognosis.

SECTION I. INFLAMMATORY PERIAPICAL RESORPTION
(Cases 1 to 6, pp. 178 to 180)

Warner et al. claim that resorption is a common pathologic occurrence that may begin at any point at which the tooth is covered with connective tissue (although it occurs more commonly in the apical region) and that all adult teeth display some minute areas of resorption, but usually with repair. This phenomenon was confirmed by Penick and later by Massler and Perreault. Radiographic evidence has shown that resorption can progress slowly, remain static, or progress rapidly and may show repair. Extensive apical resorption usually indicates severe pulp involvement, with a chronic apical periodontitis. In these situations canal debridement is essential. Seltzer and Bender reported that osteoclastic activity of the alveolar bone may be seen within a few days after odontoblastic injury. It should be kept in mind that the clastic cells do not have a preference for bone and will resorb tooth structure as well. Frank showed that the crater-shaped resorptive defect could heal by gutta percha obturation alone. Coolidge, and later Seltzer, demonstrated by histologic analysis that the resorptive areas of tooth structure healed by cemental repair. Kronfeld reported that the most important function of cementum is the repair of injuries to the root surface. Bone-like substances (osteodentin, osteoid) have also been reported to repair resorbed dentin.

Once an apex has matured, it can undergo extensive periapical resorption, which opens the canal system thereby resembling the immature apex (Fig. 7–2). The main cause of this apical pathosis is irritation from a necrotic or irreversibly involved pulp. The resorption may also be due to a combined periodontic-endodontic lesion (see Section X).

The osteoclasts, cementoclasts, and/or dentinoclasts found in the granulation tissue of the apical pathosis do not evenly resorb the tooth structure at the apical foramen. Quite often, the resorptive process proceeds

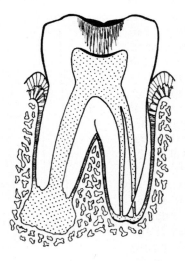

Figure 7–2 The distal root manifested significant apical resorption, which mitigated against creating an effective apical stop during instrumentation.

into the root canal a few millimeters, thereby opening up the diameter of the apex even more. This resorptive process can be halted and healing permitted by obturating the canal system, thus preventing the exchange of an inflammatory infiltrate fed by an aberrant blood supply between the canal system and the periapical lesion.

If the canals are of small enough diameter and apical fixation (stop) can be created by dropping back 2 mm from the radiographic apex during the shaping of the canal, the canals can be obturated with gutta percha. Every long-standing periapical cyst or granuloma will result in some resorption of tooth structure (Case 1). Fortunately, in most instances only the obturation of the canal with a final filling material is needed. Strindberg pointed out that the canal is generally open at the apex; thus circumstances may foster a pronounced overfilling and a consequent poor prognosis. In situations in which the canal's diameter is quite large and the periapical resorption has removed any natural apical constriction, the canals can be effectively treated with the calcium hydroxide technique (Cases 2, 3, and 4). Far too often, this inflammatory periapical resorption is associated with a previous endodontic filling that initially did not obturate the canal system, thus allowing a continuation of the resorption process (Case 5).

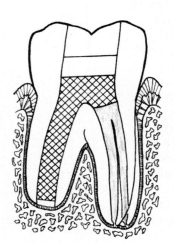

Figure 7–3 The distal canal was treated with calcium hydroxide paste as if it were an immature canal with a necrotic pulp. The mesial canals demonstrated little resorption, and it was felt that fixation could be created; therefore, the canals were obturated with gutta percha.

As in the apexification technique, one would expect osteogenic healing of the periapical pathosis to occur before sufficient thickness of the calcified barrier could be deposited, and this would allow satisfactory obturation with gutta percha (Fig. 7–3). Mitchell and Shankwalker reported on the extensive osteogenic potential displayed by calcium hydroxide. The purpose of employing the calcium hydroxide technique is to achieve biologic healing by means of canal obturation plus the antibacterial effect and physiologic healing promoted by the alkaline pH of the calcium hydroxide. Tronstad et al. suggested that calcium hydroxide actively influences resorption areas, first by arresting the osteoclastic activity and second by stimulating the repair process of the tissues.

Apical root resorption may also be the result of systemic conditions, neoplasms, erupting teeth, traumatic occlusion, excessive mechanical forces (Case 6), idiopathic causes (see Section XI), or pathosis (cysts) associated with involvement of an impacted or an involved neighboring tooth. It has been well documented that orthodontic movement can cause external root resorption, and the resorption usually occurs at the apex. These conditions alone usually do not necessitate endodontic treatment. However, if the pulpal systems of these root-resorbed teeth subsequently become irreversibly involved as a result of decay or trauma and if the cause of the resorption is eliminated, these teeth can be treated with calcium hydroxide in order to achieve an effective apical stop. If it is discovered that the vascular supply to resorbed roots has been severed during the surgical removal of pathologic tissue, neoplasms, or impacted teeth, it is recommended that a reverse amalgam filling procedure be carried out (during surgery) and that the root canals be filled with gutta percha. However, if the severance of the blood supply is not detected during the surgical procedure and the pulps subsequently become involved, calcium hydroxide treatment may be employed to generate a calcified barrier for subsequent canal obturation with gutta percha.

Chivian reported on Weiss' thesis, which showed that there is no significant difference in the amount of root resorption of endodontically treated teeth and teeth with vital pulps when both are subjected to orthodontic movement. Chivian pointed out that it is important for root canals of teeth to receive orthodontic treatment to be filled three dimensionally (with gutta percha) rather than by a solid cone technique because the apical third of the canal must remain sealed, even after resorption of the apical few millimeters of the root. Seltzer had reported that the breakdown products of silver cones are cytotoxic. Once the natural constriction of the apex and the apical few millimeters are resorbed and an exchange of tissue fluid occurs between the canal system and the periapical tissues (compounded by the cytotoxic products of the silver cone), the resorptive process is perpetuated. In retreatment of teeth containing a previous failing root canal filling, it is often difficult to create a new apical fixation; therefore, calcium hydroxide therapy stimulating an apical barrier may be the preferred treatment.

Orthodontic movement of teeth that display *active* periapical resorption and, more so, lateral root resorption is not recommended (see Case 29). Upon healing of periapical root resorption, the teeth may be considered for orthodontic movement. Moreover, Chivian pointed out that orthodontic movement is unsuccessful in instances of replacement resorption, owing to the lock-and-key adaptation of the bone.

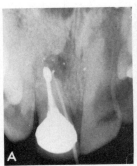
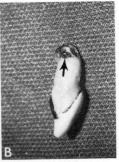

Case 1 The patient was referred with a silver point root canal filling in the maxillary left incisor and a reverse amalgam filling that had been placed several years before. A diagnostic gutta percha cone was placed in a buccal sinus tract that led to a long-standing periapical lesion (A). An exploratory surgical flap was reflected to find a resorptive defect on the *lingual* surface. Not being able to determine the extent of the resorption and considering the crown-to-root ratio that would have been left after beveling the resorptive area enough for a new amalgam reverse filling, the author elected to extract the tooth (B). The biopsy report revealed that the lesion was a periapical granuloma. This exploratory surgery was performed 7 years ago before the author realized the potential of calcium hydroxide. Today the crown, small post, and the silver cone would have been removed and the canal system would have been treated with the calcium hydroxide technique. It is felt that both the existing root canal filling and the apical amalgam restoration were not effectively obturating the canal system and the resorption was probably present at the time of the first surgery.

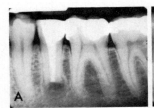
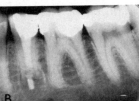
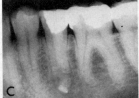
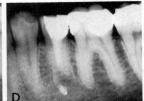

Case 2 The patient presented with a symptomatic premolar that had undergone extensive apical resorption and abscess formation. The root canal had been filled with gutta percha 10 years before the radiograph (A). Because the canal size was larger than a #140 file, it was treated with calcium hydroxide. In removing the gutta percha filling, approximately 3 mm of the gutta percha was pushed into the periapical lesion (B). When the calcium hydroxide paste was changed at the end of a 2 month period, it was found that the paste had extruded into the apical tissue, nearly occluding the lesion. The patient was comfortable until this 2 month emergency appointment, at which time he presented with severe discomfort (C). The paste was again changed at the 5 month and 10 month appointments. At the 10 month appointment the radiograph suggested periapical healing; moreover, partial apical barrier formation could be detected clinically (D). The patient has been comfortable since the 2 month emergency appointment. The calcium hydroxide treatment will be continued for approximately another 6 months in order to allow the apical hard tissue barrier to attain sufficient thickness.

Case 3 A 12-year-old patient presented with an involved right maxillary lateral incisor that had sustained a traumatic injury 2 years before *(C)*. The death of the pulp had left a wide canal system that exhibited parallel walls when compared with the contralateral tooth. The tooth probably had a blunderbuss apex at the time of pulpal death. Eighteen months after the injury, it appeared that the apex had opened even wider as a result of the periapical resorption associated with the pathosis *(B)*. Two years after the injury and 20 months after the orthopantograph *(A)* the apex shows significant periapical resorption *(C)*. A gutta percha cone was placed in the buccal sinus tract *(C)*. Calcium hydroxide is considered the treatment of choice. (Courtesy of Dr. Pataky Levent, Budapest, Hungary.)

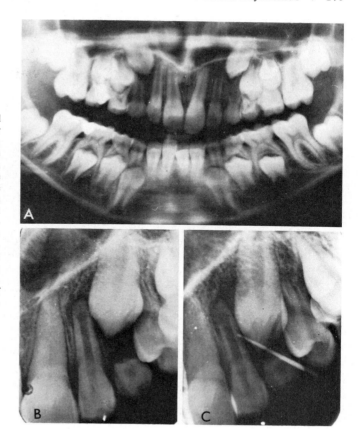

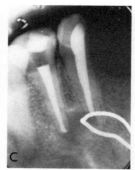

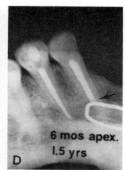

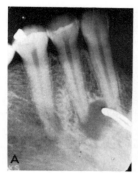

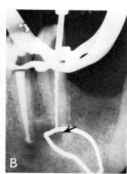

Case 4 The patient was referred with involvement of both the mandibular left cuspid and the first premolar. The patient reported a history of an automobile accident involving bilateral fracture of the mandible. Surgical osseous stabilizing wire can be seen at the apex of the cuspid *(A)*. The first premolar exhibited an apical constriction and was obturated with gutta percha. However, the cuspid had a divergent apex as a result of apical resorption *(arrow)*, confirmed both clinically and radiographically *(B)*. The canal of the cuspid was debrided and obturated with calcium hydroxide *(C)*. Calcium hydroxide treatment was continued for 6 months. A 1½ year recall showed that barium sulfate *(arrow)* had been incorporated into the apical barrier and healing of the periapical lesion had occurred *(D)*.

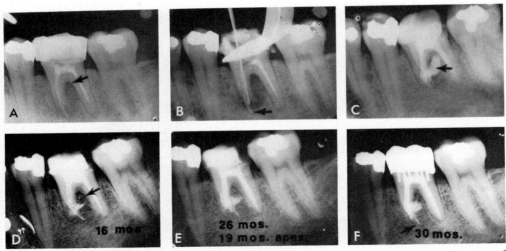

Case 5 The patient had been referred to the periodontist because of drainage of copious amounts of purulent exudate through the furcation. The periodontist, recognizing an endodontic problem, referred the patient for appropriate treatment. Apparently, the canal system had not been completely obturated at the time of gutta percha placement; the mesial portion of the apex had undergone extensive apical resorption and an endo-perio complication *(arrow)* had been established *(A)*. The gutta percha was removed from the mesial canals, but the overextended segment *(arrow)* (possibly the result of the resorption) could not be retrieved *(B)*. The mesial canals were immediately obturated with calcium hydroxide paste. Four months later, when the mesial canals were being repacked for the third time, it was again observed that the paste was still being extruded *(arrow)* from the resorbed defect *(C)*. At 16 months the radiograph revealed a healed furcation and regeneration of the lamina dura *(arrow)* *(D)*. Nineteen months after initial treatment, the radiograph suggested healing with a calcified barrier at the mesial root apices. The distal canal was re-treated, and all three canals were obturated with gutta percha, using lateral condensation. A 26 month re-call revealed a reattachment of the periodontal ligament on clinical examination or a clinically improbable junctional epithelial attachment in the furcation and an asymptomatic tooth *(E)*. Thirty months after the initial appointment a recall radiograph showed continued healing. The opaque area distal to the mesial roots represents remnants of the barium sulfate that had been incorporated into the healed osseous tissues. The overextended gutta percha point *(arrow)* of the mesial root had not deterred healing. The tooth was found to be in traumatic occlusion, apparently as a result of the large restoration *(F)*. The author does not advocate the picket fence placement of pins for restoration.

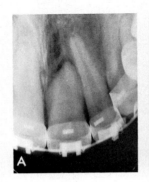
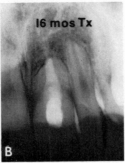

Case 6 A 16-year-old patient was referred with a history of lingual luxation of the right maxillary central incisor 2 weeks previously. The patient had been undergoing ortho-dontic treatment at the time of trauma *(A)*. The tooth demon-strated a negative response to electric pulp tests and test cavity. Upon gaining access, degenerated pulpal tissue was found along with some vital pulpal remnants in the apical few millimeters. No apical fixation could be created, even with a #140 file. The canal system was obturated with calcium hydroxide paste. A 16 month recall radiograph revealed periapical healing, and the resorption process appeared to have ceased *(B)*. Orthodontic treatment was continued for 10 months after the initial treatment with calcium hydroxide.

SECTION II. INTERNAL ROOT RESORPTION
(Cases 7 to 10, pp. 183 and 184)

Internal resorption had been described as early as 1830. Mummery published the first extensive study of pink spots in 1920. The exact etiology of internal resorption is not known, but Seltzer and Bender suggest that it may be the result of an irreversible chronic pulpitis. Pritchard, in 1931, showed histologically that internal resorption was comparable to a granuloma of the pulp. Internal resorption is the result of dentinoclastic (osteoclastic) activity nourished by a highly vascularized granulation tissue that has replaced normal pulp. This resorption may be idiopathic or may result from trauma or caries and iatrogenic procedures such as restorative preparation and/or improper restoration placement. Stanley described the mechanism of a typical chronic inflammatory response in the pulp. It is felt that if there is reinjury or the irritating factors persist, the chronic inflammation *may* lead to a resorptive process. Probably the most frequent causes of internal resorption are traumatic forces and/or traumatic occlusion. These traumatic injuries may produce foci of intrapulpal hemorrhage that will be replaced by granulation tissue, resulting in the establishment of a more permanent aberrant vascular system. Extirpation of the pulp will halt the resorptive process. Calcium hydroxide procedures such as vital pulpotomy and pulp capping can be the cause of internal resorption, especially in primary teeth. In many instances, internal resorption may be caused by improper technique or the traumatic injury to the pulp rather than the action of the calcium hydroxide itself.

Radiographically, the internal resorptive lesion of pulpal origin has a sharp, smooth margin that can usually be clearly defined and is continuous with the pulp space, as opposed to the progressive asymmetric resorption of tooth structure that originates in the periodontium. Chivian et al. and Gartner et al. emphasize that in order to evaluate the extent of the resorptive defect and determine the proper treatment plan, one needs to take several radiographs from different horizontal angles. Variations in the horizontal angle during exposure of the radiographs should confirm or deny this contiguous nature. Cathey points out that other radiolucencies (nutrient canals, foramina, or external resorptive defects) may be superimposed on the pulp cavity, but their relationship to the cavity will vary in proportion to changes in the horizontal angle. This would appear as a darker radiolucency within a radiolucency as a consequence of the varying amount of residual calcified tooth structure, which casts contrasting radiopaque shadows. Once the resorption has been detected, early treatment is necessary. These teeth are usually asymptomatic until the root is perforated. If the resorption has not perforated the root, the canal can be adequately debrided and obturated with a softened gutta percha technique (see Case 55). If the resorption has perforated the root, the periodontium will ultimately be destroyed if the tooth is not treated. During the debridement appointment, if the aberrant pulp cannot be removed with a bent tip of file, 5.25 per cent sodium hypochlorite can be left in the canal for several minutes to initiate proteolysis of the tissue. Whenever possible, mechanical debridement should be attempted, as it is doubtful that the sodium hypochlorite can accomplish complete debridement. During subsequent appointments, it is recommended that sterile water be used as an irrigant to prevent possible damage to the healing tissues.

Frank and Weine describe their treatment of perforating defects (due to internal resorption) with calcium hydroxide paste. They advocate this nonsurgical treatment because of the lack of predictability in locating and treating the defect by a surgical approach and the possibility of production of a periodontal defect as a result of placement of the alloy. The author advocates continuation of the calcium hydroxide treatment until a calcified barrier is created (Case 7); occasionally the barrier is osseous tissue formation replacing the area of perforation. When the resorption has perforated the root surface, a calcium hydroxide periodontal paste can be used to stimulate a biologic repair of cementoid or osteoid type tissue, provided the perforation is within osseous tissue (Cases 8 and 9). If it can be determined that the resorption has occurred on the facial surface of a root protruding out of the cortical plate or that the process has caused resorption of the cortical plate around a root eminence (such as a canine), calcium hydroxide treatment is not recommended, and repair of the defect by a surgical approach is preferred.

For the best prognosis, immediate calcium hydroxide therapy is required for the perforation found within bone. At the initial appointment there may be considerable hemorrhage caused by the granulation tissue profusing through the resorptive defect. It may be difficult to dry the canal completely. As the calcium hydroxide paste is condensed, special consideration should be given to obturating the resorptive defect, hopefully pushing the paste into direct contact with the periodontium. This will aid in controlling the hemorrhage and establishing an environment conducive to healing. If the canal was not completely dry at the time of initial placement of calcium hydroxide, the paste should be changed in 3 or 4 weeks. If the canal was initially dry, the paste should be changed in 6 weeks. The canal will often be dry at the second appointment, but it is not unusual to find some seepage at the second or even the third appointment. In removing the paste at the recall appointments, care should be taken not to puncture the defect, as this will disturb the healing tissues and cause hemorrhage. Usually, after the second paste filling appointment, the patient need *not* be recalled until an additional 6 weeks or 2 months before evaluation of another paste change.

The calcium hydroxide paste needs to be changed regularly at recall intervals, as compared with the procedure for treatment of root apexification. The size of the defect has a direct bearing on the number of paste changes needed to obtain the calcified matrix, as the larger the perforation, the greater the possibility of resorption of the paste. If at the first recall (6 weeks or longer) the paste is found to be the same consistency as it was when placed, the patient can be given a longer time interval of 3 months before the next recall. It is not recommended that the final filling be placed the first time the paste is found to be *dry* upon re-entry of the canal(s). Adequate time must be allowed for *sufficient thickness* of the calcified barrier to form in order to be able to withstand condensation pressures of the final obturation with gutta percha. The resorptive defect with a calcified matrix is the ideal situation in which to employ final obturation with the warm gutta percha (Schilder) technique (Case 8).

If it cannot be determined by radiographic and clinical procedures whether or not the resorptive process has perforated the root, the canal may be packed with calcium hydroxide as a diagnostic aid in determining the existence and extent of the perforation (Case 10). In instances in which the resorptive defect is quite extensive and all the pulpal tissue cannot be removed, the canal may be packed with the paste in order to obtain the necrotizing effect of the calcium hydroxide on the residual pulp tissue. This tissue may later be removed and the canal obturated with gutta percha.

Because pain is so infrequently associated with internal resorption, routine follow-up is imperative for teeth with traumatic injuries, occlusal dysfunction, deep restorations, pulp cappings, and especially pulpotomies. A wait-and-see approach is inappropriate. Electric and thermal pulpal tests are of no value in differential diagnosis because of the vitality of the pulp. The internal resorption is a progressive dissolution of dentin, enamel, and cementum and can be halted only by pulp removal or the necrosis of the pulp.

In a recent article, Frank redefined the "external-internal progressive resorption" phenomenon. He described the resorptive process as originating on the external root surface and then progressing inward, destroying and extending to the side of the root canal, but *not* invading the root canal system. Frank reported three cases demonstrating this resorptive pattern. The author agrees with Frank's treatment, as follows:

First, the apical canal space is obturated with gutta percha; then (coronal to the filling material) a round bur is used to establish a communication between the root canal space and the irregular "external-internal" resorptive defect. After this, Frank recommends filling this defect from within the root canal outward, using amalgam (in posterior teeth) or composite resin (in anterior teeth), in those cases in which the resorptive pattern is situated coronal to or level with the *crestal bone height*. The author supports Frank's philosophy that reflection of a flap and placement of an external restoration would cause more damage to the periodontium than use of the internal approach. In many instances in which the defect is above or at the bone height, a crown lengthening procedure would benefit the gingival health after restoration. However, in instances in which external-internal progressive resorption occurs just *below* the bone height, the author is concerned about the *long-term* results, as duplicated in Frank's Case 2, illustrating a sulcular communication and adjacent osseous loss. Tronstad et al. and Andreasen's studies demonstrate that, once the cementum (intermediate layer) has been penetrated, calcium hydroxide can have a beneficial effect. In this regard the author suggests the possibility that, if the defect is *below* the crestal bone level, calcium hydroxide therapy, rather than amalgam, would produce greater biologic benefit and long-term success because a periodontal pocket would be prevented in many instances.

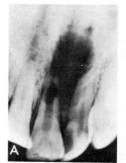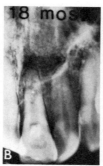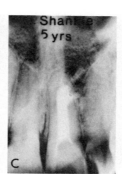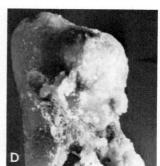

Case 7 The patient presented with a maxillary incisor with a perforating resorption and a large periapical and lateral lesion *(A)*. Periapical healing was detected after 18 months of calcium hydroxide treatment *(B)*. Calcium hydroxide treatment was continued for a total of 3 years, at which time gutta percha obturation was performed. The radiograph revealed complete healing and re-establishment of the PDL at 2 year recall after gutta percha obturation *(C)*. Subsequently, the tooth received an oblique fracture that could not be treated. A calcified callus *(arrow)* can be seen at the healed resorptive site of the root *(D)*. (Courtesy of Dr. Jack Shankle, Chapel Hill, North Carolina.)

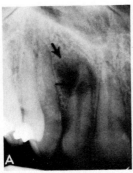
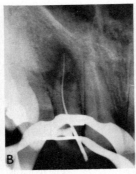
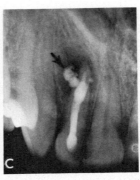
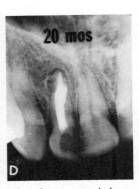

Case 8 The patient presented with a severe toothache and extraoral suborbital swelling that almost caused closure of the eye. The tooth was opened and appropriate drainage through the tooth was established. The canal yielded copious amounts of purulent exudate, followed by a serous exudate, and finally by hemorrhage (A). A working length was determined (B) and the canal was instrumented to a #70 file. At the initial debridement appointment the canal system was obturated with the calcium hydroxide paste, and extrusion of the paste (arrow) through the resorptive site was noted (C). The patient experienced much discomfort the first night but on the second day became quite comfortable. Calcium hydroxide treatment continued for 10 months, at which time a calcified barrier could be detected clinically and the paste seemed as dry as it had been when placed at the 3 month recall appointment. Gutta percha obturation was performed, using the warm gutta percha technique. A 10 month post–gutta percha recall appointment (20 months from the initial treatment) showed continuing but still incomplete healing (D).

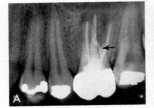
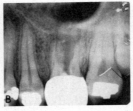
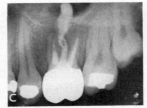
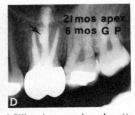

Case 9 The patient was referred with a symptomatic first molar that received a root canal filling 1 year prior. A gutta percha cone was placed in the buccal sinus tract (arrow) that led to a large periapical and intraradicular lesion (A). The gutta percha filling was removed, and extensive intraradicular root resorption could be detected radiographically. Clinically, a large defect could be demonstrated on the facial surface of the palatal root with endodontic instruments (B). A calcium hydroxide paste was condensed into the canal system, following which a large quantity of paste extruded out of the resorptive defect of the palatal root (C). After 21 months of calcium hydroxide treatment, a calcified barrier was detected in the area where the resorptive defect had occurred. The canal system was then obturated with gutta percha using lateral condensation. Six months after the permanent root canal filling (27 months from the initial treatment), the radiograph suggested osseous healing of the pathologic findings. The opaque area at the tip of the arrow is barium sulfate incorporated into the healed barrier, and the other diffuse opaque area represents remnants of the barium sulfate from the gross extrusion of the paste that became incorporated into the healing bone (D).

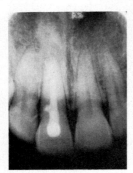

Case 10 The canal system was obturated with a radiopaque calcium hydroxide paste to determine the extent of the resorptive defect.

SECTION III. IATROGENIC ROOT PERFORATIONS
(Cases 11 to 13, pp. 186 and 187)

Iatrogenic root perforations can be managed with the same calcium hydroxide treatment as the resorptive root perforations. Persistent treatment is the key, featuring immediate placement of the calcium hydroxide followed by a change of the paste at the first 6 week recall and then when indicated. Furthermore, the defect must be below the crestal bone level to prevent dilution of the paste through an established periodontal pocket or sulcus. Often the situation goes unnoticed until symptoms or a sinus tract (fistula) develops. When a perforation is thus detected, the calcium hydroxide paste must be placed early. This lessens the chance of periodontal complications. When the perforation is on the facial surface of the root (especially in instances of facial root prominence, such as a cuspid), a surgical repair will usually yield the best prognosis. For calcium hydroxide therapy to be successful, the perforation has to be in an area that has osseous potential. If the facial perforation is in an area covered by sufficient thickness of bone, calcium hydroxide treatment would be indicated. However, when a large surface of the root has been destroyed, calcium hydroxide treatment would *not* be effective, as the calcium hydroxide would be resorbed from the canal before any organized healing process could be established (Case 11).

Probably the greatest cause of iatrogenic root perforations can be attributed to dentists' attempts to create post space by means of rotary instruments. Having deviated from the canal and having laterally perforated the root surface, the dismayed dentist may yet feel that the post will seal off the perforation. It is impossible to seal a perforation site with a post and zinc phosphate cement. This cement has one of the poorest sealing qualities of all sealing cements, and the post cannot be adapted well enough to seal the perforation effectively. If the perforation cannot be treated by a surgical approach, calcium hydroxide paste can be employed to stimulate biologic healing (Cases 12 and 13), followed by gutta percha obturation. The best treatment here is *prevention*: Create the desired post space by removing the gutta percha with hot pluggers rather than with a rotary drill.

Another common iatrogenic cause of root perforations is instrumentation of a curved root where the canal is straightened (ledged) at the lateral height of the curvature and ultimate perforation of the root. Fortunately, in most of these instances the perforation is small and relatively close to the apex. It is recommended that the canal terminus be dropped back, the instrument be carried to a few sizes larger, and the canal system be obturated with gutta percha. Evaluate the tooth at intervals, and, if healing is not detected, a surgical approach should be considered. Cases in which a perforation is caused by a large endodontic instrument (#70 or larger) and an apical stop cannot be created should be considered for calcium hydroxide treatment, especially if surgery is not feasible. A perforation in the apical one third of a dilacerated root may result in failure to negotiate or renegotiate the curvature of the root. Because a significant portion of the involved root is left, it is recommended that a surgical root tip resection be performed up to the perforation after the canal system is obturated with gutta percha (in instances of persistent periapical pathosis).

Another result of injudicious instrumentation is "canal stripping," resulting in a perforation of the furcation side of the roots. If the molar access preparation is not extended sufficiently, the file will not be able to cut the protruding enamel over the canal's orifice and the instrumentation will be diverted to the distal, thus increasing the chance of perforation (in either the furcation area or the lateral height of root curvature). "Canal stripping" can also be created by allowing the tip of a precurved endodontic file to be repeatedly dragged along the furcation side of the canal during the withdrawal motion of endodontic instrumentation. Immediate, persistent calcium hydroxide treatment can be employed to create a biologic healing process for later gutta percha obturation, provided the defect is not too large, thus allowing constant dilution and resorption of the paste before an organized healing zone can be established.

Perforations above the crestal bone height can be corrected by a restoration. On the other hand, if the defect is 1 or 2 mm below the crestal bone level, the desirable treatment is either orthodontic extrusion or apical repositioning (reduction of the periodontium below the defect) in order to allow the final restoration's margins to be properly placed. There is a good chance that if calcium hydroxide treatment were to be performed, the initial inflammation created by the paste and the technique would resorb the existing 1 or 2 mm of crestal bone, resulting in a hopeless periodontal complication.

Frank advocated immediate obturation of the canals with gutta percha at the time of the perforation, rather than waiting for subsequent periodontal breakdown to take place. The author agrees with this in instances in which the periodontium is not destroyed at the time of perforation or the perforation is of small size. In many cases, blood rushes into the canal and the periodontium is damaged beyond its ability to act as a barrier. In this situation, calcium hydroxide treatment is advocated after the canal is dried as effectively as possible (see Section VII on the control of hemorrhage).

Sinai summed up the prognosis of perforation as follows: "The prognosis for a tooth with a perforation depends on the location of the perforation, the time the perforation is opened to contamination, the possibility of sealing the perforation, and accessibility of the main canal."

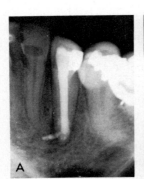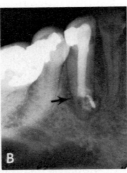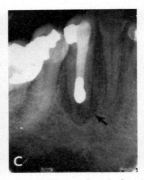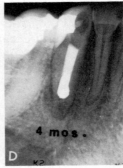

Case 11 The sixth application of calcium hydroxide paste had been placed after 10 months of treatment (A). After 1 year of treatment, the patient again presented with severe discomfort, as she had on numerous occasions before. The paste in the apical one third of the canal had resorbed (B). It was suspected that the apex protruded from the osseous tissue. A surgical flap was raised, and it was found that not only was the apex protruding from the cortical plate but that the facial surface of the apical one third of the root had been destroyed by resorption. A #6 round bur was used to remove the canal contents and any remaining facial surface in the apical one third of the root. The net result was that the root was beveled within osseous tissue and toxic irritants from the canal were removed. The purpose of this procedure was to promote deposition of cementum within the canal walls and on the exposed dentin. This served to provide a better crown-to-root ratio. A reverse amalgam filling was placed in the remaining portion of the root canal that was supported by intact root (C). At a 4 month recall, the patient was asymptomatic and the radiograph suggested osseous healing (D).

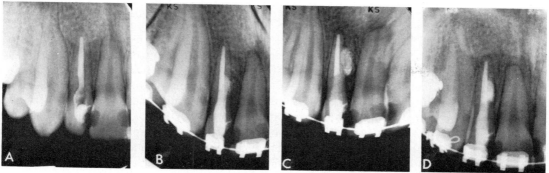

Case 12 The patient presented with a symptomatic maxillary lateral incisor. A rotary instrument that was used for post preparation had caused a mesio-lingual perforation *(A)*. After debridement of the post space, a paste of calcium hydroxide was extruded through the defect. At the first recall visit the radiograph showed that the overextended paste was resorbed and a mushy paste was found in the canal system *(B)*. A new paste was condensed *(C)*. At the fourth recall visit a fourth paste was condensed and was maintained in the canal system because of the support of a healing periodontal matrix *(D)*. The tooth is still being treated with calcium hydroxide at the University of Florida's Student Clinic.

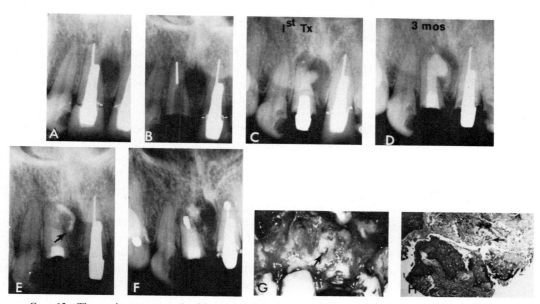

Case 13 The patient presented with a buccal draining sinus tract due to a long-standing lingual post perforation of the maxillary left central incisor. The radiographic radiolucency of the lesion suggested that both cortical plates were perforated *(A and B)*. A post puller was used to remove the post and a Hedstrom file was used to engage and remove the segmented silver cone *(B)*. The canal system was obturated with a calcium hydroxide paste, with some extrusion of the paste through the perforation site *(C)*. Three months from the initial treatment a third calcium hydroxide paste, containing one fourth barium sulfate, was condensed *(D)*. After 19 months of numerous changes of the paste, osseous tissue was detected radiographically on the mesial aspect of the root *(arrow)* in the area of the perforation. Remnants of the barium sulfate could be seen in the lateral tissue *(E)*. The paste was dry upon re-entry into the canal and a partial healing barrier could be detected. The patient was wearing a temporary treatment partial during the calcium hydroxide treatment.

A surgical flap was reflected in order to place a reverse amalgam filling in the apex of the right central incisor. Buccal cortical plate was detected over the lesion site, except for a small perforation that contained calcium hydroxide paste *(arrow, G)*. A specimen was curetted from the lesion. A reverse amalgam filling was placed in *both* incisors because the left (right in photograph) incisor's apex was protruding from the cortical plate. A surgical repair of the perforation was not attempted because the defect existed on the lingual surface of the root *(F)*. A histologic analysis of the specimen revealed new osseous formation in contact with the "spent" calcium hydroxide paste *(arrow)* *(H)*. (Histologic analysis courtesy of Dr. Harold R. Stanley, Gainesville, Florida.)

SECTION IV. FURCATION PERFORATIONS
(Case 14, p. 188)

Overzealous endodontic access preparation is the most common cause of perforations of the furcation. Hopefully, this occurs only when the pulp chamber has so diminished in size because of dystrophic changes that it is not easily detected. It should be kept in mind that the distance from the pulpal floor to the periodontal ligament (PDL) is usually less than 3 mm. Prevention is definitely the best treatment (see Chapter 1). Another common cause of furcation perforating is drilling apically in an unnegotiable calcified canal with a round bur, hoping that the underlying canal space can be negotiated.

If rapid treatment is not rendered in furcation perforations, the inevitable sequelae of periodontal inflammation in the furca may rapidly produce a noncorrectable periodontal lesion. In these situations, Frank suggested that the teeth be hemisected and restored by bicuspidation. Harris recommended sealing the perforations with Cavit. Sinai advocated an amalgam repair after a lubricated metal instrument is placed in the canal. The author has had repeated success in repairing furca perforations with amalgam, provided the defect is small. The occlusal portion of the perforation is enlarged with an inverted cone bur and a ledging (shelving) is created just above the furca opening. This provides retention form and allows one to condense the amalgam into the line angles, thus reducing the chance of amalgam extrusion during the condensation.

When the perforation is greater than 1 mm, and especially when furcation tissues are destroyed or periodontium breakdown is apparent but a periodontal communication has not been established, it is felt that calcium hydroxide paste can be employed to stimulate a biological repair (Case 14). It is of utmost concern that therapy be initiated as soon as a perforation is detected. Calcium hydroxide paste is packed to a depth of approximately 2 mm over the pulpal floor. The paste should be changed at the end of 6 weeks and then when indicated. The normal healing of the perforations takes from 3 to 9 months, depending upon the extent of damage before the initial paste placement. Expect organization of the periodontium to act as a matrix for a later amalgam or gutta percha seal.

If the canals can be "cleaned and shaped" and then obturated with gutta percha, a more predictable result will occur. The presence of an effective root canal filling would deny access of tissue fluids to the area of the calcium hydroxide paste. Of prime consideration is the time interval

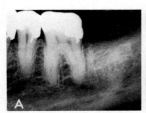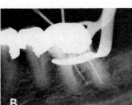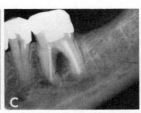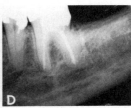

Case 14 The patient presented to the student clinic for endodontic treatment (A). The pulpal floor was perforated during an attempt to negotiate the mesial canals (B). This was not brought to the attention of the instructors until 1 month after the perforation. Significant loss of furcation bone was apparent in the 1 month interval (C). The perforation site was immediately packed with calcium hydroxide, which was changed at 6 weeks. Five months after this change, the radiograph showed evidence of bone repair with restoration of the lamina dura in the furcation area (D).

before obturating the canal system with gutta percha. If this obturation is to be postponed for more than 1 week, calcium hydroxide treatment needs to be initiated to prevent extensive furcation involvement. Again, a well-adapted intratreatment temporary filling of sufficient thickness is essential to prevent contamination to the site of perforation.

SECTION V. THE AVULSED TOOTH
(Cases 15 to 37, pp. 215 to 221)

Rationale for Reimplantation

Avulsion is the complete separation of a tooth from its alveolus. Andreasen, in reviewing the literature, reports that avulsion can occur in up to 16 per cent of traumatic injuries and is predominantly found in the age group 7 to 10 years. Andreasen theorized that after trauma the loosely structured periodontal ligament found around the developing root fosters complete avulsion, rather than other types of dental injury (Case 34).

Replantation is the return of a tooth accidentally avulsed by acute trauma into its alveolus. Replantation of an avulsed tooth has historically been considered a temporary procedure, as the retention span has varied from a few years to 10 years. Emmersten and Andreasen, in a clinical and radiographic study of 100 molars with periapical pathosis, reported that reimplanted teeth showed healing and no root resorption. However, at the end of a 13 year follow-up, only one molar in the study remained with no infection. Although there are documented exceptions to this survival time, extending up to 42 years, literature reports indicate a high but variable 80 to 96 per cent frequency of resorption of replanted teeth. Failures caused by root resorption are often seen following the reimplantation of teeth. Although this is an alarming statistic, there are sufficiently valid indications that justify the replantation procedure. In view of new experimental and clinical data, there is reason to believe that these percentages can be significantly improved upon.

External Resorption

Cementum is not a static tissue, but a biologically dynamic tissue subject to remodeling. Limited localized resorption of cementum can be considered universal, and it has been reported to occur on normal root surfaces with a frequency as high as 90 to 100 per cent. Usually there is a delicate biologic balance between deposition and resorption of cementum. Trauma in some form is the etiologic factor that causes the unfavorable shift toward resorption. Multinucleated osteoclasts (cementoclasts) are mobilized from the adjacent periodontal ligament and bone to produce the resorption.

Andreasen and Hjörting-Hansen described three types of external resorption that replanted teeth undergo: surface resorption, replacement resorption, and inflammatory resorption. Simon et al. also described similar resorptive patterns.

Surface resorption is characterized histologically by the presence of superficial resorption lacunae that may contain evidence of repair (Case 21). The resorptive areas are not necessarily confined to cementum but do usually involve a portion of the dentin. The process is self-limiting and shows new repair cementum even though the original root architecture may not have been re-established. Radiographically, this type of resorption is difficult to detect. Such resorptions can occur as a consequence of subluxations, luxations, occlusal trauma, and orthodontic movement. In a recent study, Andreasen showed that surface resorption occurs universally in replanted teeth and is self-limiting only if the resorptive cavity is shallow and does not penetrate the intermediate layer of cementum; however, if the surface resorption contacts dentinal tubules that are in communication with infected necrotic pulp tissue or an infected leukocyte zone, the resorptive process is perpetuated.

A more consequential type of resorption occurs as a postoperative complication of replanted and luxated teeth that either have not received proper endodontic treatment or have suffered death of the periodontal ligament, or both. In these instances, osteoclastic activity is intensified to produce a gradual but progressive resorption of the root with simultaneous replacement by bony trabeculae. Radiographically, the integrity of a normal periodontal ligament space is lost as the replacement bone blends imperceptibly into the adjacent alveolar bone (Case 19). This replacement resorption, or ankylosis, involves a firm fusion of tooth to alveolus. This type of resorption usually leads to loss of the replanted tooth within a few years. Andreasen postulated that an ankylosed tooth becomes a part of the remodeling phase of bone. Ankylosis may be observed 3 to 4 months after replacement. Clinically, the tooth is immobile, frequently infrapositioned, and emits high-pitched sounds upon percussion, which differ clearly from adjacent uninjured teeth. Andreasen reported that when the alveolar bone (plate) was fractured, ankylosis occurred in 80 per cent of replanted teeth.

When inflammation persists in association with resorption, the process is accentuated and becomes a self-perpetuating phenomenon that eventually advances to involve adjacent alveolar bone. The inflammatory process interferes with the elaboration of repair tissue. Upon histologic examination, the resorptive areas will be filled with highly vascularized granulation tissue that is heavily infiltrated with acute and chronic inflammatory cells (Case 22). The inflammatory reaction is initiated when the resorption establishes direct or dentinal tubular communication with a pulp cavity containing necrotic pulp tissue or an inadequate root canal filling. These portals permit free exchange of toxic, autolyzed tissue products and bacteria. This type of resorption may be detected radiographically as radiolucent areas on the root and in the alveolar bone that are due to the absence of mineralized repair tissue (Cases 15, 17, 18, and 23).

External resorption compounded by inflammation, not unlike internal resorption, can be rapidly progressive in a very brief period of time. Clinically, the tooth may be loose, extruded, and sensitive to percussion, emitting a dull sound.

When there is crushing or severing of the periodontium, the ensuing inflammation causes an initial surface resorption of the root. It is felt that if the initial resorption erodes the cementum sufficiently to allow bacteria and/or pulpal breakdown products to enter the periodontal ligament space, these irritants (coupled with invading microorganisms from saliva and the replanted tooth) will accelerate the initial inflammation and compound the later resorptive process. Lateral and accessory canals may allow irritants from the canal system to contribute to this inflammatory resorptive phase. It is also felt that if the periodontal ligament is destroyed at the time of an avulsion or if the inflammatory resorption is persistent enough to alter or eliminate the periodontal ligament, replacement resorption will occur.

Ankylosis occurs when the root surface and the alveolar bone fuse because of the loss of the PDL. Thus, in many instances the resorptive process is a *progressive cycle*; what is classified as a type of resorption is merely a period of the cycle. Surface resorption occurs first, followed by inflammatory resorption in which the PDL is infiltrated or replaced by granulation tissue (containing the clastic cells), and finally by a severe loss of tooth structure as the replacement resorption sets in. This may lead to complete loss of the root(s). As replacement resorption approaches the pulp and a toxic stimulus from the canal system contributes to the process, the resorption may convert to an inflammatory nature. Inflammatory resorption alone may cause appreciable loss of tooth structure. Rowe and Schultz recently demonstrated that in the human periodontitis lesion the proximity of the inflammatory infiltrate to the bone surface is a significant factor in the osteoclastic resorption of alveolar bone. The findings in this study could be correlated to the inflammatory infiltrate that can diffuse through the dentinal tubules after resorption of the cementum, thereby perpetuating the resorption of neighboring bone and other dental tissues by osteoclastic action.

It has been reported that inflammatory resorption can be reversed, but replacement resorption is irreversible. The key to preserving root structure may lie in *containing* the inflammatory process *before* the periodontal ligament is eliminated, thus preventing the natural osteoclastic process of resorption of mineralized tissue and replacement of root structure with newly formed osseous tissue. It is felt that the periodontal ligament, with its cellular contents, and the alveolar bone proper constitute the barrier that prevents this biologic process from occurring, whether or not the teeth are traumatized (Cases 24 and 25).

In 1975 and 1981, Andreasen expanded upon the classification of root resorption to include the characteristics of periodontal changes after replantation:

1. Normal periodontium.
2. Inflammation in the PDL without root resorption.
3. Downgrowth of pocket epithelium (below the dentino-enamel junction).
4. Surface resorption.
5. Inflammatory resorption.
6. Replacement resorption.
    a. Active replacement resorption.
    b. Linear resorption.
    c. Arrested replacement resorption.
    d. Repaired replacement resorption after initial resorption.
    e. Repaired replacement resorption without initial resorption.

Rate of External Resorption

Andreasen reports that inflammatory resorption that occurs as a result of trauma may be demonstrated radiographically as early as 3 weeks after the insult. Both inflammatory and replacement resorption are usually observable radiographically within 2 to 5 months after the injury and are most often evident after the *first* year. Kemp et al., in their evaluation of 71 replanted teeth, observed that in some cases rapid dissolution of most of the root occurred in a period of a few months; in other cases root resorption appeared to be a very slow process. Grossman and Ship reported on replanted teeth and found that within 6 months, 43 per cent of the teeth showed evidence of resorption. Only 4 per cent of the replanted teeth showed no evidence of resorption for follow-up periods of 2 years or more. They concluded that "the longer the time interval, the fewer the successes."

In baboon experiments, Hammer et al. observed within 6 months the beginning stages of cementoclastic resorption of teeth that had been replanted in less than 20 minutes and that had the PDL removed and the canal obturated with gutta percha. By the end of 1 year, a more obvious root resorption was observed that had eroded the tooth substance to expose the root canal filling. In monkey experiments, Andreasen found histologic evidence that inflammatory resorption cavities had been initiated in teeth without endodontic treatment after just 2 weeks and that a greater frequency occurred after 8 weeks. Barbakow et al. also demonstrated the first evidence of surface resorption at 2 weeks. At the end of the 8 week observation period, ankylosis was found in all their monkey specimens.

Based on recent primate experiments, Andreasen described the following histologic (histometric) resorptive patterns of mature permanent incisors with replantation after either 0 or 18 minutes and sacrifice at 1, 2, 4, or 8 week intervals: "Surface resorption was first recognized after one week and became prominent after two weeks; the frequency increased slightly after four and eight weeks. Inflammatory resorption was first recognized after *one* week and showed a rapid extension with increasing observation periods. Replacement resorption was first noted after *two* weeks, where the peak frequently occurred."

Andreasen pointed out that inflammatory resorption is quite frequent and rapid following replantation of permanent teeth in the 6- to 7-year-old age group. He explains that this accelerated process is the result of thin dentinal walls and/or wide dentinal tubules.

Andreasen concluded that there is a direct correlation between age and the rate of replacement resorption. Younger patients with a higher bone metabolism, as a general rule, will display external root resorption at a faster rate than older individuals. Deeb et al. also reported that patients younger than 17 years had significantly more root resorption than those from 17 to 30 years.

Resorptive Considerations

Research has shown that there are several factors that have a definite effect upon the resorptive potential of the exarticulated tooth:

1. Periodontal ligament.
2. Extraoral time.
3. Transportation.
4. Splinting.
5. Initiation of root canal treatment.
6. Calcium hydroxide.
7. Fluorides (possibly).

The Role of the Periodontal Ligament

The most recent studies suggest that the maintenance of the viability of the periodontal ligament is absolutely necessary in preventing progressive resorption of replanted teeth. In dog experiments, Hammer demonstrated that if the periodontal ligament was scraped off the root, root resorption continued until the tooth was lost. Healing did occur without resorption of replanted teeth in those cases in which the periodontal ligament was left adhering to the root. In a significant study, Löe and Waerhaug observed that in cases of replanted teeth either without the periodontal ligament or after being air-dried for a variable time, granulation tissue was produced in the periodontal space and normal reattachment was never regained. Ankylosis was produced within 30 days. However, in those instances in which teeth with a vital PDL were replanted, they regained a normal periodontal attachment. Similar observations have been reported by Grossman and Sherman. Van Hassel, Oswald, and Harrington confirmed the importance of a viable PDL in their study of 42 lateral incisors of monkeys, using follow-up periods of 16 to 39 months. In their study the periodontal ligament was intentionally removed from half the teeth prior to replantation. Of those 21 teeth in which the PDL was removed, all but one showed evidence of severe resorption. Of those 21 teeth in which the PDL was *left* at the time of replantation, nine were retained with a radiographically intact PDL space. It is possible that the prognosis may have been enhanced in those teeth replanted with an intact PDL because the study contained several variables, such as remodeling of the socket in some instances, manipulation of teeth by extraoral endodontic treatment, and the use of two different extraoral periods (30 to 90 minutes). In a baboon study, Hamner et al. showed that if the PDL was removed, none of the specimens demonstrated reattachment of the PDL; however, reattachment could be observed when the PDL had been left intact.

It is felt that the prime concern in treating the exarticulated tooth is *the preservation of the periodontal ligament*, cementum, and cortical bone of the socket (Case 24). There are many factors of concern, such as out-of-the-mouth time and proper splinting (passive), but these relate directly to preserving the attachment apparatus. Hammer and Andreasen pointed out that the survival prognosis was proportional to the number of viable periodontal fibers preserved.

Nasjleti et al. concluded from their radioautographic studies that the periodontal ligament left attached to a replanted tooth showed healing activity, and it was apparent that the PDL maintained its vitality either by a rapid re-establishment of the vascularity or, more probably, by diffusion of nutrients via the ligament's severed interface.

Löe and Waerhaug showed that even if periodontal fibers had been devitalized, when such teeth were replanted with portions of the PDL still attached, those portions resorbed more slowly than the denuded root surfaces. Melcher, and later Grant and Bernick, suggested that the PDL acts as an osteodepressive to prevent ankylosis.

Recently Andreasen demonstrated that root resorption was primarily related to the amount of damage to the PDL remaining on the root surface.

Topography of Root Resorption

Andreasen demonstrated the topography of resorption by measuring (histometrically) the cross-sections of replanted monkey incisors after 8 weeks. His results indicated that inflammatory resorption is strongly linked to "corner" surfaces of replanted incisors *without* endodontic treatment; moreover, in these same corner surfaces of endodontically treated teeth, surface resorption was most evident. This may be due to the more severe severance of the PDL from the cementum in these corner surfaces during the rotating process of extraction. Andreasen also showed in the same study that the natural concavities of the root showed little inflammatory resorption. This may be linked to the existence of a greater amount of PDL tissue left on the root. In another article, Andreasen demonstrated similar findings, emphasizing the preference of both *surface* and *inflammatory* resorption for the rounded labial and lingual corner surfaces rather than for the flat or concave proximal surfaces. He attributed these responses in the periodontium to areas in the PDL and/or the root surface that were injured by the avulsion extraction or by extended drying. In a third study, Andreasen found the *replacement* resorption had the same significant preference for the rounded labial and lingual corner surfaces rather than for the flat or concave surfaces. In addition, replacement resorption was found more in the apical portion of the root than in the coronal portion.

Initial Periodontal Healing after Replantation

Andreasen, in reviewing Hammer's histologic healing sequence after experimental tooth replantation in dogs, demonstrated that immediately after replantation, a coagulum was found between the two parts of the torn periodontal ligament. The line of separation of the PDL was most often located in the middle but could occur at the insertion of Sharpey's fibers into either cementum or alveolar bone. After 3 to 4 days, the space in the periodontal ligament (coagulum) was invaded with young connective tissue. New collagenous fibers developed by 2 weeks, and complete repair of the periodontal ligament occurred after 4 weeks. Recently, Andreasen found that healing of the PDL, as assessed histologically or via mobility testing, was almost complete 2 to 4 weeks after replantation.

An appreciation of the normal healing of the periodontium allows one to arrive at a rationale for the timing for splinting and initiation of endodontic treatment. Andreasen found that gingival fibers showed repair in the majority of replanted teeth after 1 week. This finding of united gingival fibers implies that the tooth has some support in its socket after 1 week. This was supported by the work of Nasjleti et al. However, Loe and Waerhaug, and later Andreasen, reported that in contrast to the normal healing of the PDL, large amounts of granulation tissue may form, replacing the PDL and resorbing tooth structure and bone. This type of healing resulted in tooth loss.

Role of the Socket

The tooth is anchored in the socket by means of Sharpey's fibers, which are embedded in the cementum on one side and the alveolar bone on the other (Case 25). In instances of exarticulation, these fibers and remnants of the periodontal ligament, with some cellular contents, remain attached to the wall of the socket. Andreasen demonstrated that when avulsion occurs, the line of separation is most often situated in the middle of the PDL, leaving fibers attached to the root surface and to the bone of the alveolar socket. These remnants of the PDL remain viable because they are bathed in a blood clot; quite often, they have the potential for regeneration of the torn ligament. One should be cautious when treating the socket in order to prevent damage to this viable tissue. Curettage should *not* be performed. The author recommends that the best treatment of the socket is gentle aspiration of the blood clot just before replantation in order to allow proper seating of the tooth. If the blood clot cannot be removed by aspiration alone, sterile water or saline irrigation should be employed to aid in removal of the clot. Failure to remove the clot will result in a marked increase in the hydraulic pressure, which, in and of itself, may favor initiating a resorptive process, but certainly will make repositioning and retention of the tooth in the alveolus most difficult.

Oswald et al. found that teeth replanted in an intact socket had a slightly better prognosis than teeth in which the socket had been removed before replantation.

In a significant study, Morris et al. observed the influence of socket tissue changes in delayed tooth transplantation. They showed (in monkeys) that teeth out of the mouth for 20 minutes and autotransplanted to sockets vacated for 2 hours showed more ankylosis and root resorption than teeth out of the mouth for 2 hours and autotransplanted to sockets vacated for 20 minutes. They concluded that the undisturbed bony socket must have a part in the healing process. Their results confirmed Morris et al.'s hypothesis of "periodontal homeostasis," in which the root surface and periodontal ligament tend to inhibit osseous activity and in that way help preserve the integrity of the periodontal space.

In a recent experiment in which the labial socket wall was removed before replantation, Andreasen found that new alveolar bone was formed when the replanted teeth had a vital PDL, in contrast to the replanted teeth that had a damaged, and possibly necrotic, PDL. Teeth with a damaged PDL demonstrated labial root absorption.

In another study using histometric analysis, Andreasen indicated that the major decisive factor determining periodontal repair without root resorption was the preservation of the *cemental* portion of the PDL. He concluded that the length of the extra-alveolar period seemed to exert some influence upon the socket, enhancing the development of replacement resorption.

In yet another study, Andreasen speculated that *longer* periods of socket vacancy could result in an organized blood clot in the socket that might provide resistance, thereby further injuring the PDL upon replanting the tooth.

The removal of or traumatic damage to a socket may delay the remodeling phase of osteogenesis. However, unless the inhibiting influence of the periodontal ligament is present, the remodeling phase of a regenerating socket wall will affect *odontogenic* structures after a sufficient period. If a socket is removed, this space will be replaced by healing granulation tissue containing osteoclasts that will not have the inhibitory influence of a healing periodontal ligament and intact cortical bone. The process of ankylosis and resorption is one of osseous tissue and its precursor tissues. Therefore, areas of ankylosis may form where the remodeling of the socket occurs more quickly than regeneration of the PDL and cortical bone.

Missing Cortical Plate

In a significant primate study, Andreasen demonstrated that, after surgical removal of the socket's facial cortical plate, a vital periodontal ligament in replanted mature teeth was able to induce the formation of new alveolar bone. Avulsed teeth that may seem hopeless because of a fractured or avulsed cortical plate should be replanted. The tooth should be positioned as closely as possible to the socket wall near the intact cortical plate opposite the injured bone. Luxated and avulsed teeth with the facial cortical plate missing as a result of traumatic injury have been treated, and at recall appointments facial healing was found. Kristerson described an auto-transplantation of a tooth to a socket in which the adjacent bone was missing, and after 18 month recall, a thin bony plate was found that attained almost normal occlusal level.

Out of the Mouth Time

Loe and Waerhaug demonstrated that the extraoral period had the greatest bearing on the success of replantation. A normal PDL was never found in teeth replanted after a prolonged drying period, in contrast to the finding of functionally oriented PDL fibers after a *short* drying period. The literature has shown that extended extra-alveolar intervals are responsible for extensive root resorption. The earlier the tooth is replanted, the more favorable the prognosis, as there is less chance of necrosis of the PDL and cementum. The best prognosis is achieved by replanting the tooth within 30 minutes. A short extra-alveolar period favors retention of viable periodontal ligament cells, which, in turn, limit external root resorption. Soder, by counting labeled cells from tissue cultures of the periodontal ligament and measuring the uptake of neutral red in vital staining, was unable to show any viable PDL cells after the tooth was out of the mouth for 2 hours and incubated at 37°C. In two recent histologic studies, Andreasen again confirmed that teeth replanted 90 minutes and 120 minutes after dry storage showed extensive root resorption. After a 60 minute drying period, very few vital cells were found on the root surface, and no viable cells could be demonstrated after 120 minutes. After 30 minutes of dry storage, inflammatory root resorption was very prominent, and after 60 minutes of dry storage, there was a high incidence of replacement resorption.

An interesting finding by Kemp et al. in their evaluation of 71 replanted teeth was that only 14 per cent of the teeth were replanted within *one* hour after accidental avulsion. Therefore, according to the literature, root resorption would be expected in the vast majority of replanted teeth. Accordingly, treatment should be initiated early to prevent this occurrence.

Transportation and Storage

Numerous studies have demonstrated that prolonged dryness of the root preceding replantation leads to extensive root resorption. Andreasen reported that keeping the tooth in the oral cavity is the best means of transportation. Dry storage resulted in severe ankylosis. Saline was a much better storage medium; however, saliva was the best. Extra-alveolar time has a crucial influence on the viability of the PDL.

In a recent monkey experiment, Andreasen confirmed Cvek's clinical study in which dry storage of teeth before replantation resulted in a marked increase in inflammatory and replacement resorption. Despite increased extra-alveolar periods, storage in saline or saliva greatly reduced the frequency of replacement resorption, compared with dry or tap water storage. Andreasen postulated that saliva and saline were better storage media than tap water because of the significant differences in electrolyte concentration and osmolarity of these substances. In a recent significant study, Blomlöf confirmed his previous experiments demonstrating that milk was superior to saliva as a storage medium. It was found that 50 per cent of human PDL cells were viable after 12 hours' storage in milk, whereas no PDL cells were viable after 3 hours' storage in saliva. A combination of brief storage in saliva with subsequent storage in milk was better than storage in saliva only. In an earlier study, Blomlöf reported that saliva was hypotonic, whereas milk had a more suitable osmolarity for human PDL cells.

Camp recommended that the avulsed tooth be replaced immediately in the socket whenever possible, and the patient should then go to the dentist's office for evaluation and stabilization. Mullaney recommended that an avulsed tooth that is going to be transported intraorally should be wrapped in the center of a wet handkerchief (or cloth) and then only the portion of the handkerchief containing the tooth should be placed in the mouth, thereby preventing swallowing of the tooth during transportation.

The vitality of the PDL can be better maintained (when milk is unavailable) by placing the tooth in the patient's own saliva for the following reasons: the components of saliva are similar to blood chemistry, the tooth is maintained at body temperature, and the cell physiology is more compatible with what occurs in the socket. In summary, the most suitable means of transportation of the avulsed tooth is immediate replacement in the alveolar socket; the second choice would be milk; a close third choice would be an intraoral placement of the tooth (wrapped in a moist cloth); the fourth choice would be transportation via a cup of saline; and the least desirable medium is tap or creek water. The most detrimental means of transportation is dry storage.

Andreasen expanded upon a previous experiment by Hammer involving the delay of replantation after autotransplant submucosal storage in order to prevent root resorption. In instances in which the PDL was damaged as a result of drying for 120 minutes, it was found that the submucosal storage did *not* prevent resorption. However, in instances of submucosal storage of teeth with a vital PDL, Andreasen found that osteogenesis took place adjacent to the periodontal ligament in approximately half the teeth. He postulated that the root's vital periodontal ligament remnants contain osteoprogenitor cells, which induce the surrounding tissue to form osseous tissue.

Endodontic Treatment Before Replantation

An interesting study by Andreasen, based on a computer analysis conducted in Denmark, showed that the prognosis for replanted teeth was best when performed by patients or physicians and poorest when performed by dentists. Dentists tend to manipulate the root physically, thus damaging the vital periodontal ligament, and/or they may delay the replantation procedure by performing root canal treatment before replanting the tooth, thus worsening the prognosis. Even more disastrous, dentists scrape or place caustic disinfectants and other chemicals on the root. These caustic drugs may kill the cementocytes and coagulate the collagen fibers of the PDL. Hammer (and later Loe and Waerhaug and recently Van Hassel et al.) has shown that intentional removal of the periodontal ligament is followed by extensive replacement resorption and ankylosis.

Neither pulp extirpation nor root canal filling with gutta percha should be performed before replantation. Andreasen feels that immediate replantation and postponement of pulp extirpation and canal obturation is the preferred treatment for avulsed teeth. His study indicated that leaving the pulp tissue for this period may lead to an increase in the extent of inflammatory resorption, but he suggested that treating the canal system with calcium hydroxide would arrest this resorptive process. The results of Andreasen's study showed that the use of gutta percha–Kerr sealer root canal fillings consistently increased the frequency of surface and replacement resorption, compared with use of pulp extirpation or with nonextirpation. It was conjectured that the filling procedure and/or the material itself (especially the eugenol from the sealer) may have injured the periodontal ligament in the apical zone.

Andreasen and Kristerson demonstrated that root canal treatment and canal filling with calcium hydroxide *before* replantation resulted in more replacement resorption than occurred in control teeth. They speculated that the increased resorption may be due to a diffusion of the calcium hydroxide through the apical foramen, thus injuring the periodontal ligament.

Endodontic treatment should not be performed before replantation, whether the canals are filled with calcium hydroxide or not. The canal system should be filled with calcium hydroxide eventually in order to retard or prevent inflammatory resorption. However, based on the results of this study, this author disagrees with the conclusion that postponement of calcium hydroxide obturation until *after* 2 weeks may be the preferred treatment. A study involving obturation of the canal system with calcium hydroxide *one* week after replantation would resolve the question. Because the endodontic treatment was performed *before* replantation and because group II teeth (filled with gutta percha) showed replacement resorption in 10 of 11 teeth, whereas group III teeth (filled with calcium hydroxide) showed replacement resorption in 8 of 8 teeth, this author wonders what effect just the manipulation of the root and the endodontic treatment had on the prevalence for resorption.

Coccia followed up 129 avulsed teeth; 72 teeth had their pulps extirpated before replantation or within 48 hours after replantation, and these teeth did not receive calcium hydroxide treatment until inflammatory root resorption was evident. Subsequently, Coccia felt that the initial occurrence of apical replacement resorption could not be attributed to pulp retention. Because, in Coccia's study, calcium hydroxide was not introduced until some time later, the resorption could not be attributed to this material.

Studies have reported the occurrence of resorption in the periapical region upon replantation. In their studies of periapical tissue reaction to instrumentation, Seltzer et al. and Bhaskar and Rappaport demonstrated that resorption of the cementum occurred initially after instrumentation. Van Mullem et al., in a monkey study, showed that resorption stimulated by instrumentation occurred not only in the periapical cementum but also in the cortical bone at the periapex. They distinguished between infected and noninfected groups of teeth and concluded that the presence of resorption in their 7 day and 42 day groups without bacterial infection was the result of instrumentation. Van Mullem et al. demonstrated that after 42 days the resorptive reaction was still active but was counteracted by a reparative process.

The root canal filling should be delayed until after splinting not only to preserve viable periodontal tissue remnants of teeth out of the mouth for prolonged periods, but also to maintain the maximum healing potential of the socket.

Under no circumstance should reverse amalgam (or other materials) fillings be used before replantation. Invariably these reverse fillings end up as islands of foreign material in the periapical tissues as resorption takes its toll (Cases 16 and 19). Also, these reverse plugs prevent the full effectiveness of the calcium hydroxide.

Apex Removal

The rationale for removing the apex is to provide room for the blood clot after the tooth has been seated into its original position or possibly to aid in preventing extrusion when edema of the PDL occurs. However, both Massler and Heithersay point out that the removal of the apex is not necessary in order to obtain satisfactory repositioning. This procedure is not recommended, because, in most instances, proper splinting will prevent incisal displacement and aspiration will remove the blood clot. If the tooth still will not seat, irrigation with sterile water or saline solution will often dislodge the most stubborn blood clots. If the apex is removed, the blood clot will be replaced with granulation tissue and may promote apical resorption. Andreasen has shown that the adaptation of the tooth to the socket appears to have little influence on resorption, however. Every attempt should be made to maximize repositioning. Moreover, the historical technique of trephination after reimplantation is no longer considered a necessary procedure.

Endo-Osseous Implants

Heithersay points out that the use of Vitallium or other metallic endodontic implants (which extend from the root canal beyond the apex) for support of a tooth undergoing resorption is an "illusion." He points out that, as a result of ankylosis, these teeth are firm until their eventual loss. The author also does not recommend their use, for these solid cones do not effectively obturate the canal system. Once resorption removes the apex, thus allowing a tissue fluid exchange between the root canal and the periodontium, the resorptive process will most likely be accelerated.

Mobility

In a study by Andreasen, replanted teeth initially showed very high mobility values but demonstrated normal levels 3 weeks after replantation. After 2 weeks, the teeth were only moderately mobile. Ankylosis was detected clinically 5 to 6 weeks after replantation, but radiographic demonstration was not detected until 8 weeks after trauma. In instances of transient replacement resorption, clinically (and in a few cases radiographically) lowered mobility values were exhibited in the period from 6 to 52 weeks after replantation. In only one instance did the transient ankylosis last for 6 weeks, whereas the remaining cases showed a longer duration. The concept of transient ankylosis was that it occurred as a normal part of repair and could be eliminated by functional stimulation during the resorptive process. Teeth that displayed transient replacement resorption had a significantly shorter extraoral period compared with teeth with permanent replacement resorption. Thus, mobility testing can be of great value in the early diagnosis of replacement resorption, for this would allow earlier treatment attempts to eliminate or retard this resorption. This study's macroperiodontometer results correlate with what Andreasen found previously, namely, that after replantation, there is rapid healing of the periodontal ligament up to the 3 wk period.

Barbakow et al. cited similar findings, and recently Barbakow found that ankylosis occurred by the end of 8 weeks in all replanted monkey teeth in their experiment, whether the extra-alveolar time was 30 or 120 minutes.

Splinting of Traumatized Teeth

Stabilization of the injured tooth by splinting prevents further damage to the periodontium during the healing phase. Andreasen, in 1975, recommended that splinting of an avulsed tooth be minimized to a period of approximately *one week* in order to reduce the possibility of ankylosis. In 1975 Andreasen showed histologically, in monkeys sacrificed after 8 weeks, that in teeth replanted after a prolonged period (120 minutes), splinting time made no significant difference. However, he found that in replanting teeth out of the socket for a short period (18 minutes) a significant *decrease* in the frequency and extent of replacement resorption occurred in either nonsplinted teeth or teeth with a minimal splinting period (2 weeks). He concluded that splinting exerted a harmful effect upon periodontal healing of replanted teeth after a short extraoral period. He found that the extent of replacement resorption was significantly related to splinting time. An unexpected finding in this experiment was that functional stimuli may prevent or eliminate replacement resorption. Andreasen hypothesized (based on the findings of Clark and Haynes) that functional stimuli may depress osteogenesis and enhance fibrous healing. He also speculated that eventual prevention of replacement resorption does not mean that resorption or some ankylosis did not occur initially, but that in instances of fixation the ankylosis becomes irreversibly established. He further pointed out that the reason for the prevalence of replacement resorption in the 120 minute extraoral group may be the result of damage to the root surface (such as drying of the PDL). Using monkey studies, Barbakow et al. showed that after 8 weeks it was not possible to find any significant difference in root resorption between untreated teeth and teeth obturated with gutta percha. These investigators immobilized the teeth for a 4 week period. They also suggested that the prolonged splinting may be responsible for the increased amount of ankylosis.

Scott and Zelikow pointed out that "evidence is convincing that splinting can contribute to ankylosis, and that splinting should be the minimal period that allows the tooth to become sufficiently firm to be retained without the splint." Splinting is necessary initially. Andreasen and Kristerson postulated that a certain amount of functioning for replanted teeth during the healing period enhances those beneficial resorption processes that eliminate existing (transient) ankylosis sites.

However, Andreasen and Kristerson recently showed in instances of nonvital PDL that nonsplinted teeth displayed slightly more resorption activity than the splinted teeth in the *osseous cervical* region. Andreasen also recently found that active replacement resorption was more common in the experimental group of monkeys with *no splinting* or *traumatic occlusion* as compared with the splinted group in replanted teeth with nonvital periodontal ligaments. He concluded that the presence and extent of root resorption are related to the degree of occlusal function.

Andreasen suggested that in instances in which rigid types of splints are used, the incidence of resorption increases. Massler recommended loose splinting. Stabilization (of avulsed and luxated teeth) should be done with a *passive* splint; that is, the splint should allow normal physiologic tooth movement without acting as an orthodontic appliance (Case 42). Slight mobility of a tooth during the healing period will help eliminate small areas of ankylosis and allow for functional arrangement of the healing periodontal fibers. The PDL remains functional only if in function. Cathey pointed out that any tooth mobility beyond normal physiologic limits causes irritation and resultant inflammation, which delays healing and/or induces root resorption. Andreasen indicated that ankylosis is not always permanent, for in 25 per cent of cases it disappears spontaneously. The severance of the PDL of the involved tooth will easily allow a displacement movement of the tooth if the slightest force is incorporated into the splint. Splinting under pressure also causes increased inflammation, which in turn contributes to the resorption. Also, traumatic occlusion must be avoided in the splint design, as it could encourage root resorption.

Splinting Methods. Acceptable splinting methods include the acid-etched composite resin technique or use of the acid-etched composite resin with orthodontic wire reinforcement. The author has found that Nuva-seal splints do not hold up but that Nuvafil may be satisfactory. When orthodontic banding is employed, care must be taken not to incorporate undesirable forces. Interdental wiring and the arch bar splint are irritating to the gingival tissue. Because these two splints have the tendency to accumulate plaque, there may be a delay in the healing of the gingival reattachment. Vanek pointed out that in the management of several loosened teeth, tightening of the interdental wires may displace the teeth. The cold-curing acrylic splint is unesthetic, bulky, and does not permit good oral hygiene; however, it usually provides a better splint than many other splinting methods.

Camp recommends that the splint be simple and biologically acceptable to the healing gingival tissues. Therefore, he disapproves of the commonly used arch bar splint ligated around the cervix of each tooth. He has found orthodontic ligature wire, acid-etched to the facial surface, to be advantageous in that it is easily and directly applied, nonirritating to the gingiva, stable, hygienic, and esthetic. It allows access to the root canal system and is easily removed without damage to the remaining tooth structure.

Camp's splinting technique is useful in several situations: when there is no adjacent tooth, when a large diastema exists (often occurring in young patients), when there has been little damage to the socket, or when the proximal tooth has full coverage (Case 26). In uncomplicated avulsions, when proximal teeth are soundly supported, the author has found an acid-etched interproximal splint to be effective, provided the etching material is kept high in the contact area away from the interproximal gingiva, sufficient bulk is placed, and the splint is utilized for the *minimum* splinting period (Case 43). In the acid-etched interproximal splinting technique, a shorter splinting period is recommended because this method often does not allow for the necessary physiologic tooth movement that the orthodontic wire reinforcement splint does.

Splinting Technique. The tooth or teeth are apically repositioned in the socket and aligned in accordance with the adjacent teeth and the contour of the arch. After repositioning the teeth in the patient's normal anatomic position, they are checked for occlusal interference in all excursions of the mandible, especially extrusive movement, thus minimizing further trauma to the periodontal ligament.

If considerable plaque, blood, and other debris are found, the crowns should be cleaned before etching. Be cautious in using a prophy paste, as it may contaminate the socket and act as a foreign body. It is more important to minimize the post-traumatic manipulation than to ensure clean enamel surfaces for etching. Neaverth and Goerig recommended a plain flour pumice because prepared pastes contain certain additives that interfere with adhesion of the splinting material.

The author recommends the application of a rubber dam whenever possible. During application, the dam should not cause movement of the injured teeth. Therefore, a very large hole should be cut, encompassing several teeth and including sound, well-supported adjacent teeth (for example, the hole should be stretched cuspid to cuspid if several anterior teeth are involved). This would aid in preventing salivary contamination. Boxing wax may be placed over the gingiva and the most distal tooth for isolation and protection.

To allow physiologic tooth movement the proper gauge orthodontic wire is needed. A splint in this situation is comprised of two components: (1) stainless steel wire and (2) composite resin. Waldron stated that the flexibility and the rigidity of this splint are directly related to the cross-sectional diameter of the wire and the amount of free wire between the composite retention. In young adults or older patients with proximal contact, a size 0.016 or 0.018 inch round wire or 0.016 × 0.016 inch square wire is the desired width. In the young patient with interproximal distances of more than 1 mm, a larger gauge is needed, such as 0.030 inch round wire or 0.018 × 0.025 inch rectangular wire. A stainless steel orthodontic wire is recommended, and it need not be tempered if the wire is adapted to the teeth before the composite is applied. The more closely the wire is adapted to the teeth and the greater the amount of composite that covers the wire, the more flexible the wire may be. Therefore, the smaller gauge wires will be quite stable. Adequate amounts of composite are necessary to secure the wire to the labial surface of the teeth; however, it must be remembered that the more wire incorporated in composite, the less flexible the splint — regardless of wire size. In case of emergency, a paper clip may be used; however, it may not permit the desired physiologic tooth movement. In instances of horizontal root fractures requiring orthodontic wire (because of diastemas) a size 0.030 or 0.036 inch round wire is recommended, and it must be adequately covered with composite.

The dried facial enamel surface is then etched with orthophosphoric acid (30 to 50 per cent) for approximately 1 minute. It should be remembered that the more surface in a mesio-distal direction that can be incorporated, the better the mechanical bond. Watson, as reported by Heithersay, demonstrated that the amount of enamel affected by the etching procedure is approximately 15 to 25 microns.

The acid is rinsed away with water; then the area is air dried and evaluated — a chalky surface indicates that adequate etching has occurred.

The composite is mixed and then either painted or applied (with a plastic instrument) to the etched portion of the teeth and overlying wire. It is usually not necessary to flow the material onto the lingual surfaces. After setting, the unwanted excess can be removed with white stones, flame-shaped diamond burs, or fluted composite finishing burs. An advantage of the acid-etched splint is removal can usually be accomplished by removing the bulk of material in fragments and chipping the remainder off. Neaverth and Goerig have described in detail the acid-etched splinting technique and the rationale for splinting.

Splinting Periods. The author recommends a span of *one* to *two* weeks time for splinting avulsed and luxated teeth, depending upon the mobility of the tooth immediately after replantation. This mobility is, in turn, directly proportional to the amount of crushing of the periodontium and adjacent alveolar bone at the time of impact. Therefore, stabilization is utilized only for a time period sufficient to allow reattachment of the periodontium. In instances of a minimally traumatized socket, Nasjleti et al. showed that in *seven* days both continuity of the periodontal ligament and a new junctional epithelium were re-established. Andreasen found that teeth splinted for only 1 week tended to reach normal mobility levels 3 weeks after replantation.

In instances of luxation or avulsion in which the cortical plate(s) have been fractured, the recommended time for stabilization is 4 to 6 weeks, depending on the degree of bone mobility. Of course, any time a splint is removed and there is still significant movement (Class II or III mobility) of the teeth or cortical plates, the splint should be reapplied for a brief period. Clark and Hayes reported that teeth insufficiently splinted because of bone fractures depressed osteogenesis and enhanced fibrous healing.

The luxated or avulsed tooth is *stabilized* to allow physiologic movement (Case 26), whereas the horizontally fractured tooth (root) is *immobilized* by rigid fixation in order to allow a better prognosis for calcified healing at the fracture site. The horizontally fractured tooth that maintains a viable pulp is stabilized for a period of 4 to 8 weeks, depending upon the root level of the fracture. In the case of a horizontally fractured tooth in which the pulp of both segments is irreversibly involved and calcium hydroxide is being employed to stimulate a calcified healing of the fracture site, immobilization of the segments is usually required for a period of 4 to 12 *months* in order to allow sufficient time for the organization and formation of the calcified barrier. Often the splinting time depends upon the level of the horizontal fracture. The acid-etched composite resin splint *without* orthodontic wire reinforcement is the preferred technique for a horizontal fracture because this method offers the best probability for immobilization of the occlusal segment. In instances of horizontal fractures with open contacts (diastemas), a 0.030 inch or larger orthodontic wire is recommended, and the composite should cover the entire length of the wire on the facial surface of the splinted teeth, thus giving more rigidity to the splint.

Contributory Role of Canal Contents to Resorption

In replanted teeth, pulpal necrosis may cause periapical inflammation and/or resorption as well as inflammatory lateral root resorption. Gurney, and later Shovelton and Andreasen, established that bacteria can be found throughout the entire canal system and particularly in the dentinal tubules.

Andreasen has suggested that inflammatory root resorption may be induced and sustained by the diffusion of toxic substances or bacteria from the root canal via the dentinal tubules to the periodontal ligament space. In 1981, in a significant histologic study using monkeys, Andreasen found active inflammatory resorption sites to be connected with either necrotic pulp tissue or an infected leukocyte zone in the pulp in every section studied. These pathways were via communicating dentinal tubules. Torneck, and later Bergenholz and Makkes et al., reported that sterile necrotic tissue elicits only a mild inflammatory response compared with the strong response elicited by necrotic bacterial-infected tissue. In instances of avulsion, it would be difficult to prevent bacterial contamination of replanted teeth, especially if caustic chemicals are not to be used on the PDL and endodontic treatment before replantation is contraindicated.

A recent study by Andreasen demonstrated that inflammatory resorption of replanted teeth without endodontic treatment was initiated after a 2 week observation period and that bacterial invasion into the dentinal tubules rarely occurred. However, in every tooth that was examined in the 2 week group, the pulp tissue subjacent to the dentinal tubules leading to an area of inflammatory resorption contained bacteria. After the inflammatory resorption had begun (at 8 weeks), a rapid bacterial invasion was seen in the dentinal tubules communicating with external inflammatory root resorption sites. In no instance was vital pulp tissue found in relation to *active* inflammatory resorption. These findings then led Andreasen to the following hypothesis for surface and inflammatory resorption:

> Damaged periodontal ligament and root surface areas are attacked by a resorption process. Inflammatory resorption or surface resorption will then occur, depending on the pulpal status and the depth of the resorption cavity. If the resorption cavity penetrates the intermediate layer of cementum and contacts dentinal tubules that are in communication with infected necrotic pulp tissue or an infected leukocyte zone, inflammatory resorption will take place as a result of the diffusion of toxic elements from the pulp canal to the resorption cavity. However, in the presence of an infected necrotic pulp, if the resorption cavity does not penetrate the intermediate layer of cementum, only surface resorption occurs.

In a recent study, Andreasen's histologic findings indicated that an interaction might occur between inflammatory and replacement resorption.

A major factor in healing of the periodontal ligament is elimination of any existing necrotic tissue and/or bacterial toxins exiting from the canal system. Woechile demonstrated that periapical inflammation was present in replanted dog teeth after pulp extirpation or without endodontic treatment, but was not found in these teeth after the canals were filled with gutta percha. Root canal treatment is generally recommended within 2 weeks to avoid the resorptive process and abscess formation. Removing the pulp at the earliest possible time decreases the early resorptive process (Case 23). Andreasen demonstrated that when the pulp tissue of replanted teeth was not removed for a period of 2 weeks or longer, significant pulpal necrosis and autolysis occurred. Breakdown products from the necrotic pulp caused inflammation in the apical periodontal ligament, and this, in turn, resulted in failure of healing and eventually complete resorption of the root. Andreasen reported that the presence of bacteria was registered in all sections of nonfilled teeth, whether the pulp was extirpated or not. Teeth with extirpated pulps showed a narrow zone of necrotic pulp tissue in most areas. In this experiment, one would expect that the teeth were not completely debrided because the mandibular lateral incisors were instrumented only to the equivalent of a #10 file and the maxillary incisors to a #50 or 60 file. Add to this the fact that the monkeys' teeth were not completely mature. Seltzer's electron microscopic studies showed similar results of vital and necrotic tissue zones after endodontic instrumentation.

Chronic inflammation is associated in the pathogenesis of localized bone loss and specific local factors that might be involved include bacterial endotoxins, prostaglandins, and osteoclast-activating factor. However, a root canal can seldom be completely debrided or disinfected. What is the effect of the Tomes' processes and/or bacteria left in the dentinal tubules (especially in young patients) after replantation and after the initial resorption process has penetrated the different cemental layers? Are these small concentrations of toxins sufficient to perpetuate the resorptive phenomenon? Calcium hydroxide may benefit the environment by rendering bacteria and residual necrotic debris remaining in the root canal system innocuous in a more physiologic manner.

Cementum Barrier

Avny et al., in their autoradiographic studies, showed that radioactive aqueous parachlorophenol can penetrate through dentin from the pulp chamber and root canal to at least the cemento-dentinal junction. Anderson and Ronning, using recently extracted teeth, demonstrated dye penetration through the dentinal tubules to the tooth's periphery. Taylor et al., in an in vivo autoradiographic study, showed that radioactive aqueous 2% parachlorophenol can also diffuse through the dentinal tubules into the periodontal ligament. Linden reported a significant difference in the permeability of dentin of young and old permanent teeth to water and saline solution. This may be related to the differences in the diameter of the dentinal tubules of mature and immature teeth. Such evidence suggests that fluids may penetrate across the cemental barrier. However, at the very least, a tissue fluid exchange would be allowed between the canal system and the periodontal ligament in the event that resorption of cementum had occurred. In a recent study, Andreasen found that surface resorption occurred in replanted teeth irrespective of the extra-alveolar period and the type of storage medium used. Andreasen suggested that once the initial resorption after replantation had eroded the *intermediate* layer of cementum, diffusion of toxic elements from the pulp may cross over into the PDL. His histologic evidence seems to support the concept of the protective action of this intermediate layer of cementum after the regular cementum has been resorbed.

The pH Phenomenon

Cohen-Scali reported that calcium hydroxide expands to 2.5 times its initial volume when it comes into contact with water. When placed in a canal, calcium hydroxide (Ocalexic) should absorb the water molecules in the canal and tubules and penetrate not only the secondary canals but even the dentinal tubules. Blaha, utilizing dye penetrations, demonstrated the effective penetration of calcium hydroxide into dentin. Pashley pointed out that once the cementum is lost, a pathway for movement of solutes and solvents through the dentinal tubules is established. The rate of permeation of substances through dentin depends on the molecular size, the surface area available for diffusion, the patency of dentinal tubules, and the thickness of the remaining dentin. Substances as large as albumin readily permeate dentin.

It is plausible to assume that the cessation of resorption can be mediated by a change in the environmental pH. Kawahara et al. showed that, as calcium hydroxide paste becomes dispersed into a medium, the local environment changes from neutral to a pH of over 9.8. It has been postulated by many investigators that the pH of calcium hydroxide influences the inflammatory resorptive process of teeth by the diffusion of calcium hydroxide's ions through the dentinal tubules; however, this correlation was not established until the significant study by Tronstad, Andreasen, Hasselgren, Kristerson, and Riis. They correlated findings in untreated teeth with pulpal necrosis, demonstrating a pH range of 6.0 to 7.4 in the pulp, dentin, cementum, and also the periodontal ligament. The optimal conditions for resorption of hard tissues is an acid pH in order to allow the necessary enzymatic activity to occur. When they obturated the canal system of replanted and nonreplanted teeth with calcium hydroxide, the peripheral dentin (next to the cementum) revealed a pH range of 7.4 to 9.6 in replanted teeth and 7.4 to 8.0 in nonreplanted teeth. However, the cementum was not influenced by the calcium hydroxide. Tronstad et al. postulated that once the surface resorption has eroded the cementum, the calcium hydroxide may have a beneficial influence because, in their study, exposed dentinal tubules (denuded of cementum) showed an alkaline pH when treated with calcium hydroxide. The immature teeth (with their wide dentinal tubules) showed a consistent pH of 8.0 throughout the entire dentin.

It has been demonstrated that there is an increase in acid phosphatase activity in areas of resorption and inflammation. Conversely, it has been shown that there is an increase in alkaline phosphate activity in the areas of repair and active calcification. Tronstad et al. further emphasized that at an acid pH there is demineralization of the mineral component of the hard tissues because of the activation of acid hydrolases. They pointed out that the neutralization of the local environment (by calcium hydroxide) may be specific in inhibiting the osteoclastic acid hydrolase activity and already existing acid products such as lactic acid. The repair process in the local environment may be further benefited when brought to an alkaline pH, as it is thought that this may encourage hard tissue formation by activating alkaline phosphatases. Binnie and Mitchell found a high level of alkaline phosphatase in the cells of the fibrous capsules surrounding subdermal implants of calcium hydroxide in rats.

Other Possible Benefits of Calcium Hydroxide

Tronstad et al. theorized that calcium hydroxide may have other beneficial effects in regard to arresting inflammatory root resorption and stimulating healing. These include (1) the presence of calcium ions, being necessary for the activity of the complement system in the immunologic reaction, may activate the calcium-dependent adenosine triphosphatase (ATP-ase), which is associated with hard tissue formation; (2) calcium hydroxide's ability to denature proteins (in the root canal), rendering them less toxic; and (3) calcium hydroxide's antibacterial effect. Obturation of the canal system with calcium hydroxide will place abundant calcium and hydroxide ions in the local environment, possibly allowing some of these modes of action to occur.

Calcium Hydroxide Therapy

Very little literature is available on the use of calcium hydroxide to prevent, reverse, arrest, or retard external root resorption but several clinicians such as Andreasen, Camp, Cathey, Chivian, Cox, Heithersay, and Tronstad have been advocating such use for several years. In 1971 Andreasen was the first to report healing, by calcium hydroxide treatment, of the roots of replanted immature teeth that displayed progressive external root resorption.

Cvek, in 1973, described the arrest of pre-existing external root resorption of *luxated* upper incisors presenting with pulpal necrosis and treated with calcium hydroxide. However, in comparing the percentage of arrested external root resorption, he found no statistically significant difference between those teeth treated with calcium hydroxide (98 per cent) and those immediately obturated with gutta percha (94 per cent). Cvek concluded that the arrest of external root resorption is related exclusively to the removal of necrotic pulp and the antibacterial treatment of the root canal. He did find the frequency of progressive resorption to be 11 times higher in teeth treated with an intracanal medicament containing formalin than in teeth not treated with a formalin-containing medicament. Andreasen, in 1972, suggested that the calcium hydroxide obturation of immature teeth can be effective in preventing inflammatory root resorption of replanted teeth. In 1976 and in a more recent article, Andreasen stated that pulp removal and introduction of calcium hydroxide into the canal will prevent inflammatory resorption and permit re-establishment of the periodontal ligament.

Heithersay and Tronstad reported that calcium hydroxide is useful for an extended period as a temporary root canal filling in controlling resorption. In 1980, Coccia's study of 129 avulsed teeth in children, which utilized different modes of treatment, demonstrated that the use of calcium hydroxide arrested or decreased the rate of inflammatory resorption after 3 months when compared with canals filled with gutta percha. Coccia speculated that the mechanism of repair is similar to that of apexification.

Time Sequences of Endodontic Treatment. In instances of avulsed teeth with completed root formation (closure), there is little hope in re-establishing a viable pulp, and the ultimate result will be pulp necrosis followed by invasion of microorganisms. Therefore, endodontic treatment should be initiated to prevent later complications. Root canal treatment is generally recommended within 2 weeks to avoid the resorptive process and abscess formation. In a recent primate study of 50 samples, Andreasen found that when mature permanent incisors were replanted immediately and after 18 minutes delay, pulp necrosis was prominent in *all* teeth after 2 weeks.

A patient presenting with a dental trauma usually is uncomfortable, anxious, and needs suturing of soft tissue lacerations. Therefore, the tooth should be splinted immediately, and the patient should return when the dentist can adequately perform the endodontic therapy. After the tooth has been repositioned and stabilized, the patient should be seen in approximately 7 days, and at the same appointment the dentist should establish sufficient endodontic access, biomechanically clean and shape the canal system, and obturate the canals with calcium hydroxide paste. Often the splint can be removed at this same appointment, preferably after the root canal treatment.

If the canal is debrided and filled with calcium hydroxide shortly after replantation, this will serve to minimize root resorption, mobility, and pain (compare Cases 23 and 27). The reason for a *seven* day limit before calcium hydroxide treatment is to prevent necrotic pulp tissue products and microorganisms from penetrating through the dentinal tubules. This will allow the beneficial actions of calcium hydroxide to take effect once the surface resorption has eroded the cementum enough to allow an ionic exchange to the resorptive sites. Andreasen showed that soon after replantation, large amounts of granulation tissue are formed, replacing the periodontal ligament and resorbing the hard dental tissues and bone. Nasjleti et al. and Andreasen demonstrated changes toward root resorption as early as 14 days after replantation. Loe and Waerhaug observed that ankylosis occurred within 30 days in instances of a damaged periodontal ligament.

Calcium Hydroxide Technique. The same principles of calcium hydroxide treatment as described in the technique section are employed in treating luxated and exarticulated teeth. It is recommended that the canal system be cleaned and shaped and then filled with a dry calcium hydroxide paste approximately 1 week after the injury. The paste should be *changed* approximately 6 weeks after the initial placement and subsequently changed whenever it is found to be diluted or resorbed out of the canal system. At the 6 week recall appointment, the paste will often be found to be dry upon re-entry; however, this is such a critical time, that it is essential to replace the paste with a fresh mix. Particular attention should be paid to obturating the canals with the paste. In avulsion cases the patient should be recalled at approximately 2 month intervals for the first year. For best results, it is wise to change the paste at the 6 month recall, even though it is determined by radiographic and clinical signs that the paste need not be changed. At this 6 month recall, upon entering the canal system, the clinician will often find various portions of the paste wet, despite a radiographic appearance of a dense filling. In instances of avulsion or luxation, after the first 6 weeks paste change, it should be a routine procedure to change the paste every 4 to 6 months. Of course, any time the paste is seen to be diluting or there is swelling, other symptoms, or resorption is detected, the paste should be changed immediately.

In instances of avulsion, it is suggested that calcium hydroxide therapy be continued for 1 to 2 years (or more). The duration of calcium hydroxide therapy can often be estimated at the time of initial treatment by factors such as the out-of-mouth time interval and the condition of the periodontal ligament before replantation. However, one must keep in mind that individual host susceptibilty to reimplantation may foil the prediction. In the earlier months of treatment, the dryness of the paste upon each reentry into the canal and the amount of external resorption that has already occurred will aid in estimating the time frame of treatment.

Supposedly, if a tooth has been out of the mouth for 2 hours or more, there is a 95 per cent chance that external resorption will occur. Keeping in mind this statistic, whatever can be accomplished for these teeth to prevent this external resorption should be employed (Cases 28, 29, and 30). Approach these cases cautiously; explain to the patient that the calcium hydroxide therapy will retard and may prevent external resorption. Every clinician who follows such patients with traumatic injuries has observed numerous cases in which the teeth have been out of the mouth only a very brief period or have been only partially luxated and have still undergone invasive resorption (Cases 15 to 20). With this kind of prognosis, the author recommends that *every* exarticulated tooth with a *closed apex* that is to be replanted receive *calcium hydroxide therapy,* regardless of the out-of-mouth time interval. For a discussion of instances of immature teeth, see the latter portion of this section.

Dentists have a tendency to watch and wait until obvious resorption or pathosis occurs before initiating treatment (Case 23). Numerous cases of avulsed teeth, already displaying external resorption, have been referred to the author weeks or months after the injury (Case 31). In these instances, it was found that in approximately half (or less) of these cases, the external resorption had been halted and/or repair initiated. Therefore, it is of utmost importance to obturate the canal system with the calcium hydroxide paste within the first 2 weeks after the trauma.

In many instances, teeth with prolonged extraoral time, even though they are appropriately treated with calcium hydroxide therapy, will initially undergo some external resorption or root remodeling. If appropriate calcium hydroxide treatment is employed, the involved teeth will (in most cases) display a reversal of the resorptive process. This is especially true if the resorption is of an inflammatory nature. However, once the periodontal ligament space is lost and bone has fused to the tooth structure, the most that can be hoped for is a slowing down of the resorptive process. This can be done with fresh mixes of calcium hydroxide to promote a basic pH in the local environment that retards or prevents the clastic action from taking place. The healing root may not regain the original contour, but when healing has occurred, a periodontal ligament space should be radiographically visible around the entire root, even though the space may follow scalloped-out areas of the root. Continue calcium hydroxide therapy for 1 year after healing has occurred, or for at least 1 year in those instances in which resorption was never evident.

Camp reports that many of these teeth, after the final filling, reinitiate or undergo the resorptive process. Therefore, continuation of a 6 month recall procedure for a few years is imperative. If recurrent external resorption is noted after gutta percha obturation, it is recommended that the filling be removed and calcium hydroxide therapy again be initiated (unless the patient is old enough for fixed replacement and desires this treatment). If recurrent resorption occurs, recalling the patient for evaluation of paste dilution should usually involve a longer time period (such as 3 to 6 months) after the first routine 6 week paste change.

The benefits of calcium hydroxide therapy could be shown if one were to compare Case 32 with Case 33. According to the literature, the prognosis for Case 32 would be very favorable. The tooth was immediately replanted by the patient's mother and then splinted, and 2 weeks after the injury the canal was obturated with gutta percha. The prognosis for Case 33 would be extremely unfavorable: The tooth was air-dried for approximately 90 minutes, and the periodontal ligament was then removed. Actually, in Case 32 massive external resorption occurred within the first year; the tooth did *not* receive calcium hydroxide treatment. On the other hand, in Case 33 very minimal external resorption occurred after 2 years; the tooth received calcium hydroxide treatment 5 days after replantation.

Cases 28 and 30 represent two examples of teeth that were out of the socket for more than 2 hours and should have provided more than a 90 per cent chance for progressive external resorption within the first year. The teeth were exarticulated for approximately 3 hours and 7 hours, respectively, and both cases were treated with calcium hydroxide shortly after replantation. At recall appointment, the radiographs display very minimal external resorption in both cases.

Fluorides

In 1961, Hudson reported that nearby resorbing cells were specifically inhibited by fluoride. Likins et al. demonstrated the direct effect of fluoride on bone, cementum, and dentin that changes the hydroxyapatite into fluorapatite, which was more resistant to resorption. Coccia, in a 5 year study of 129 avulsed teeth in 82 children, showed that the use of 2% neutral sodium fluoride solution seemed to decrease the rate of replacement resorption. If the extraoral period exceeded 7 hours, the rate of resorption was more severe in the sample not treated with fluoride. In addition, after 3 years the amount of resorption was even more evident in the same sample not treated with fluoride.

The roots of exarticulated teeth that have been out of the mouth for more than 2 hours and teeth that have not been transported in a compatible liquid medium or in which the PDL has been destroyed should be treated with a fluoride solution before replantation. In such instances, Camp recommended that when progression of the resorptive process is inevitable, the roots be painted with a fluoride solution. Coccia treated the teeth for 5 minutes with 2% *neutral sodium fluoride* and postulated that the mechanism of fluoride inhibition on root resorption might be similar to its action on other mineralized tissues.

Despite the conflicting evidence in regard to the application of topical fluoride to roots of replanted teeth, there appears to be no irreversible damage to the roots that have had the PDL removed or in which the PDL is nonvital. However, if there is any possibility of retaining or regaining the vitality of the PDL, the author does not recommend such treatment. Thus, topical fluoride treatment for replanted teeth should be considered a last resort therapy.

Cervical Resorption

The author has noted in his following of patients with luxated or avulsed teeth that most of these teeth not receiving proper treatment exhibit external resorption in the cervical crown/root structure (Cases 15, 17, 18, 19, 20, 29, and 32). This may be due to the severe crushing of the periodontium in this area because the crestal bone acts as the fulcrum line in the event of trauma. Cell death in this area, coupled with ready access of bacterial invasion to the cervical area before reattachment or the walling off of the root by healing tissues, may compound the inflammatory process. It had been reported that a massive early infection during the postoperative period interferes with the repair of the periodontal membrane. It is thought that normal reattachment in the cervical area *may* not occur, owing to the persistence of inflamed granulation tissue; however, in this cervical region, the resorptive process usually occurs first in the bone just apical to the crestal bone level. Once the resorption is initiated and establishes a periodontal communication, the resorptive process is further expanded. Quite often this area goes unnoticed because the resorption may easily be mistaken for radiographic burnout. It is noted only after extensive resorption. Loe and Waerhaug reported resorption in the gingival third of nearly all replanted teeth, most often found buccally and lingually.

Once the resorptive process has invaded the canal system and the resorption is at or above the existing crestal bone level, calcium hydroxide treatment would be to no avail. The key to preventing or retarding this resorption would be to treat the tooth with calcium hydroxide soon after replantation. Canal debridement and gutta percha obturation may not be sufficient, as demonstrated in Case 17. Periodontal probing for detection of this granulation tissue must be part of the recall procedure. However, the results of Simon, Andreasen et al., and Line et al. showed that initial healing of the gingival attachment during the first few months after replantation may not allow probing of a resorptive defect. Kemp et al. have demonstrated that, as time passes, there is a greater chance for resorption to occur in this area. If significant pocket depth and/or granulation tissue is detected, deep scaling and curettage are indicated, or a surgical flap must be reflected in order to eliminate this tissue. Replacement resorption located above the crestal bone height is not a possibility; therefore, treatment of this area with calcium hydroxide obturation in order to prevent or reduce inflammatory resorption appears to be the therapy of choice.

Harrington and Natkin observed cervical resorption when they bleached seven teeth that required endodontic treatment as a result of trauma. Four cases that were reported revealed a traumatic history that might lead to root resorption. It was interesting that six of the teeth were bleached more than 6 years after the root canal fillings. It is possible that the cementum could have been resorbed after the occurrence of trauma and that, because the existing cervix was above the cementum-producing area, the dentinal tubules had been left patent and exposed. Thus, application of the caustic bleaching agents reinitiated the inflammatory resorption. The resorptive process often occurs in the cervical area, and, because this area is not capable of cemental and other periodontal repair, the resorptive potential may be prevalent throughout the patient's life. As a result of Harrington and Natkin's findings, one might consider full coverage for *discolored* teeth that have had a history of trauma. However, the very least one might do is place a white base (IRM or ZOE) over the gutta percha that is obturating the cervix, thus preventing penetration of superoxol into the cervical periodontium.

One should keep in mind that splinting techniques that cause accumulation of plaque and further prevent good oral hygiene and proper stimulation of the gingival tissues may promote resorption in the cervical area. A constant irritation in this area after replantation may prevent gingival fibers from reattaching and allow an ingress of bacteria and toxins into the periodontium, thus amplifying the existing resorptive process.

The Immature Apex

Kaqueler and Massler found that replantation of mature teeth was uniformly less successful than that of immature teeth. Ohman found that the replantation of a young child's tooth with incomplete root formation had a much better chance for revascularization and re-establishment of viable elements within the pulp. Skoglund et al. demonstrated the possibility of survival of the original pulp tissue if there is partial revascularization within a 4 day period.

Avulsed teeth with closed apices should be treated within 1 week with a calcium hydroxide paste, regardless of the time period out of the socket. The possibility of revascularization is extremely small, and the chance of external resorption is a greater probability. However, in instances of avulsed teeth with very immature apices, the author advocates that these teeth *not* be endodontically treated initially; rather, the teeth should be replanted and splinted for the appropriate time. The more open (divergent) the apex, the greater the chance of revascularization and long-term retention, provided that the tooth is replanted within 30 minutes (Case 34). However, the author agrees with Heithersay that teeth out of the mouth for 2 hours or more should be replanted in order to achieve a possible re-establishment of viable tissue within the root canal. If transported in a suitable liquid medium, some teeth *may* re-establish their pulp vitality when exarticulated up to 1 hour or more. These young teeth should be followed weekly or, at the most, biweekly because if they do become involved, the *thin* roots may resorb completely within a few weeks. Skoglund and Tronstad showed that external root resorption started as early as 4 days post-reimplantation. The thin dentinal walls and wide dentinal tubules may allow a faster ingress of toxins into the PDL and intensify the resorptive process (Case 36). When reimplantation is a success, apexogenesis will occur in some instances; in other instances the tooth may remain vital and functional but because of damage to Hertwig's root sheath, the root formation ceases (Case 35).

Based on dog experiments, Anderson et al. and later Monsour reported that the pulp can respond in several ways, i.e., formation of either regular or irregular dentin and osteodentin or, alternatively, the pulpal space may fill in with bone attaching to the root via an intrapulpal periodontal ligament. Fish and Meyer-Bardowicks had reported cases in which traumatized teeth underwent stenosis or obliteration of the root canals by hard tissue. Skoglund and Tronstad, in a recent study of replanted and autotransplanted immature dog teeth, demonstrated by angiographic and histologic techniques that the original pulp tissue survived in only a few teeth. Rather, in the majority of teeth, the pulp became necrotic after the procedure and repair occurred by means of ingrowth of a well-vascularized, cell-rich connective tissue that reached the pulp horn after 30 days. After 180 days, the pulp tissue was greatly reduced and the original pulp cavity was replaced, mostly by a hard tissue resembling bone or cementum. These findings confirmed previous studies.

If immature teeth *do* present with root resorption and/or pulpal or periapical involvement, the pulp should be removed and the canal system obturated with calcium hydroxide paste. Many of these immature teeth that become involved may not sustain long-term retention. However, the treatment is for the purpose of maintaining the space, hopefully long enough to allow a permanent fixed replacement when the adjacent teeth have erupted far enough to allow adequate placement of the margins of the restoration (Case 36). Heithersay suggested that in instances in which pulp necrosis occurs, calcium hydroxide treatment may allow further root development and calcification. Camp reported that in teeth replanted in a mixed dentition, the extent of external resorption occurring on a replanted tooth with pulpal involvement was potentially greater if the replanted tooth is adjacent to a deciduous tooth (which is undergoing apical resorption by the erupting permanent tooth).

Primary Teeth

Andreasen does not recommend the replantation of primary teeth, as this may present complications to the permanent tooth bud, which is in such close relationship to the primary tooth. The crucial aspect in treatment of an avulsed or luxated primary tooth is that if the cervical loop is destroyed, the potential for formation of the permanent tooth is lost. Final mineralization of the enamel may be altered if only the reduced enamel epithelium is damaged. If the injury occurs later in tooth development and Hertwig's epithelial root sheath is disturbed, root development may be incomplete or altered. If the primary tooth is lost very early, the eruption of the permanent tooth will be delayed approximately a year. If it is lost very late, the permanent tooth will erupt prematurely.

Management of the Avulsed Tooth

Telephone Instructions. If the accident is described on the telephone and the accompanying adult has a reasonable knowledge of dental anatomy, the tooth should be handled by the crown and, if the root is grossly contaminated, the tooth should be briefly rinsed with water (with a stopper in the sink). If the tooth cannot be replanted, it should be transported in a cup of milk or between the lips and teeth in a wet handerchief, as described previously. The patient should be transported to the dentist's office immediately.

Office Emergency Treatment. Rinse the tooth only if necessary, because it has not been ascertained whether rinsing the avulsed tooth in tap water is detrimental (owing to osmolarity) to the PDL. When there is resistance in seating the tooth into its proper position, gently aspirate the clotted blood from the socket. Reinsert the tooth into the socket slowly and gently to allow for the escape of fluids from the socket. After properly seating the tooth, hold it with firm digital pressure and compress the expanded cortical plates with firm pressure for a few minutes. To prevent the possibility of stabilizing the tooth in malposition (Case 37) take an immediate radiograph in order to verify the normal position and to detect a possible fracture of the alveolar bone. Also, study the radiograph for embedded tooth fragments and foreign objects. Digital pressure should be applied for 5 minutes after repositioning any large bone fragments.

Splinting. Stabilize the tooth with a passive splint for approximately _one_ week, utilizing acid-etched composite resin with orthodontic wire reinforcement. Avoid placing the tooth in traumatic occlusion, since this increases active replacement resorption. Bend round wire (0.018 inch) to conform to the arch configuration. It should be long enough to cover one to two teeth on either side of the avulsed tooth. Clean the teeth and dry the area. Acid-etch the labial surfaces, then place the arch wire in close proximity to the teeth. Stabilize the wire by placing boxing wax on the most distal teeth. Mix the composite and apply to the teeth, nearly covering the arch wire. Take care to keep the composite away from the gingiva, because if gingivitis is allowed to develop around the tooth, reattachment will be prevented (see subsection on splinting technique).

Cleanse (lavage) and suture any soft tissue lacerations after palpation of the injured tissues. A periodontal pack should be adapted in instances of dehiscence and/or fracture of the alveolar bone.

History. The time and condition of the traumatic injury plus any prior treatment of the injury should be recorded. Also, any previous injury to the area should be recorded. Notation of the out-of-mouth time and the manner of storage and treatment of the PDL will aid in predicting the prognosis of the replanted tooth. A proper medical history should also be taken. Contemplated orthodontic treatment should be taken into account when the plan of treatment is made.

Use of Drugs. Pearson and Nicolazzo do not recommend anesthesia until the physical and neurologic status of the patient has been determined. Neaverth and Goerig caution against the use of epinephrine in tissue, as it may retard the essential flow of blood, especially in instances of a fracture of the alveolar plate. Routine antibiotic coverage is not recommended except in instances of gross contamination, fracture of the alveolar plate, or indication in the patient's medical history. Although there are usually no specific contraindications to the use of supportive antibiotic therapy, the relative infrequency of *immediate* acute infections as a consequence of tooth replantation makes this procedure questionable. Perhaps it would be more rational to reserve the use of antibiotic therapy for those cases in which it is specifically indicated. Anti-tetanus prophylaxis is mandatory when there has been contact of the tooth with soil. Moreover, the patient should be supported systemically by the use of human tetanus immune globulin and/or a course of tetanus toxoid, whichever is appropriate to the individual's history of immunization.

Diagnosis. Quite often, when an avulsion occurs, the patient does not seek treatment within the "magic" time limit of 30 minutes. Frequently the tooth is not transported in a suitable medium to maintain maximum vitality of the PDL. These occurrences reinforce the need to consider measures to prevent or retard external resorption. Decreasing the probability of root resorption and ankylosis will enhance the prognosis of the replanted tooth.

Post-operative Instructions. Instruct the patient to avoid extreme hot or cold foods, maintain a soft diet for the first 2 weeks, avoid chewing on the injured tooth, and rinse with warm saline solution as much as possible the first week.

Treatment. When the root apex is *closed* or nearly closed, the pulp should be extirpated and the root canal biomechanically prepared and then obturated with calcium hydroxide paste approximately 1 week *after* replantation. Also, the splint should usually be removed at this appointment. If the root apex is *immature* (divergent), the tooth should be evaluated at the end of 4 to 6 weeks for vitality. Only after diagnosis of pulp necrosis is the immature tooth treated with calcium hydroxide.

In approximately 6 weeks the calcium hydroxide paste should be removed. Irrigation should be accomplished with sterile water or saline. A new calcium hydroxide paste filling is placed after the canals are dried (see Section V, subsection on calcium hydroxide treatment). Temporize carefully.

Also, at the 6 week appointment the neighboring teeth need to be evaluated, because traumatic injuries often involve more than the obviously injured teeth.

Recall. The traumatized teeth should be reviewed by radiographs, checked for symptoms, and probed for periodontal pockets at 3 month intervals for the first year. After the first year the teeth should be checked at 4 to 6 month intervals until the permanent root canal filling is placed. The paste is changed when appropriate after the first 6 weeks' change (see Section V, subsection on calcium hydroxide treatment).

Permanent Fill. After approximately 1 year of calcium hydroxide treatment *without* evidence of root resorption, the canal system should be obturated three dimensionally. The patient should then be recalled 6 months and 1 year after obturation of the canal system with gutta percha.

Prevention. In conclusion, the dental profession needs to encourage *preventive* measures, such as the greater use of mouthguards in sporting activities, in order to decrease severe injuries to teeth. Results achieved by the use of mouth protectors in sports have been quite favorable.

Text continued on page 222

Case 15 The patient's maxillary central incisor had been luxated toward the palate 3 years prior to this radiograph. Calcium hydroxide was contraindicated because the resorption was above the crestal bone height when the patient was referred.

Case 16 The patient was referred 9 months after avulsion of both maxillary central incisors. Reverse amalgam fillings were placed at the time of replantation. Reverse fillings are contraindicated because manipulation of the tooth causes damage to the periodontal ligament. Invariably, at recall appointments the amalgam is observed by radiograph to be floating in the periapical tissues.

Case 17 The maxillary right central incisor had been luxated 1 year prior to the radiograph. Shortly after the trauma, the root canal system had been obturated with gutta percha. The patient was referred for consultation 1 year later. Calcium hydroxide treatment was contraindicated because of the extensive cervical resorption.

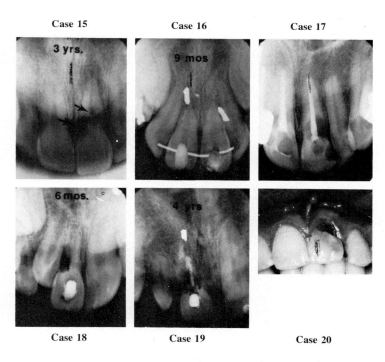

Case 15 / Case 16 / Case 17 / Case 18 / Case 19 / Case 20

Case 18 The maxillary left central incisor had been avulsed 6 months prior to the radiograph. The patient was then referred for consultation. Again, calcium hydroxide treatment would be to no avail because of the extensive resorptive area that communicated with a periodontal pocket.

Case 19 The patient presented with a history of avulsion 4 years prior to the radiograph. A reverse amalgam filling was placed before replantation and later the canal was obturated with gutta percha. Replacement and inflammatory resorption had removed most of the root.

Case 20 Internal resorption of a tooth that was traumatized a few years before. No calcium hydroxide treatment was performed in any of the above six cases.

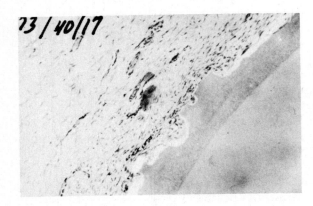

Case 21 Histopathologic specimen of early cemental root resorption. This is typical of the surface resorption, which is too minimal to be seen radiographically. (Courtesy of Dr. Harold R. Stanley, Gainesville, Florida.)

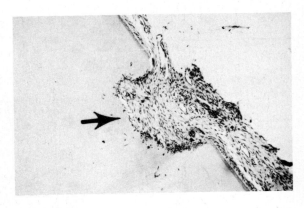

Case 22 Histopathologic specimen of a resorptive bay invading the dentin, which is representative of inflammatory root resorption. (Courtesy of Dr. Harold R. Stanley, Gainesville, Florida.)

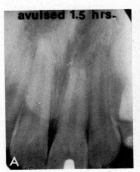
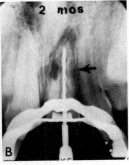

Case 23 In a 12-year-old patient the maxillary right central incisor was exarticulated for approximately 1½ hours before replantation (A). The patient was not referred for treatment until 2 months later. At that time the radiograph revealed extensive inflammatory resorption that had invaded the canal system (B).

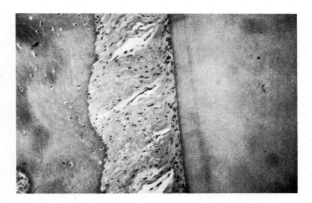

Case 24 Histologic specimen of a normal periodontal ligament in man. The undifferentiated mesenchymal cells next to the hard tissues are believed to differentiate into either blastic or clastic cells. (Courtesy of Dr. Harold R. Stanley, Gainesville, Florida.)

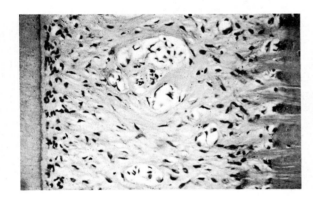

Case 25 Histologic specimen of the periodontal ligament from an animal study. Sharpey's fibers can be seen embedded in osseous and cemental tissue. (Courtesy of Dr. J. F. Knoché, Paris, France.)

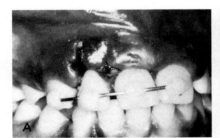
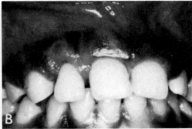

Case 26 A splint of orthodontic rectangular wire was acid etched to the facial I surfaces of the teeth, thus stabilizing the maxillary left lateral incisor (A). Two weeks after the traumatic avulsion, only the slightest mobility existed (Class I)(B). The splint was left on for 1 week. Obturation of the root canal system with calcium hydroxide was performed 5 days after the trauma.

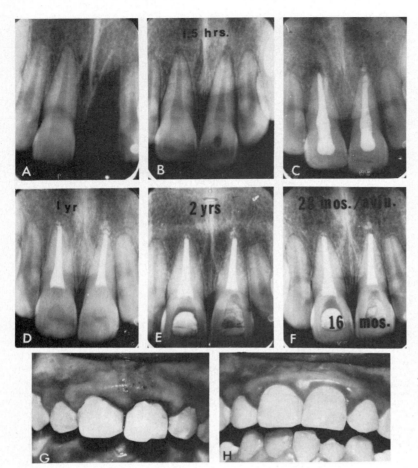

Case 27 A 13-year-old patient presented with an avulsed maxillary right central incisor (A). The tooth was replanted after being out of the socket for approximately 1½ hours (B and G). The canal was obturated with calcium hydroxide 1 week after the injury. A 3 month radiograph suggested minimal resorption. The left central incisor had been luxated; therefore, it was also treated with calcium hydroxide (C). A 9 month clinical examination revealed good esthetics and function of the teeth (H). After 1 year, the radiograph suggested minimal root resorption. For this reason the paste was removed and the canal system of both central incisors was filled with gutta percha. The access openings were filled with a tooth-colored restorative material (D). Two year and 28 month recall radiographs suggested minimal root resorption (E and F). The patient then moved from the area and the author does not know why another practitioner entered the access fillings.

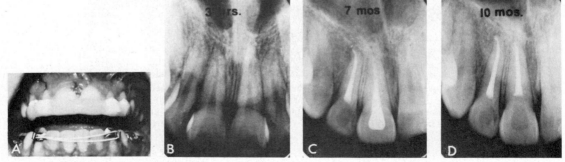

Case 28 Stabilization of the maxillary left central incisor was accomplished with an acrylic rim splint covering the incisal surfaces of the anterior teeth. It was cemented with white IRM (A). The tooth was replanted after approximately 3 hours (B). The lateral incisor, which had been only subluxated, was obturated with gutta percha while the avulsed central incisor was treated with calcium hydroxide. A 7 month recall suggested only minimal resorption (C). At the 10 month recall, the radiograph showed re-establishment of the periodontal ligament. The calcium hydroxide paste was removed, and the root canal system of the central incisor was filled with gutta percha (D). (Splinting was performed by Dr. Hank Tabeling, Gainesville, Florida.)

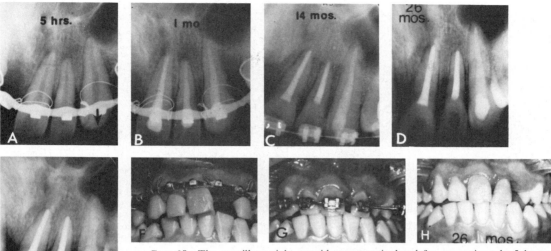

Case 29 The maxillary right cuspid was exarticulated for approximately 5 hours before reimplantation, and the right central and lateral incisors were luxated to the point of lying flat on the palate. The teeth were stabilized by an oral surgery arch bar and ligated with orthodontic wire (*A* and *F*). The patient was referred 1 month after the injury, at which time the canal systems of all three teeth were filled with calcium hydroxide (*B*). The calcium hydroxide was removed from the central and lateral incisors, which were then filled with gutta percha 10 months after the trauma. Orthodontic treatment was initiated 1 year after the injury. Fourteen months after the accident, and after 2 months of orthodontic treatment, the radiograph suggested minimal resorption of the cuspid and apical orthodontic movement resorption of the central and lateral incisors (*C*). A clinical photograph showed the progress of 7 months of orthodontic movement (*G*).

A radiograph taken 26 months after the initial trauma (including 14 months of orthodontic treatment) suggested some distal resorption of the cuspid (*D*). The orthodontic bands were removed at 26 months (*H*). A 30 month recall suggested periapical healing of the central and lateral incisors and some distal resorption of the cuspid (*E*). At the 30 month recall, the canal of the cuspid contained a wet calcium hydroxide paste in the cervical area; however, the paste was dry apical to that point. At 3 year recall, resorption in the cervix was confirmed by reflection of a surgical flap. The fact that the inflammatory resorption occurred despite the calcium hydroxide treatment may be due to the orthodontic forces applied to the avulsed cuspid, or it might be that calcium hydroxide does not always exert a positive influence in the cervical region. However, in light of the fact that no other treatment can provide a better prognosis, it is recommended that calcium hydroxide treatment be employed in these instances along with curettage of the cervix when resorption is noted here. It should also be pointed out that the cervical resorption was not detected until after 14 months of orthodontic treatment.

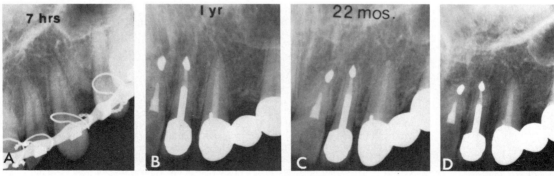

Case 30 A 25-year-old patient avulsed the maxillary right cuspid as a result of a small plane crash. The tooth was not reimplanted until approximately 7 hours later (*A*). The patient was referred 1 week later, at which time the cuspid was treated with calcium hydroxide paste. The maxillary right lateral and central incisors were only luxated, but the pulps became necrotic. They were filled with gutta percha. Periapical surgery (with reverse amalgam fillings) was undertaken on the two incisors 4 months after the trauma. The central incisor was still symptomatic 3 months after partial canal obturation (because of a calcified canal system).

One year after the avulsion of the cuspid, little external resorption has occurred (*B*). Twenty-two months after the accident, there was slight resorption in two areas (one on the mesial and one on the distal) (*C*). The radiograph suggested minimal resorption 3 years after the trauma (*D*). The calcium hydroxide paste was changed approximately every 6 months after the initial change at 6 weeks. Because of the patient's availability, the canal system still contained calcium hydroxide paste after 40 months.

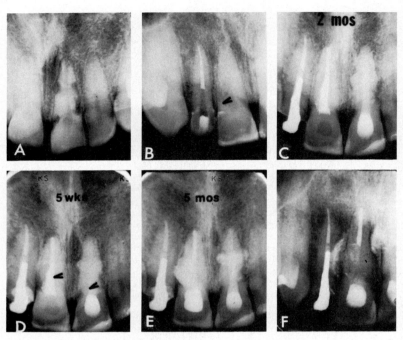

Case 31 A 29-year-old patient presented for his first appointment 8 months after trauma to the anterior teeth as a result of a small plane crash. It is believed that the maxillary central incisors were only luxated. The maxillary right central incisor displayed extensive external resorption, whereas little resorption was noted in the left central incisor (A). The right central incisor was obturated with calcium hydroxide paste that day. During an appointment 1 month later, the maxillary left lateral incisor was found to contain vital pulp tissue; however, it was filled with gutta percha because of an oblique fracture below the bone level. A post and core were required for final restoration. No significant external resorption was noted in the left central incisor at this time (arrow) (B). Two months after the initial appointment, the maxillary left central incisor (containing a necrotic pulp) was obturated with gutta percha, using the vertical condensation technique. The calcium hydroxide paste was changed in the right central incisor (C).

Five weeks after the gutta percha placement in the maxillary left central incisor, extensive external resorption was noted on the distal aspect of the tooth, just below the bone height. No change was noted in the mesial external resorptive area located just below the bone height of the right central incisor, which has been treated with calcium hydroxide (D). The gutta percha filling of left central incisor was removed to the apical extent of the external resorption and filled to that level with calcium hydroxide paste 1 month after noting the extensive resorption. Five weeks later the calcium hydroxide was changed. A massive amount of the paste may be observed radiographically to be extruded through the large distal resorptive area of the left central incisor (E). The paste was changed for the third time in the right central incisor, 5 months after the initial calcium hydroxide treatment (E). After 22 months of calcium hydroxide treatment of the left central incisor, the radiograph suggests resolution of its distal resorptive area (F).

This case should be compared with Case 30, in which the tooth was treated with calcium hydroxide 1 week after the trauma.

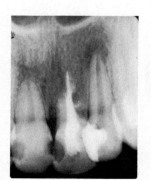

Case 32 The patient was referred for consultation of the right maxillary central incisor 1 year after avulsion. The tooth was immediately replanted by the patient's mother and then splinted by the referring dental clinic after the injury. The root canal was obturated with gutta percha approximately 2 weeks after the accident. Because at the time of referral the external resorption had invaded the cervix and the remaining root-to-crown ratio was minimal, extraction of the central incisor was recommended, and the lateral incisor was filled with gutta percha.

The central incisor's periodontal ligament was not removed intentionally, and the tooth was replanted within a few minutes; however, extensive external resorption occurred. The author recommends calcium hydroxide treatment of every avulsed tooth that has a closed apex to prevent or retard external resorption.

Case 33 An 18-year-old student was referred 5 days after avulsion of the maxillary left central incisor. The periodontal ligament was scrubbed off by the referring dentist because it was covered with black dirt *(A)*. The tooth was again traumatized 3 weeks after the initial avulsion. The root canal of the incisor was filled with calcium hydroxide 5 days after the initial accident. A degenerating ischemic infarcted pulp was removed during the instrumentation of the canal system. At a 2 year recall, the root had undergone minimal resorption *(B)*. The canal system is still being treated with calcium hydroxide paste. Clinically, the tooth is ankylosed. The paste is being changed approximately every 6 months. Despite the fact that the periodontal ligament had been intentionally removed, there seems to be minimal root resorption of the calcium hydroxide–treated tooth.

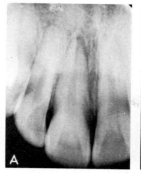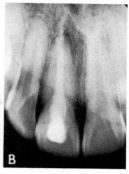

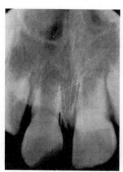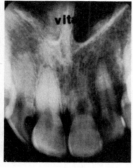

Case 34   **Case 35**

Case 34 The crown of the left maxillary central incisor was fractured as a result of traumatic injury. This stage of root development often lends itself to complete avulsion, owing to the short crown-to-root ratio and loosely structured periodontal ligament. The divergent apex allows a greater possibility for revascularization in instances of avulsion.

Case 35 A patient in her 20's was referred for consultation regarding her immature right maxillary central incisor. All vitality tests yielded a normal response, and the tooth was only slightly mobile. No treatment was indicated at this time. In instances of avulsion, Hertwig's root sheath may become damaged, preventing continued root development. The pulp may revascularize, maintaining the original pulp tissue; however, more likely, the pulp will first be replaced with granulation tissue and then a portion of the pulp space will be replaced by hard tissue (osteodentin).

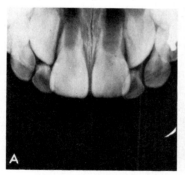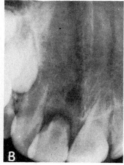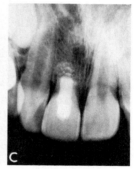

Case 36 The first radiograph represents a routine examination recall taken 1 week before avulsion of the maxillary left central incisor *(A)*. The patient, 8 years of age, was referred because of pain 6 months after avulsion. The tooth had a Class III mobility. A purulent exudate was found in the pulp chamber *(B)*. Proper drainage was established; then the canal system was debrided and obturated with calcium hydroxide paste (see Section XI). The paste was changed three times over the course of a year. A 1 year recall showed periapical healing, and the tooth demonstrated only a Class I mobility *(C)*. The purpose of treatment was space maintenance, hopefully long enough that the space could be replaced with a fixed prosthesis.

Case 37 The maxillary central and lateral incisors were luxated approximately 9 mm toward the palate. The teeth were repositioned and stabilized on the day of the trauma. A radiograph was not taken until 3 days later, when it was recognized that the teeth were not repositioned in the sockets *(A)*. Repositioning was attempted at this time by the referring dentist with limited success *(B)*. It is speculated that, after 3 days, the blood clot and the healing tissues would not allow proper repositioning. The need to confirm repositioning of replanted teeth by a radiograph cannot be overemphasized. The teeth are now being treated with calcium hydroxide therapy.

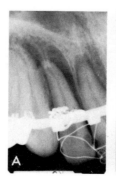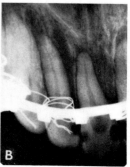

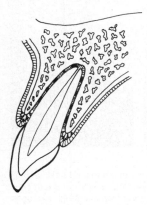

Figure 7–4 Subluxation injury without severing the periodontal ligament but with hemorrhage in the ligament.

SECTION VI. THE LUXATED TOOTH
(Cases 38 to 43, pp. 226 and 227)

Luxation is described as the dislocation of a tooth from its alveolus that might result from acute trauma or a pathologic process. In most luxation injuries, the traumatic forces are absorbed by the periodontium without apparent damage to the tooth structure. A distinction is made between the subluxated (concussed) tooth and the partially luxated tooth. Andreasen refers to the concussion injury as one that does not result in abnormal loosening of the teeth, whereas the subluxation injury is one that results in abnormal loosening of the teeth *without* displacement (Fig. 7–4). In discussing treatment, these two divisions (concussion and subluxation) will be placed in one category, *subluxation*. Often it is very difficult to distinguish between these two divisions. Luxation will be described in this section as a tooth with a partial dislocation from its alveolus (Figs. 7–5 and 7–6). Extrusive, intrusive, and laterally luxated teeth will be placed in one category, *luxation*. Andreasen reports that luxation injuries make up about 20 to 40 per cent of traumatic injuries affecting the permanent teeth, but these injuries occur more commonly in the primary teeth. The treatment to be described here will be for permanent teeth. Usually, the appropriate therapy for luxation injuries of deciduous teeth is extraction, especially in the intruded cases in order to prevent possible damage to the underlying permanent tooth buds. Luxation injuries of permanent teeth, as in avulsed teeth, most frequently involve the maxillary central incisors.

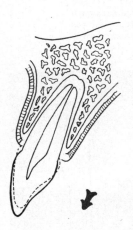

Figure 7–5 Extrusive luxation injury with severing of the periodontal ligament.

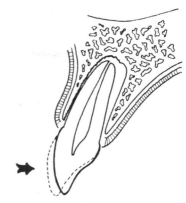

Figure 7-6 Lateral luxation injury with severing of the periodontal ligament. The prognosis for a luxated tooth can often be improved by treating the canal system with calcium hydroxide.

Subluxation

Often in instances of subluxation, but more so when luxation occurs, the trauma compresses the blood vessels at the apex long enough to shut off the blood supply, leading to an anoxic condition of the pulp. When the blood supply resumes, it does not occur soon enough and many degenerative (ischemic) changes in the pulp result. The subluxated tooth is *not* completely severed from the periodontal ligament, but hemorrhage will occur in the ligament space and the accompanying osseous tissue as a result of the traumatic injury. The tooth may undergo some surface resorption but usually will not undergo significant inflammatory resorption unless a long-standing necrotic canal system is left untreated. The subluxated tooth may have some mobility, but usually this is not significant enough to require intraocclusal splinting. At the initial appointment, the traumatized tooth should be categorized into one of the two above-mentioned divisions as the basis for the type of treatment to be rendered. Sometimes it is difficult to make this distinction, especially if the patient does not present for treatment until a few weeks after the trauma.

In some instances the pulp of the subluxated tooth does not respond to vitality testing initially after trauma but will elicit a response at a later date. Conversely, a pulp may elicit an initial positive response, and at some time after the trauma, the pulp may become necrotic and yield no response. In instances of an ischemic infarct, one would not expect a response to pulp testing initially or at a later date, owing to the severance of the nerve and blood supply. Pulp test results are recorded at the time of trauma, and the patient is given an appointment in approximately 1 month for pulp re-evaluation. If this evaluation indicates a vital pulp, the patient should then be recalled at 3 months, 6 months, and 1 year for further evaluation. When there is an initial pulp vitality response but no response at a later date, this tooth becomes a candidate for endodontic treatment. In the true subluxation (concussion) injury, external resorption is usually not of the same concern as in the luxated tooth. If the subluxated tooth becomes involved, it is usually manifested in one of three ways: pulpal necrosis, internal resorption, or pulpal calcification to approximate complete canal closure. Calcium hydroxide treatment is usually not indicated in the true subluxated injury unless the internal resorption has perforated the root (see Section II). Most cases of subluxation can be treated successfully by canal obturation with gutta percha.

Luxation

In instances of luxation, the periodontal ligament generally is severed along with the vascular supply to the canal system (Case 38). Many of the same principles apply to luxated teeth as to avulsed teeth, except that the prognosis is better with luxated teeth. The severance of the periodontal ligament is of major concern in the displacement of teeth. The severe inflammatory reaction occurring in the periodontium results from the tearing of the periodontal ligament fibers and crushing of the adjacent osseous tissue. The net results are islands of resorption of the root surface. This is usually perpetuated by necrosis or irreversible pulp involvement when there is stretching or severance of the vascular supply at the apex and/or lateral canals. The exact mechanism of external resorption is not known, but it is postulated that initial cemental resorption on the root surface exposes the dentinal tubules, thus allowing toxic products (issuing from the necrotic pulp and Tomes' fibers) to pass outward through dentinal tubules and lateral canals to the root surface. Surface resorption is not usually observed radiographically, but it most likely occurs as part of the severe inflammation in the periodontal ligament.

There is probably a higher incidence of resorption than is generally recognized. Often the resorptive process is not manifested until a few months or even years later. Resorption in the cervical area often goes unnoticed because it can easily be mistaken for radiographic cervical burnout. Careful probing of the sulcus and exploration of the tooth structure are needed to detect this situation during follow-up appointments. If periodontal pockets are detected, the granulation tissue must be curetted and toxic canal material must be eliminated by canal obturation — preferably with an initial calcium hydroxide paste treatment. Gutta percha obturation will not stimulate the healing process, as will calcium hydroxide (see Case 17). Once the external resorptive process has perforated into the canal system and established a communication between canal and crevice, the calcium hydroxide treatment will be of no benefit. The key for a good prognosis is *early* treatment with the calcium hydroxide paste in order to prevent or retard this inflammatory resorption. Hopefully, if the surface resorption occurs at the cervix, the canal obturation with calcium hydroxide will stimulate a healing response before the resorption has perforated into the canal system. The prognosis can be further enhanced by curettage of the granulation tissue at the same time as obturation with the calcium hydroxide paste.

It is felt that a luxated tooth has a better prognosis than an avulsed tooth because the periodontal ligament is bathed in a blood clot or is maintained in some areas by the capillary plexus surrounding the tooth. Replacement resorption does not seen to occur as often when the periodontal ligament is maintained; instead, inflammatory resorption is the main problem and this can be controlled by calcium hydroxide treatment (Case 39). If the local inflammation from the initial trauma is so severe that it causes complete resorption of the periodontal ligament and the ligament's attachment to the tooth before any organized healing occurs (especially if the canal is not obturated), replacement resorption can proceed. Therefore, early treatment to remove the toxic stimulus from the root canal system is of prime importance.

Many investigators believe that displaced (luxated) teeth should not be repositioned, as this promotes ankylosis. In many instances a soft tissue and/or osseous dehiscence occurs as a result of increased pressure placed on the periodontium of the displaced teeth (Cases 40, 41, and 42). Those who fear ankylosis advocate natural eruption in intruded cases and orthodontic extrusion for treatment of laterally displaced teeth. The author advocates the repositioning of luxated teeth followed by calcium hydroxide treatment of the canal in order to prevent or retard this resorptive process and diminish the chance of dehiscence (Case 43). When repositioning a tooth, the root needs to be placed within the confines of the cortical plate and the cervix needs to be positioned at or below the bone height.

In treating any traumatic injury, especially avulsions or luxations, the adjacent teeth need to be evaluated, as they frequently sustain a subluxation (concussion) injury. If the alveolar cortical plate is fractured, it should be reduced (repositioned) or removed if it cannot be stabilized. Antibiotic therapy is indicated when the alveolar fracture communicates with the oral environment. If there is no cortical plate fracture, antibiotics are not indicated, as it is comparatively rare to have an immediate acute infection following traumatic injuries. As with avulsed teeth, intraocclusal splinting is applied for 1 to 2 weeks. If an alveolar fracture is present, however, the splinting may be applied for up to 6 weeks. The calcium hydroxide treatment should be initiated within 1 week and changed at the 6 week interval. Treatment is monitored as described in the technique section. The minimum recommended period of calcium hydroxide treatment for luxated teeth is 6 months. There should be 1 year of calcium hydroxide treatment, and after that year, if no resorption can be detected along the root surface by clinical or radiographic means, the final gutta percha filling may be placed. After the canal is obturated with gutta percha, the patient should be recalled at 6 month intervals for the next 2 years. If external resorption then becomes evident, the gutta percha should be removed and the calcium hydroxide therapy continued until the resorption has ceased and healing occurs.

Summary of Generalized Treatment for Dislocation Injuries

  I. Subluxation: Abnormal loosening with displacement.
  A. Splinting: Not normally indicated.
  B. Treatment: Recall the patient initially in 4 to 6 weeks for pulpal evaluation testing. In instances of pulp involvement, gutta percha obturation is indicated.
 II. Luxation: Partial dislocation from the alveolus with severance of the periodontal ligament.
  A. Splinting: Tooth repositioned and a passive splint placed for 1 to 2 weeks.*
  B. Treatment: Calcium hydroxide obturation within 7 days and treatment continued for approximately 1 year with appropriate paste changes. The final obturation is with gutta percha.
III. Avulsion: Complete separation from the alveolus.
  A. Splinting: Tooth reimplanted and a passive splint placed for 1 to 2 weeks.*
  B. Treatment: Same as luxation.

---

*Note: In instances of cortical bone fractures, a more rigid splint is recommended for a period of 4 to 6 weeks.

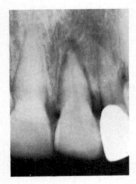

Case 38 The patient presented a few days after a luxation injury. The immediate indicated treatment was stabilization, canal preparation, and obturation with a calcium hydroxide paste.

Case 39 The patient presented 3 months after a luxation injury. The radiograph reveals inflammatory resorption (*arrows*) of both maxillary central incisors. At the time the radiograph was taken, only the right incisor had received the calcium hydroxide paste (*A*). The left incisor received the paste at the same appointment. The teeth were treated with calcium hydroxide for 1 year. An 8 month post–gutta percha obturation recall (20 months from initial treatment) suggested that cementogenesis had occurred, for an intact periodontal ligament can be observed on the radiograph (*B*).

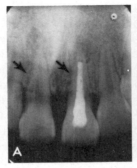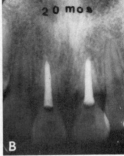

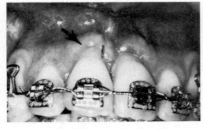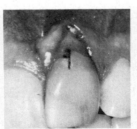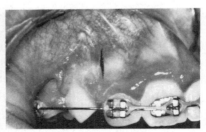

| Case 40 | Case 41 | Case 42 |

Case 40 The patient was referred a few months after the labial luxation of the maxillary central incisors. The teeth were repositioned orthodontically. Facial dehiscence of hard and soft tissues was the result of not repositioning the teeth immediately after the luxation injury.

Case 41 The patient presented 1 year after the labial luxation of the right central incisor. The tooth was not repositioned. The canal was filled with gutta percha and no calcium hydroxide treatment was performed. Facial dehiscence and a root perforation from external resorption resulted.

Case 42 The patient was referred a few weeks after a subluxation injury. He was wearing orthodontic appliances at the time, and the trauma must have activated the appliance to cause labial movement of the left lateral incisor. The tooth was sore and the labial soft tissues were stretched taut across the root. Palpation of the root revealed that it had broken through the cortical plate. The patient was immediately referred to his orthodontist for appliance adjustment.

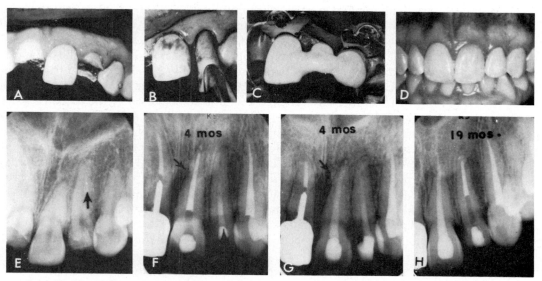

Case 43 The patient was referred the same day as multiple injuries were sustained. A sedative restoration had been placed over the exposure on the left central incisor, caused by an oblique fracture of the crown. The right lateral incisor also had sustained a subosseous oblique fracture. The right central incisor had been slightly sub-luxated (A). The radiograph revealed an intruded (arrow) right lateral incisor (E). This tooth was extracted and intentionally repositioned above the fracture (B). A rubber dam was placed and the tooth was stabilized by acid etching an acrylic splint (C). The splint was removed 2 weeks later. The left central incisor received a temporary crown while the crown of the right lateral incisor was built up by acid etching. At this time the left and right central incisors received gutta percha root canal fillings. The right lateral incisor received a calcium hydroxide paste filling a few days after the trauma. Three months after the initial trauma the right cuspid was found to have a necrotic pulp and was treated and obturated with gutta percha.

Four months after the initial treatment the right central incisor, which had been very slightly subluxated and had received a gutta percha filling, was starting to undergo lateral root resorption (upper arrow). It is significant that the right *lateral* incisor, which had been intentionally repositioned and had received calcium hydroxide treatment, had undergone minimal resorption (F). The gutta percha filling was removed from the root canal of the right central incisor, and the canal was obturated with calcium hydroxide, some of which extruded through the resorptive perforation (arrow). The paste was changed for the second time in the right lateral incisor (G). After 19 months of calcium hydroxide treatment in this tooth, no significant lateral resorption was detected. For this reason the paste was removed and the canal was obturated with gutta percha, using lateral condensation. Post space was prepared in this right lateral incisor, and 1 month later a post, core, and crown were cemented (D). The right central incisor is still being treated with calcium hydroxide (H). (The fixed prosthodontics was performed by Dr. Anthony Gegauff, Gainesville, Florida.)

SECTION VII. THE HORIZONTAL ROOT FRACTURE
(Cases 44 to 52, pp. 232 to 236)

Austin, in 1930, found that 31 of 40 teeth with cross fractures of the roots gave positive responses to vitality tests. Kronfeld, in 1933, suggested that root fractures have the ability to heal themselves provided that the fragments are in close apposition and immobile in the position. A high percentage of horizontal intraosseous root fractures do not need endodontic treatment if the fracture is diagnosed early and maintained by the appropriate alternative therapy (Figs. 7–7 and 7–8). This assumes that there is no chronic periodontal complication. If microorganisms or epithelium invades the fracture site, the prognosis is poor for the occlusal segment (Case 44). The site of fracture determines the degree of tooth mobility. The prognosis is most favorable for maintaining a viable pulp if the horizontal fracture is in the apical third of the root and least favorable if the fracture is in the cervical third. This probably relates to a natural stabilization by the osseous tissue of those fractures in the apical third. However, Andreasen and Hjörting-Hansen stressed that no significant difference in prognosis exists between fractures located in the apical, middle, or coronal third of the root provided that the teeth are immediately repositioned and are firmly immobilized. Extrusion of the coronal fragment and inadequate splinting seem to increase the frequency of pulp necrosis. Usually, complications occur within 2 months of injury. The majority of early detected horizontal fractures undergo repair if treated by reduction of displaced fragments and firm stabilization by interocclusal splinting for a period of 6 to 8 weeks (Case 45).

After studying 65 anterior teeth receiving root fractures, Michanowicz et al. concluded that the integrity of the periodontal membrane is the essential requisite in root repair. They further observed that cementum will be deposited at the fractured ends of the two segments and the continuous deposition of cementum will join the segments. Andreasen reviewed the process of multiple hard tissue (dentin, osteodentin, and cementum) that can form the uniting callus between the root fractures. He further described that, in most cases, the innermost layer of repair is dentin and the more peripheral part of the fracture line is incompletely repaired with cementum.

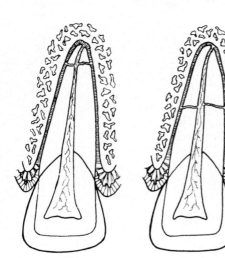

Figures 7–7 and 7–8 The vital pulps of teeth that have sustained a horizontal fracture of the root can often be maintained by tooth stabilization.

Figure 7–7   **Figure 7–8**

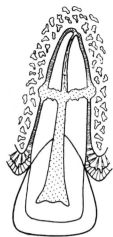

Figure 7–9 When the incisal portion of the pulpal system becomes irreversibly involved, only this segment needs treatment.

Degering pointed out the difficulty of diagnosing a suspected fine fracture of a root and/or supporting bone. His study showed that dark-density films increased the latitude of the diagnostic range and that two additional radiographs should be taken of the questionable area with a plus and minus 15 degree vertical angulation in relation to the original tube position. The dentist should not misinterpret radiographically what appears to be a double fracture, for in most instances one is viewing a single oblique root fracture in which the buccal and lingual fracture lines are recorded side by side on the radiograph (Case 46). Andreasen notes that after healing of the fractured segments with callus formation, the fracture line is generally discernible on the radiograph because of the lower radiopacity of cementum.

If there is only partial involvement of the pulpal system, it is usually confined to the incisal (occlusal) portion, as the apical segment remains vital in the vast majority of instances (Fig. 7–9). It is conjectured that the traumatic forces are dissipated at the fracture site without severing the blood supply to the apical segment while displacing the incisal segment enough to sever the vascular supply to that segment. Many horizontal fractures do not respond to vitality testing immediately after the traumatic injury. Vitality testing is not reliable initially. Therefore, it is advisable to wait at least 2 months after the trauma before treating the incisal segment as irreversibly involved. The pulp of the incisal segment may have been severed initially, but collateral circulation may be re-established through the fracture site. In instances in which the *incisal* pulpal segment becomes involved, only this portion needs treatment. If the pulp has increased secondary dentin deposition (as usually occurs in older individuals), it may be possible to ledge the dentin intentionally in the incisal segment and obturate the canal with gutta percha.

Traumatic injuries occurring in children less than 11 years old have a tendency to be subluxated or avulsed. Unfortunately, the majority of horizontal fractures occur in young individuals (ages 11 to 20) whose canal system is very wide. Since there is a great possibility of a gutta percha filling overextension, it is recommended that the incisal portion be treated with calcium hydroxide (Case 47). This serves the dual purpose of arresting the inflammatory resorption occurring at the fracture site and creating a calcified barrier that will ultimately allow the incisal canal to be obturated properly. If the *apical* segment of pulp is presumed to be vital, this segment should never

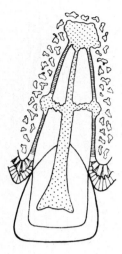

Figure 7–10 If the entire pulp becomes involved, both segments require endodontic treatment.

be instrumented. The incisal segment of the pulp system is instrumented and treated with calcium hydroxide paste as if it were an apexification treatment. After *approximately* 1 year of treatment, if a sufficient calcified barrier has been generated (Fig. 7–11), the calcium hydroxide should be removed and the incisal portion obturated with gutta percha.

If both segments of the root are involved (Fig. 7–10), treatment is needed for both portions. If the root segments are widely separated or if the roots are greatly displaced, it is recommended that surgical endodontics be performed, removing the apical segment and placing a reverse amalgam filling in the incisal segment. Of course, the incisal segment must be of sufficient length to allow osseous stabilization. Permanent interocclusal splinting can be employed to aid in stabilization, when needed. The author does not recommend intraosseous implants for stabilization, as it is often difficult to obturate the canal system with the implant.

Horizontal and oblique crown-root fractures in the cervical area or just below (2 mm) the crestal bone pose a clinical problem to the restorative dentist. In the past, these nonrestorable roots have been extracted, or a crown lengthening procedure has been achieved by periodontal surgery. At times, the extraction of the root has left an osseous defect not conducive to a pleasing fixed prosthesis. Moreover, when apical repositioning of a flap and

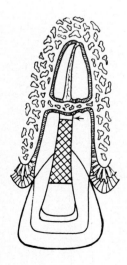

Figure 7–11 The incisal portion of the canal system in Figure 7–8 can be treated with calcium hydroxide to stimulate a calcified barrier.

ostectomy (if needed) are performed to allow for sufficient exposure of the remaining root, the result may be adverse periodontal changes to the neighboring teeth or an unpleasing gingival contour of the involved tooth (compared with the adjacent teeth).

The attempt to bury margins of restorations in order to secure sound tooth structure usually results in a poor gingival response. Therefore, in extrusion of a tooth, approximately 3 mm of root above the crestal bone height is needed to allow for sufficient periodontal attachment. Ingber et al. described the "Biologic Width" as the combined dimension of the connective tissue attachment and the epithelial attachment. They arrived at 2.04 mm as the dimension of the "Biologic Width," and a minimum of 1 mm coronal to the epithelial attachment of sound tooth structure must be available to place a margin for the final restoration. When esthetics is a concern, the orthodontic extrusion can be accomplished by hollowing out the pontic of a three unit bridge if the neighboring teeth need full coverage (Case 48). Otherwise, the natural crown or an acrylic denture tooth that has had the lingual portion of the crown removed to resemble a pontic can be acid etched to adjacent teeth to prevent the need for preparing these teeth for restoration. An operative pin or hook is placed on the lingual surface as close to the incisal edge as the occlusion will allow. A small orthodontic elastic is run from a temporarily cemented post in the root canal to a hook on the natural crown, the denture tooth, or inside the pontic. The author advocates a period of 1 to 2 months to extrude the root, thereby diminishing the possibility of promoting external resorption, and a period of approximately 2 to 4 weeks for stabilization after the root has been extruded.

Andreasen stressed that *immediate repositioning* and *fixation* are the two most important factors in the treatment of root fractures. Dislocation of the coronal segment negatively influences the prognosis to a significant degree if the segment is improperly repositioned. Digital manipulation can reposition the displaced segment, and rigid fixation can best be accomplished by an acrylic splint and reinforced with orthodontic wire if open contacts exist (see Section V). Frank states, "the first consideration following the traumatic injury would be the reduction of the displaced coronal fragment. The closer the apposition of the fractured portions, the more likely the possibility that healing will occur." He was referring to healing by a vital pulpal system. If, however, the pulpal system is irreversibly involved or necrotic and there is no separation (or less than approximately 1 mm of separation) between the fractured segments, calcium hydroxide may be introduced to promote a calcified union in the fracture site (Fig. 7–12).

In instances when both segments are involved, if the displaced segments can be aligned in close proximity, calcium hydroxide is the treatment of choice. When digital pressure alone cannot reposition the malalignment, a rubber dam is placed around the involved and neighboring teeth and the largest possibile size endodontic instrument is introduced into the canal for exploration and stabilization of the segments until they are properly aligned (Case 49). Once the segments are realigned, interocclusal splinting is placed while the endodontic instrument remains in place. The canal system is properly prepared and obturated with calcium hydroxide. The author has found that in treating both fractured segments with calcium hydroxide, the splint normally needs to remain in position approximately *four months to one year*, depending upon the mobilization of the fractured segments. This extended stabilization time helps to immobilize the segments, which is

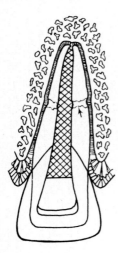

Figure 7–12 In Figure 7–9, in which the two root segments are in close proximity, a more predictable calcified deposition forms between the fractured segments if the canal system is treated with calcium hydroxide.

essential for calcified healing of the fracture site. The calcium hydroxide is changed and monitored as in the apexification technique. Once the healing callus (Case 7) has formed, the root canal system should be obturated with gutta percha. It is *not* recommended that the two fractured segments be reinforced by an internal (intraradicular) rigid material, because solid core material would in all likelihood not completely obturate the canal system of both segments and the calcific barrier would most likely be porous. These circumstances would permit fluid exchange between the canal system and the periodontium and would cause ultimate failure (Case 50). It is interesting to note that the literature abounds with descriptions of cases concerning endodontic implants, whether they be intraosseous or intraradicular. Long-term, successful recalls are rarely displayed. If the fractured tooth does not have sufficient osseous support, permanent interocclusal splinting (fixed prosthodontics) should be employed (Case 51). By saving a fractured tooth (as opposed to extraction), the crestal bone can be maintained and a more esthetic result can be achieved.

Andreasen and Hjörting-Hansen have histologically demonstrated that horizontal root fractures heal by means of one of four tissue categories: calcified, connective, a combination of osseous and connective, or granulation tissue. Successful healing (of the first three categories) occurred in 54 per cent of the fractures. Inflamed granulation tissue was found between the tooth segments when the pulps of one or both segments became necrotic. When calcium hydroxide is properly placed in the canal system, the prognosis for a *calcified* healing of the involved segments is much better (Cases 50 and 52).

Text continued on page 237

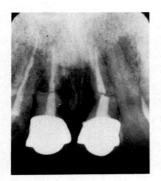

Case 44 The patient was referred 1 year after traumatic injury and placement of gutta percha root canal fillings. The teeth were not adequately splinted before or after the fillings. Periodontal complications are well established and calcium hydroxide treatment is contraindicated at this time.

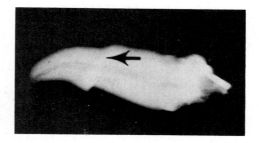

Case 45 The tooth sustained a horizontal fracture and was extracted several years later for prosthodontic reasons. Healing had occurred along the fracture site *(arrow)* even though the segments were slightly displaced. No endodontic treatment was performed. (Courtesy of Dr. J. F. Knoché, Paris, France.)

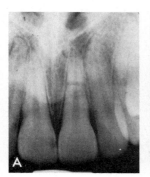 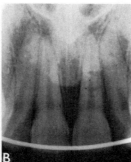

Case 46 The patient was referred immediately after a traumatic blow to the maxillary anterior teeth. The radiograph reveals an oblique fracture to the right central incisor *(A)*. The segments were immediately reduced and splinted with a passive orthodontic wire supported by acrylic acid etching. At the 2 week recall the segments were still properly aligned *(B)*. The splint remained for approximately 1 more month, since the segments remained vital. If either segment had become involved, approximate calcium hydroxide treatment would have been initiated and the splint would have been employed up to 1 year, depending upon which segment(s) were involved.

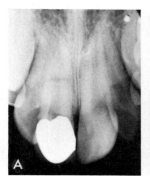 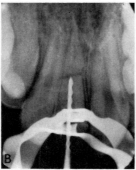 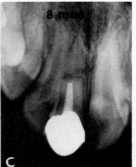 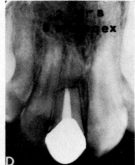

Case 47 An 11-year-old boy presented with a symptomatic maxillary left central incisor 3 months after a traumatic blow *(A)*. The tooth had not been splinted. It was felt that only the incisal segment was involved, and this segment was instrumented *(B)* and treated with calcium hydroxide for 8 months. At the end of 8 months of calcium hydroxide treatment *(C)*, a calcified barrier could be felt just short of the fracture. Radiographically, a periodontal ligament space could be seen encompassing both root segments, suggesting that resorption at the fracture site had ceased. The incisal segment was then obturated with gutta percha. A 2 year recall examination revealed an asymptomatic tooth with an intact periodontal ligament, as observed radiographically. The tooth had normal physiologic mobility *(D)*. If mobility is of concern, it is recommended that a permanent intraocclusal splinting be accomplished. If the pulp in the apical segment becomes irreversibly involved, the treatment of choice following a successful apexification procedure would be to surgically remove the apical segment. Most likely, the pulp remains vital because the apical segment retains a blood supply from the apex and there is revascularization from the periodontium at the fracture site.

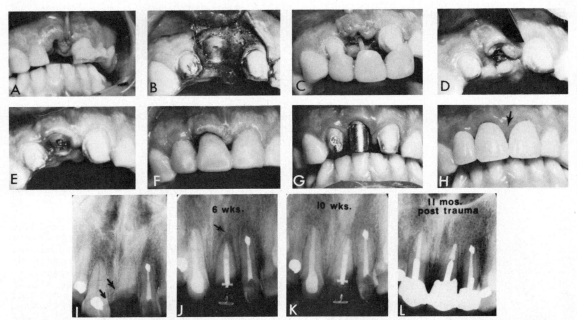

Case 48 The patient presented after an automobile accident that caused a horizontal fracture just below the crestal bone level of the maxillary left central incisor (right in the radiographs) *(A* and *I)*. The occlusal segment was lost at the time of trauma. The maxillary right central incisor was subluxated, and the left lateral incisor presented with gutta percha and reverse amalgam fillings. A flap was raised, and the canal of the fractured root was debrided and filled with calcium hydroxide paste *(B)*. The patient's mouth was filled with gauze pads to prevent possible aspiration of endodontic instruments. The top three layers of a Radix-Anchor (post) were cut off, and the remaining post with its one top layer was temporarily cemented. A temporary bridge was constructed with a wire hook quick cured inside the occlusal segment of a hollow pontic. The hook and post may be seen in the radiograph *(J)*. A Hummingbird orthodontic band was placed between the post and the hook for orthodontic extrusion *(C)*, and the bridge was temporarily cemented. This technique allowed the root to erupt into the hollowed-out pontic and alleviated the esthetic problem of a missing crown.

The extrusion process took 6 weeks until the remaining root margins had erupted enough for placement of the crown margins. The radiographic socket demonstrated the amount of extrusion achieved *(J)*. The hyperplastic tissue accompanying the extrusion process was surgically removed *(D)*. Five days later *(E)* the root with its post was stabilized with quick-cure acrylic between it and the hollowed pontic *(F)*. The root was stabilized for 10 weeks to allow healing of the periodontium *(K)*. After 4 months of orthodontic treatment, the calcium hydroxide paste was removed from the root canals of the extruded root and the right central incisor. These canals were then obturated with gutta percha, post space was prepared, and post and core restorations were made *(G)*. An 11 month recall radiograph demonstrated the functioning root *(L)*. By orthodontically extruding the root, it was possible to maintain the crestal bone level, thus providing a more esthetic bridge *(H)* than would have been possible with the osseous defect that would have resulted from extraction of the fractured left central incisor root *(A)*.

The right central incisor was treated with calcium hydroxide because it was subluxated (see Section VIII). The left central incisor was treated with calcium hydroxide not because of the trauma of the horizontal fracture but because of the added traumatic forces of orthodontic extrusion. More important, because the remaining root was initially below the crestal bone level, it was felt that the endodontic treatment in a nonsterile field (without a rubber dam) was not the desired treatment. Calcium hydroxide paste was utilized as an intracanal medication because of its bactericidal effect and its ability to render proteins less toxic. Obturating the canal with the paste prevented a tissue-fluid exchange, which also promoted healing of the periodontium as the root was extruded. (Prosthodontic treatment performed by Dr. Junhei Fujimoto, Tokyo, Japan.)

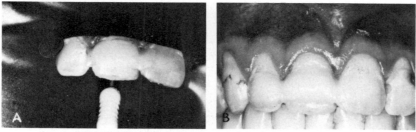

Case 49 The patient was referred after displacing the coronal tooth segment of a maxillary left central incisor as a result of refracturing an improper splint. The pulpal systems of both segments were involved. Smaller endodontic instruments were employed to negotiate the two segments and were carried to larger sizes until the segments were realigned and the files bound in the root canals *(A)*. A new acrylic acid-etched splint was placed that took into account both strength and gingival health. The canal system was obturated with calcium hydroxide. A 2 month recall after the placement of the new intraocclusal splint is shown *(B)*.

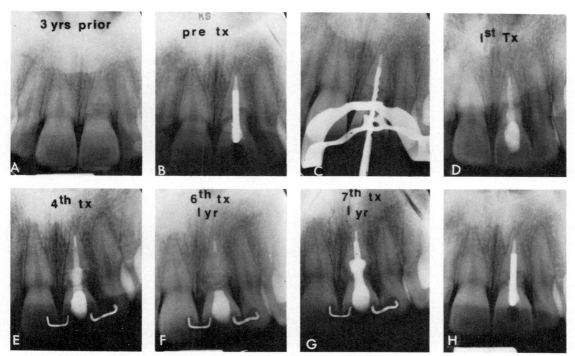

Case 50 The patient was referred with a symptomatic maxillary right central incisor that had an intraradicular Vitallium post placed 2 years previously for treatment of horizontal fractures *(B)*. A radiograph was obtained showing the patient's condition *three* years ago *(A)*. The post was removed and the canal instrumented to an existing radicular gutta percha filling *(C)*. The canal above the gutta percha was obturated with calcium hydroxide paste *(D)*. The tooth was stabilized by dovetail lingual preparations and acrylic intraocclusal splinting reinforced by orthodontic ligature wire. At the outset of the first four calcium hydroxide treatments, the paste was wet upon re-entry. Hemorrhage and granulation tissue were found invading the fracture sites. Barium sulfate could be seen diffusing outward from the fractures *(E)*. After 1 year of calcium hydroxide paste treatment, the barium sulfate was observed to be incorporated into the healing tissues. No hemorrhage or tissue fluid was found in the canal *(F)*. Periodontal probing did not reveal a communication with the fractures. A high ratio of barium sulfate was incorporated into the seventh paste application in order to determine whether any communication existed at the healed fracture sites *(G)*. A comparison can be made between the two radiographs above: *G* shows 1 year healing by calcium hydroxide treatment and *H*, the initial film, shows 2 year treatment with an intraradicular post. (Intraocclusal splinting performed by Dr. Robert Boyd, San Francisco, California.)

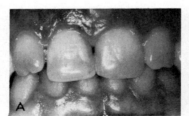
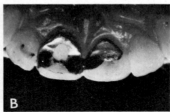

Case 51 Lingual gold pinledged intraocclusal splinting with an access opening for endodontic treatment of a horizontal fracture *(A and B)*. (Splinting performed by Dr. Stephen Rosensteil, London, England.)

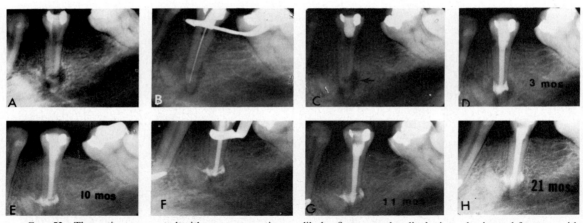

Case 52 The patient presented with a symptomatic mandibular first premolar displaying a horizontal fracture with both segments involved *(A)*. The patient had a history of an automobile accident in which he sustained a bilateral fracture of the mandible. Both segments were instrumented *(B)*, and the canal system was obturated with calcium hydroxide paste, without including barium sulfate at the initial appointment *(C)*. The paste was changed only once, 3 months from the initial appointment. Barium sulfate was added to the paste at that time *(D)*. At a 10 month recall the calcium hydroxide–barium sulfate paste could be seen radiographically, diffusing out of the canal system *(E)*. At the fitting of the master gutta percha cone before adding root canal sealer, the opacity observed in the fracture site is the barium sulfate, which became incorporated into the healing calcified tissues *(F)*. At the same visit the canal system was obturated, using the lateral condensation technique when slight extrusion of the cement was noted *(G)*. A 21 month recall from the initial treatment revealed continued healing of the periodontium *(H)*.

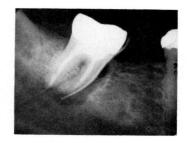

Case 53   The patient was referred with a vertically split mesial root manifesting a chronic endo-perio lesion. The root was probably split several years ago during the filling procedure. It is felt that calcium hydroxide treatment would yield a poor prognosis.

SECTION VIII. VERTICAL ROOT FRACTURES
(Cases 53 and 54, p. 237)

In the majority of vertical root fractures, the ultimate prognosis is poor and extraction is necessary to preserve the supporting periodontium of adjacent teeth. In these instances, a perio-endo lesion is established and is perpetuated by the communication from the canal system and the periodontium via the crack (Case 53). Many attempts have been made to try to fill canal systems of vertically fractured teeth with gutta percha, but they have been to no avail. Stewart has demonstrated treatment of vertical fractures

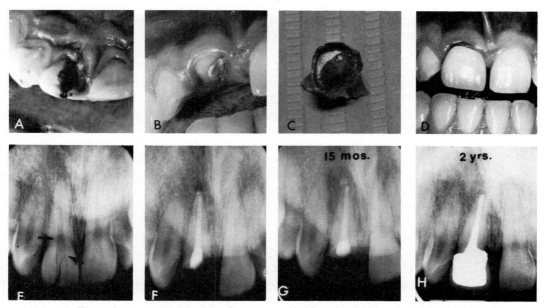

Case 54   The patient presented the day after a traumatic blow that had resulted in a vertical fracture of a maxillary central incisor. The radiograph suggests that the fracture extends below the crestal bone level *(E)*. Probing the canal with an endodontic explorer reveals that the fracture extends to the mid root portion. There was actually a double fracture: one vertical fracture and one oblique fracture just above the crestal bone level. The portion of the crown with the oblique fracture was removed *(A)* and the remaining clinical crown was reduced out of function. The canal was instrumented and treated with calcium hydroxide *(F)*. The missing crown space was replaced with a temporary partial denture. At the end of 15 months of treatment *(G)*, the sulcus was again probed to detect a possible perio-endo communication. The sulcular depth ranged from 2 to 3 mm, and this compared with the sulcular depth of the neighboring teeth *(B)*. Following removal of the paste, the canal was obturated with gutta percha and post space was prepared. A post was constructed with a core that encompassed and supported the remaining root *(C)*, and the final restoration was cemented in place *(D)*. At the recall appointment 2 years after initial treatment and 6 months after the final restoration, the sulcular depth remained the same and the radiograph did not suggest a vertical fracture pattern in the periodontium *(H)*. (Fixed restoration by Dr. Boyd Welsch, Gainesville, Florida.)

with calcium hydroxide. However, it is not certain whether or not an endo-perio communication was established before calcium hydroxide treatment.

If a tooth with a vertical root fracture is diagnosed in the early stages before a periodontal communication is established, it is felt that this root can be a candidate for calcium hydroxide treatment (Case 54). It is important to remember that there will be no dentin repair, since the odontoblastic zone was removed in endodontic instrumentation. Optimally, there will be a cementum (cemento-osteoid) repair. Emphasis should be placed on the final restoration, which must encompass the root, like bands around a barrel. This calcified deposition over the fractured site is a very thin zone that is susceptible to refracture by lateral forces.

SECTION IX. INTRACANAL MEDICAMENTS
(Cases 55 to 57, pp. 240 and 241)

Heithersay advocated calcium hydroxide as a temporary root canal filling in the treatment of involved pulps with periapical pathosis. There are endodontists who routinely place calcium hydroxide as an interim medication for most of their endodontic treatments. Because of studies such as Littman's, showing that quite often the clinician is ineffective in completely debriding a canal during instrumentation, calcium hydroxide is considered to be beneficial as an intracanal medication. Salinas reported that the liberated hydroxyl ion has a bactericidal and disinfectant activity equal to I_3OH and is three times more diffusible, plus the fact that calcium hydroxide produces complete lysis of residual canal tissue and of bacterial bodies. The ability of calcium hydroxide to denature proteins, rendering them less toxic or nontoxic, may aid in improving an endodontic prognosis.

For the sake of expediency, commercial preparations of calcium hydroxide can be used as an intracanal medication. Canal obturation is not the goal of a routine intracanal medication, but when calcium hydroxide is employed for controlling hemorrhage or for treatment of an apical abscess or cyst, canal obturation with the paste (advocated in the technique section) would be beneficial. The time span for the routine employment of calcium hydroxide as an intracanal medicament would be the same as one's usual between-appointment interval.

Hemorrhage Control. Calcium hydroxide can be very effectively employed as an intracanal medicament to control hemorrhage when the canal system contains granulation tissue (Case 55). This tissue, when served at or near the apical foramen, may continue to hemorrhage into the canal system, particularly if the natural foramen has been violated. Overinstrumentation or apical resorption of the foramen produces a larger diameter foramen, which interferes with the formation of a normal blood clot. An immediate coagulation necrosis will occur of any vital tissue that contacts the calcium hydroxide. When placing the calcium hydroxide, particular attention is needed to fill the apical foramen and/or lateral root perforation. An average of 2 to 4 weeks of calcium hydroxide treatment is needed for hemorrhage control.

Apical Abscess. Calcium hydroxide may also be employed in the "hot tooth" syndrome (Cases 8, 36, and 56). If calcium hydroxide is used in this circumstance, it cannot be overemphasized that the canal system must be *completely* debrided. Also, proper drainage through the apex or through an incision in the mucosa must be established. Weine describes the drainage sequence as first a purulent exudate, followed by a serous exudate, and finally by a hemorrhagic exudate. The principle involved is that the thoroughly debrided canal must be temporarily obturated with calcium hydroxide in order to reduce tissue fluid exchange between the periapex and the canal system. This allows the host resistance to deal favorably with the inflammation and/or infection. Such patients must be followed for the next few days, and, if this procedure does not reduce the existing cellulitis or localized swelling, drainage must be re-established either by removing the calcium hydroxide paste from the canal or by the method of incision. The author has treated numerous patients with the above procedure and has not found it necessary to remove the paste for drainage. However, every patient is followed on a daily basis for that possibility. In cases of cellulitis, a culture is taken, a disc sensitivity test is performed, and the patient is placed on antibiotics. If there is only a localized swelling, the patient is not placed on antibiotics unless the medical history warrants prophylactic use. The advantage of the method of calcium hydroxide obturation is that the paste is easy to remove from the canal if so indicated. An average of 2 to 4 weeks of calcium hydroxide treatment is needed for treatment of an apical abscess.

Apical Cyst. Calcium hydroxide may be employed as an intracanal medication in treating a true cyst, as described by Simon (Case 57). Simon described a "bay cyst" as one that is connected to the periapex and would probably heal by obturation of the root canal system. Simon further described a "cyst" as one that is completely separated from the canal system and may *not* be affected by endodontic instrumentation and obturation. Seltzer et al. suggested that overinstrumentation allows drainage of the cystic fluid, which then allows degeneration of the epithelial cells by strangulation because of fibroblastic and collagen proliferation squeezing the capillary supply to the cystic lining. Bhaskar suggested that cystic linings can be broken up by acute inflammation created by overinstrumentation. Packing the canal system with calcium hydroxide is an alternative to overinstrumentation. The initial inflammation created by obturating the canals with calcium hydroxide may be sufficient to disrupt the cystic lining. Ideally, in cases of large cystic lesions (if this can be ascertained by radiographic diagnosis, as suggested by Worth and others), the calcium hydroxide is extruded into the periapical (or lateral) lesion to ensure inflammation and possible cystic break-up. Violating a natural apical constriction is not suggested, but a constriction is frequently missing in a large periapical lesion owing to resorption of the apex. If some natural constriction is present and the calcium hydroxide is confined to the root canal system, it is possible that the inflammation created by the diffusion of the calcium hydroxide through the apical foramen may be sufficient to cause break-up of the cystic epithelial lining. If after 6 months of treatment the periapical lesion does not respond to therapy, it is recommended that the apical constriction be violated with a #25 file and the calcium hydroxide be extruded into the lesion. Although it is recognized that inflammation is created by the root canal sealer, a more predictable result is achieved if the canal system is packed with calcium hydroxide at interims. An average of 6 months is needed for calcium hydroxide treatment of apical cysts. The paste should be changed at the end of 6 weeks and used until there is radiographic evidence of break-up of the cyst and periapical healing.

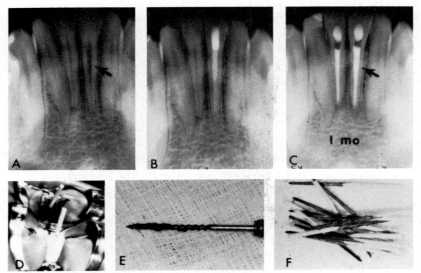

Case 55 The patient presented with a nonperforating internal resorption *(arrow)* of the right mandibular central incisor *(A)* and, upon extirpation of the pulp *(E)*, the canal continued to bleed *(D)*. Numerous premeasured paper points were applied, with no diminution of the continuous drainage *(F)*. The canal system was packed with calcium hydroxide *(B)*. After 1 month, the calcium hydroxide was removed and no hemorrhage was elicited into the canal system. The canal system was then obturated with gutta percha *(C)*. The adjacent tooth, which did not have a hemorrhage problem, was instrumented, medicated routinely, and 1 week later filled with gutta percha *(C)*.

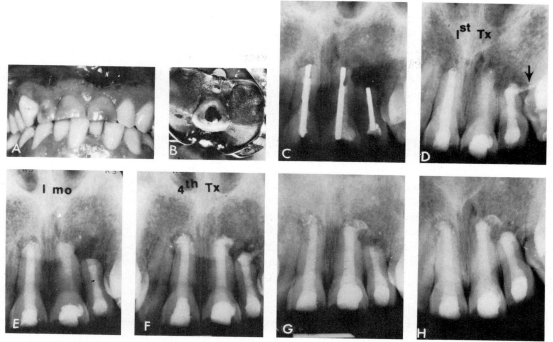

Case 56 The patient was referred with symptomatic maxillary anterior teeth that had had inadequate silver cone root canal fillings placed several years prior to this first appointment *(C)*. Not only the tooth crowns but the overlying mucosa was discolored from leakage of corrosive breakdown products of the silver cones. Three draining sinus tracts and a semilunar surgical scar were observed on the labial mucosa *(A)*. When access to the three canals was established, an immediate discharge of exudate was encountered *(B)*. The canal systems were debrided, dried, and immediately filled with calcium hydroxide. The paste may be seen following one of the tracts *(arrow, D)*. The patient remained comfortable until 1 month after placement of the paste *(E)*. At this time, when the canals were reopened, the paste was found to be wet, owing to ingress of tissue fluids through the apex. During the next three paste changes the paste was found to be wet, and hemorrhage into the canals occurred. Five months from initial treatment the (fourth) paste fillings and canals were found to be dry *(F)*. After 1 year of calcium hydroxide treatment, the radiograph suggested periapical healing *(G)*. The dry pastes were removed and partially calcified barriers could be detected at the apices. New calcium hydroxide was placed in the canals and slight apical extrusions were noted *(H)*.

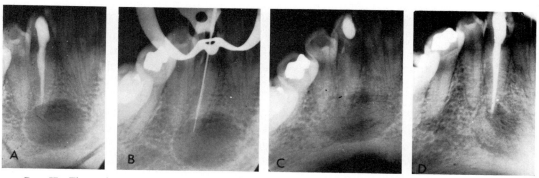

Case 57 The patient was referred with a root canal filling that had been placed in the mandibular canine 7 months previously. The radiograph showed that a large periapical lesion with well-defined borders was still present *(A)*. A diffuse swelling was observed in the buccal vestibule in the area of the canine, and the tooth was extremely sensitive to touch. The tooth was opened, and cystic fluid drainage was established through the apex *(B)*. The canal system was obturated with calcium hydroxide. Two months later, the tooth was reported to have remained comfortable, and remnants of the paste could be seen in the lesion *(C)*. The existing paste was removed and new paste placed. After 7 months of calcium hydroxide treatment there was obvious radiographic evidence of osseous healing. The paste was removed, and the canal was obturated with gutta percha at this time *(D)*.

SECTION X. ENDODONTIC–PERIODONTIC LESIONS
(Cases 58 and 59, p. 244)

Hiatt pointed out that pulpal and periodontal problems are responsible for more than 50 per cent of tooth mortality and that the interrelationship by which one of these diseases may progress to the other tissue results in a distinct and more complex pulpal-periodontal lesion. Most acute *endo-periodontic* complications (of pulpal origin), if treated in the early phases, will respond to root canal obturation alone. The endodontic-periodontic lesion, in the present context, has a pulpal etiology with a communication between the pulpal pathosis and the gingival sulcus. In contrast to this, the periodontic-endodontic lesion has a periodontal etiology but has affected the root canal system because of either periodontal treatment or a chronic periodontal pocket. Ingle and Beveridge define the "true" combined lesions as developing "when a pulpally induced periapical lesion exists on a tooth that is also periodontally involved and the infrabony defect occurs when the two lesions merge." The interrelationship of these systems can be established through the communication of the apical foramen as well as through lateral, accessory, and/or furcation canals. Studies have shown that more than 46 per cent of all molars have furcation canals, which would allow an easy exchange of microorganisms, toxins, and other tissue irritants and could cause complications in either system. It has been shown that furcation lesions could be created and maintained by inflamed and necrotic pulps, not only through furcation canals but also through dentinal tubules. Weine has displayed a photomicrograph of a lateral canal showing a communication of inflammatory infiltrate between the pulp and the periodontal ligament. If the cementum has been removed from the dentin by periodontal procedures or the cemento-enamel junction is denuded of its coating, the exposed tubules can provide a direct communication between the pulp and the oral cavity.

The dental papilla and dental sac (which differentiate into the attachment apparatus) are of a common mesodermal origin, separated initially by the epithelial root sheath. The close relationship of the pulp to the attachment apparatus is further established by their common blood supply. It has been demonstrated that the vascular supply to the periodontal ligament originates from the alveolar artery via several channels. The blood vessels course through the marrow spaces and form a plexus around the root. This plexus supplies the periodontium and the pulp via the apex and lateral canals. It has been reported that any portion of the periodontium can become affected by pulpal inflammation. It has also been reported that periodontal disease may be a causative factor in pulpal disease.

Seltzer et al. extracted 85 periodontally involved teeth and found that only 6 per cent of the teeth were pulpally *uninvolved*. Thirty-two of these teeth had no caries or restorations and, of these, 37 per cent exhibited atrophic changes, 37 per cent were inflamed, and 9 per cent were completely necrotic. This evidence strongly suggests that periodontal lesions produce a degenerative effect on the pulps. The studies of Langeland et al. showed that periodontal disease can cause pulpal inflammation, calcification, and resorption. Sinai and Soltanoff helped confirm the belief that periodontal effects on the pulp occur less frequently and at a later time interval than pulpal effects on the periodontium. Occlusal imbalance is a co-factor in many periodontal lesions and may inhibit healing of endodontic lesions. Casullo suggested that extreme occlusal trauma can result in irreversible pulpitis and, if long-standing, may even result in necrosis of the pulp. Periapical or periodontal inflammation may cause eruption of the tooth in its socket due to swelling in the adjacent tissue, which may, in turn, result in secondary occlusal trauma. In such instances, the periodontal ligament loses some of its protective defensive ability and breaks down with advancing disease.

Sharp summed it up nicely: "Pulpal disease may contribute to periodontal disease and periodontal disease may often cause pulpal inflammation." Seltzer explained that the effect of periodontal lesions on the pulp may be caused by interference with the nutritional supply, inducing atrophic and other degenerative changes and resulting in gradual death of the pulpal tissue. He also stated that inflamed or necrotic pulps, produced from periodontal lesions, can perpetuate the periodontal lesion. Deep scaling and especially surgical periodontal procedures expose large areas of cementum and may sever blood vessels, particularly in the furcation regions, resulting in a cessation of circulation to portions of the pulp. Feldman et al. state that it is not necessary to completely sever the pulpal vessels to cause irreversible pulpal damage. Ingle and Beveridge state that the prognosis in lesions with a primary periodontal etiology is not as favorable as if the primary lesion is of endodontic etiology. Prichard predicts a better prognosis if the infrabony defect contains three walls. Weine points out that periodontal and pulpal diseases have some common clinical symptoms (tenderness to percussion and swelling) and that either disease may mimic the other (clinically and radiographically). To arrive at the correct course of treatment, an accurate diagnosis of the etiologic factors is needed. Feldman et al. and Hiatt provide a comprehensive examination for the differential diagnosis and treatment of the endodontic and periodontic lesions. Harrington and Chacker also give a good basis for differential diagnosis of the endo-perio question.

A generalized summary of the appropriate treatment for combined lesions is as follows:

1. Primary endodontic lesions: The sinus tract (fistula) heals by canal obturation alone.

2. Primary periodontal lesions: An acceptable result may be gained by periodontal therapy alone. If root amputation is needed, canal obturation should precede periodontal therapy.

3. Endodontic-periodontic lesions (primary endodontic lesions with secondary periodontal complication): Canal obturation alone will often heal the communication between the canal system and the gingival sulcus. If the lesions are of long duration, combined therapy may be needed. Canal obturation should precede periodontal therapy.

4. Periodontic-endodontic lesions (primary periodontal pocket(s) with secondary pulpal involvement): Combined therapy of canal obturation and periodontal treatment is needed. The canal obturation should precede periodontal therapy because the canal system's reservoir of toxic irritants may prevent periodontal healing.

5. "True" combined lesions (concurrent primary periodontal complications and primary pulpal lesions): Treatment is the same as for the perio-endo lesions.

Simon et al. have shown that the endodontic lesion will heal if the cause of the condition is primarily endodontic and if the canal system is properly

Case 58 The patient presented with periapical furcation and extensive mesial root involvement of the first molar. An 8 mm mesial root periodontal pocket could be probed *(A)*. There was some divergence of the apices, but it is felt that intentionally ledging the canals with larger instruments would allow for gutta percha obturation. The canals, in this instance, were filled with calcium hydroxide to stimulate faster osseous healing. After 3 months of calcium hydroxide treatment, the mesial and furcation pockets could

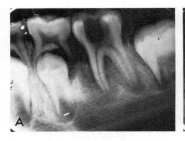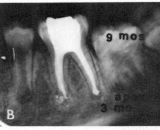

not be probed. The calcium hydroxide was removed, and the canals were obturated with gutta percha. Six months after the gutta percha fillings, the lamina dura could be observed in the furcation and along the mesial root. Some remnants of calcium hydroxide paste are noted at the apex of the mesial root *(B)*.

obturated. If a favorable prognosis for a combined lesion is to be achieved with canal obturation alone, the periodontal complication cannot be allowed to become chronic with persistence of destructive plaque, calculus, and flora, which are components of the true periodontal pocket. Preferably, these cases are treated first with calcium hydroxide to promote a faster remission of the pathosis affecting the periodontium (Cases 58 and 59). Since the calcium hydroxide promotes healing and osteogenic regeneration is faster in these large osseous defects, there is an earlier reattachment of the periodontal ligament (or formation of a clinically unprobeable junctional epithelium attachment) as a seal against the oral environment and the ingress of microorganisms.

Although the major emphasis here is to treat the endodontic-periodontic lesion before establishment of the chronic periodontal lesion, one should not hesitate to treat the periodontic-endodontic lesion for the same reasons as stated above (see Case 5 for an example of calcium hydroxide treatment of a well-established, combined lesion with inadequate canal obturation and extensive resorption of osseous and tooth structure). However, when the initial etiology of a combined lesion is endodontic and the tooth has undergone severe chronic periodontal destruction and/or traumatic occlusion, periodontal therapy is usually needed for a favorable result.

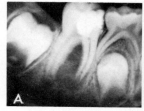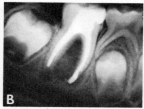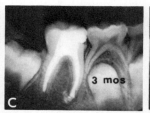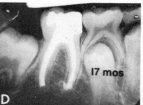

Case 59 The patient presented with periapical and extensive furcation involvement of the first molar. The furcation could be probed almost to the mesial apices. Incomplete root development with divergent apices was apparent on both roots *(A)*. The canal system was debrided and packed with calcium hydroxide paste, with some extrusion beyond the apex of the mesial root *(B)*. At the 3 month recall, furcation healing and reattachment were noted, since there was no communication into the furcation. Remnants of the extruded calcium hydroxide paste can be seen *(C)*. The paste was removed and apical barriers were detected. The canal system was obturated with gutta percha. Seventeen months after the gutta percha filling, complete healing was evidenced by re-establishment of the lamina dura. The overextruded calcium hydroxide paste had continued to resorb *(D)*.

Note that the divertent portions of the apices were obturated with gutta percha in both cases. It would have been difficult to confine the filling to the canal system if some apical barrier had not been formed.

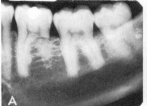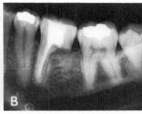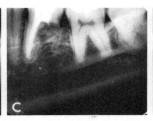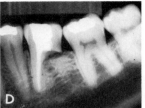

Case 60 The patient presented with an aggressive idiopathic resorption of the distal root of a vital mandibular molar; unfortunately, the resorption was just below the crestal bone height. This circumstance dictates a guarded prognosis, regardless of the type of resorption *(A)*. The canal system was obturated with calcium hydroxide *(B)*. Six months later the final paste was removed and replaced by a gutta percha filling *(C)*. Two and one half years later the radiograph suggested some continued resorption *(D)*. At this point no communication with the distal root could be detected by probing. The patient will be followed, and when a communication is established, the distal root will be amputated and the tooth contoured for patient oral hygiene maintenance. (Endodontic treatment performed by Dr. John F. Bucher, Gainesville, Florida.)

SECTION XI. IDIOPATHIC RESORPTION
(Case 60, p. 245)

Idiopathic external root resorption generally is seen as a blunting of the apices of tooth roots. It is thought that the resorptive process is of systemic origin, operating in the presence of vital pulp tissue. Fortunately its occurrence is infrequent, as apparently treatment to correct this condition is limited. In encountering what one considers idiopathic resorption, one must rule out factors that may be insidious, such as traumatic occlusion, history of trauma, bruxism, opening of the bite due to a fixed or removable appliance, orthodontic movement, deep periodontal curettage, or an involved pulp that elicits *false* pulp test results. In the last instance, there may be suppurative fluid in the canal system that conducts the electrical stimuli to the periodontium, registering a false positive response. Moreover, in multiple rooted teeth, the pulps of one or more canals may be irreversibly involved and elicit no response, whereas the pulps of another canal may be vital.

It is not certain that calcium hydroxide will prevent this resorption, but in light of the fact that there is no other predictable treatment, the author advocates calcium hydroxide treatment for the aggressive idiopathic resorptive lesions (Case 60). Because resorption optimally occurs in the environment of an acid pH and since calcium hydroxide establishes a basic pH, it is felt that the local cellular environment is neutralized or placed on the alkaline side. Also, as suggested by Tronstad et al., the calcium hydroxide may promote healing by stimulating the repair processes of the tissues and by making osteoclastic activity less likely.

SECTION XII. PERMANENT ROOT CANAL FILLING AND CEMENTS

Root Canal Filling

Many investigators advocate calcium hydroxide as a permanent root canal filling. If such a technique is employed, it is recommended that calcium hydroxide be mixed with a vehicle that would not allow easy resorption of the paste. The author's chief concern is that in nearly every clinical case that he has treated, he has found some resorption or dilution of the calcium hydroxide paste. In many instances he has found that the paste needed to be changed several times in the 1 or 2 year course of treatment. If dilution of the paste occurs in this short a time span, what will happen over the lifetime of a tooth that has supposedly been treated permanently with calcium hydroxide? Once a sufficient amount of the paste is resorbed, a portion of the canal becomes empty, thus fostering an exchange of tissue fluids and ingrowth of granulation tissue and microorganisms.

Tronstad believed that the calcium hydroxide left in the canal is converted to $CaCO_3$. Salinas reported that CO_2, liberated by lysis of organic tissue, reacts with $Ca(OH)_2$ to form $CaCO_3$ and water. Stanley described calcium hydroxide that has lost its effectiveness as "spent" calcium hydroxide. Seltzer and Bender also pointed out that calcium hydroxide can react with the atmospheric carbon dioxide to form ineffective calcium carbonate. If the paste is not changed, the calcium hydroxide may be converted, losing its effectiveness and allowing a reversal of the healing process.

Some investigators may change the paste until a calcified barrier is created and then permanently obturate the canal with a calcium hydroxide paste. It is believed that the prognosis is *greatly* enhanced by using this procedure; however, the author is still concerned about what may occur several years subsequently. Histologic studies show that the formed calcified barrier is porous. Because of this, there may be a gradual dilution of the paste, possibly resulting in a resorption of the calcified barrier and thus allowing a more significant tissue fluid exchange. In using the apexification technique the author has, on a few occasions, observed formation of a calcified barrier after a period of approximately 1 year and at the last change has found the canal to be filled with dry paste to the barrier. In order to ensure sufficient thickness of the barrier to withstand gutta percha condensation forces, the author decided to leave the paste for another 3 months. However, the patients were not available for their final appointment until 6 months to 1 year later. Upon entering the canals at this later date, the author found a wet, mushy paste in place of the dry paste previously existing. Therefore, because of these clinical impressions, the author does not recommend the routine use of calcium hydroxide as a permanent root canal filling material. There may be immediate healing, which is verified radiographically for a few months or years, but what will happen subsequently is questionable.

Root Canal Sealers

Investigators, searching for a more biocompatible cement that would at the same time stimulate hard tissue closure of any communication between the canal system and the periodontium, advocate mixing calcium hydroxide with their root canal sealers to cement gutta percha fillings. However, there is concern that in instances in which the natural apical constriction has been resorbed or violated or a large secondary canal exists, dissolution of the calcium hydroxide may occur at a faster rate than that of the sealer. This process may open the interface between the gutta percha and the canal wall, thus allowing tissue fluid and toxin exchange to occur before the formation of the hard tissue repair and perhaps even preventing the desired healing process. A second concern would be to determine what effect the eugenol component of the zinc oxide sealer would have on the calcium hydroxide. It is possible that the beneficial effect of the calcium hydroxide would be lost.

Calciobiotic,* a new commercial root canal sealer containing calcium hydroxide, contributes properties (according to manufacturer's specifications) that render the root canal sealer highly workable and biocompatible. It has less eugenol content, but the sealer does contain eucalyptol. The concerns are, first, that the mixture of the ingredients may neutralize the calcium hydroxide's beneficial effects and, second, that the possible dissolution of the calcium hydroxide may have a detrimental effect over a longer span of time than the comparatively short 20 day to 6 month recalls utilized in the manufacturer's radiographic study. Definitely, more research needs to be performed with the sealer.

Kennedy et al. and later Moriya et al. used calcium hydroxide in association with other root canal filling materials. Holland and de Souza point out that zinc oxide–eugenol cements initially cause bone resorption accompanied by a persistent localized chronic inflammation of the periodontal ligament, usually without biologic sealing. However, when calcium hydroxide is used alone, there are fewer inflammatory cells, which disappear after 15 days. The investigators employed a cement of $Ca(OH)_2$ (5 grams), zinc oxide (2 grams) and glycol propylene (5 ml). In an earlier study, Holland and Nery showed that root canal filling with zinc oxide–eugenol did not induce healing but that the addition of $Ca(OH)_2$ to the filling did show healing and biologic sealing with hard tissue apposition.

Calcium phenolate (Dycal) has the potential to be a very effective cementing agent because, when set, it forms a rigid mass that is not nearly as rapidly resorbed as pure calcium hydroxide. Stanley and Lundy demonstrated that the final product of Dycal remains hard for a time and liberates calcium hydroxide solutions of varying concentrations without its rigidity being affected. Weiss et al. and Tronstad also showed the holding qualities of calcium hydroxide. Several investigators have reported that Dycal is not as irritating as pure calcium hydroxide. Holland et al. demonstrated the beneficial effects that calcium hydroxide has on any pulp remnants after vital pulp extirpation. Goldberg and Gurfinkel, in a multiple phase study, demonstrated that Dycal is an effective root canal sealer when used with gutta percha in the lateral condensation technique. By means of a microscopic study, they showed that the Dycal completely occupied any irregularities and, in addition, established a firm adherence at the interface between gutta percha and the dentinal wall. They found that Dycal cement diminishes the prevalence of postoperative pain and that overfilling with Dycal has no influence on the immediate postoperative symptoms. This correlates with the results that Holland and de Souza found histologically. Goldberg and Gurfinkel also demonstrated that the alkalinity of Dycal persists after mixing for up to 8 months. They concluded that the persistence of an alkaline pH has a definite antimicrobial effect and stimulates the formation of apical and periapical hard tissue.

---

*Witech Laboratory, P.O. Box 3058, Erie, Pa., 16508.

A new capping agent that may also have potential as a root canal sealer is *Life*.* Life contains a resin that would aid against its dissolution as a sealer. The only concern is that the catalyst would be detrimental to tissues, as was that of Hydrex. However, a clinical and histologic study by Cox et al. showed that Life not only stimulates bridging of reparative dentin over noninflamed pulp exposures but also over *inflamed* pulp exposures. In their monkey study, they found that Dycal was not able to induce bridging over *inflamed* pulp exposures. The author is not sure that calcium hydroxide sealers improve the prognosis of endodontic treatment, but feels that more research is needed to investigate that viable possibility.

Periapical Plugging with Calcium Hydroxide

Kuttler, Tronstad, and Baume et al. showed that after pulpectomy dentin chips could be plugged at the apex to facilitate root canal obturation and to achieve a better biologic acceptance of the filling material. The dentin chips were well tolerated by the tissues. However, Holland et al. showed that if the dentinal chips were infected, they produced very unfavorable results. Dimashkieh advocated that in cases of adult teeth with apical resorption or iatrogenic overinstrumentation, oxidized cellulose sponge (which is resorbable) should be condensed into the apical portion of the canal and then amalgam should be condensed into it in order to prevent extrusion of amalgam beyond the apex of the filling. The concern here would be that if the cellulose were not adapted properly, amalgam could be pushed into the periapical tissues.

An alternative techique would be to pack the periapical osseous defect or the apical pulp stump (in instances of vital pulpal tissue) with a very firm, dry calcium hydroxide paste. Afterward, without irrigation, lightly backfile the canal walls and with positive aspiration remove the loose calcium hydroxide from the canal. Prefitted endodontic pluggers, marked to the desired filling length, would be utilized to firmly pack the apical barrier of calcium hydroxide before and after removing the paste from the canal walls. Emphasis is placed upon a dense condensation of the paste at the apical foramen. This provides an apical stop for gutta percha obturation, utilizing the technique of the operator's choice. The calcium hydroxide paste will be resorbed with time.

The author recommends this technique only in instances in which the patient would not be available for apexification therapy. The possible shortcoming of this technique is similar to that of utilization of calcium hydroxide cements. In those cases in which the canal system is divergent or resorption has occurred in the canal, all of the paste may not be effectively removed prior to gutta percha obturation. When later resorption of the paste occurs, the canal system would then be open and would be vulnerable to tissue fluid exchange.

Acknowledgements

This chapter is dedicated to Dr. John F. Bucher and Dr. Fred L. Cox, whose friendship, encouragement, and invaluable support and advice have inspired the

---

*Kerr/Sybron Pulpcapping Agent.

author to pursue the academic field. The author is indebted to and particularly appreciative of his good friend Dr. Gerald M. Cathey for his advice in documenting the scientific aspects of this investigation. A very special thanks to Dr. Harold R. Stanley for his review of the biologic principles of this chapter and Dr. John F. Bucher for his extensive help in editorial assistance. The author wishes to thank and acknowledge the invaluable assistances of Dr. Sonia I. Pena for drawing the most beautiful and detailed illustrations and Mrs. Jenny E. Wallace and Mrs. Marilyn V. Green for their numerous proof typings of this chapter. The author would also like to acknowledge Dr. Jens Ove Andreasen for all his innovative research in the area of traumatic injuries, which provided the basis for a rational approach to the treatment of such injuries.

BIBLIOGRAPHY

American Association of Endodontists: An annotated glossary of terms used in endodontics, 3rd Ed. J.O.E., Special Issue, March 1981.

American Association of Periodontology: J. Periodontol. 48:(Suppl.)15, 1977.

Anderson, A. W., Sharav, Y., and Massler, M.: Periodontal reattachment after tooth replantation. Periodontics 6:161–167, August 1968.

Anderson, A. W., Sharav, Y., and Massler, M.: Reparative dentine formation and pulp morphology. Oral Surg. 26:837–847, 1968.

Anderson, D. J., and Ronning, G. A.: Dye diffusion in human dentine. Arch. Oral. Biol. 7:505–512, 1962.

Andreasen, J. O.: Luxation of permanent teeth due to trauma. A clinical and radiographic follow-up study of 189 injured teeth. Scand. J. Dent. Res. 78(3):273–289, 1970.

Andreasen, J. O.: Etiology and pathogenesis of traumatic dental injuries. A clinical study of 1,298 cases. Scand. J. Dent. Res. 78(3):329–342, 1970.

Andreasen, J. O.: Treatment of fractured and avulsed teeth. J. Dent. Child 38(1):29–48, 1971.

Andreasen, J. O.: Effect of pulpal necrosis upon periodontal healing after surgical injury in rats. Int. J. Oral Surg. 2:62–68, 1973.

Andreasen, J. O.: Traumatic Injuries of the Teeth, 2nd Ed. St. Louis, C. V. Mosby Co., 1974.

Andreasen, J. O.: The effect of splinting upon periodontal healing after replantation of permanent incisors in monkeys. Acta Odont. Scand. 33(6):313–323, 1975.

Andreasen, J. O.: Periodontal healing after replantation of traumatically avulsed human teeth. Acta Odont. Scand. 33(6):325–335, 1975.

Andreasen, J. O.: Presentation, American Association of Endodontists, 33rd Annual Session, Hollywood, Fla., April 28, 1976.

Andreasen, J. O.: A time-related study of periodontal healing and root resorption activity after replantation of mature permanent incisors in monkeys. Swed. Dent. J. 4:101–110, 1980.

Andreasen, J. O.: Analysis of topography of surface and inflammatory root resorption after replanatation of mature permanent incisors in monkeys. Swed. Dent. J. 4(4):135–144, 1980.

Andreasen, J. O.: Analysis of pathogenesis and topography of replacement root resorption (ankylosis) after replantation of mature permanent incisors in monkeys. Swed. Dent. J. 4(6):231–240, 1980.

Andreasen, J. O.: Delayed replantation after submucosal storage in order to prevent root resorption after replantation. Int. J. Oral Surg. 9:394–403, 1980.

Andreasen, J. O.: The effect of pulp extirpation or root canal treatment on periodontal healing after replantation of permanent incisors in monkeys. J.O.E. 7(6):245–252, 1981.

Andreasen, J. O.: Relationship between surface and inflammatory resorption and changes in the pulp after replantation of permanent incisors in monkeys. J.O.E. 7(7):294–301, 1981.

Andreasen, J. O.: Interrelation between alveolar bone and periodontal ligament repair after replantation of mature permanent incisors in monkeys. J. Perio. Res. 16(2):228–235, 1981.

Andreasen, J. O.: The effect of excessive occlusal trauma upon periodontal healing after replantation of mature permanent incisors in monkeys. Swed. Dent. J. 5(3):115–122, 1981.

Andreasen, J. O.: Effect of extra-alveolar period and storage media upon periodontal and pulpal healing after replantation of mature permanent incisors in monkeys. Int. J. Oral Surg. 10(1):43–53, 1981.

Andreasen, J. O.: Periodontal healing after replantation and autotransplantation of incisors in monkeys. Int. J. Oral Surg. 10(1):54–61, 1981.

Andreasen, J. Ö.: Relationship between cell damage in the periodontal ligament and subsequent development of root resorption. A time-related study in monkeys. Acta Odont. Scand. 39(1):15–25, 1981.

Andreasen, J. O., and Hjörting-Hansen, E.: Replantation of teeth. I. Radiographic and clinical study of 110 human teeth replanted after accidental loss. Acta Odont. Scand. 24(3):263–286, 1966.

Andreasen, J. O., and Hjörting-Hansen, E.: Replantation of teeth. II. Histological study of 22 replanted anterior teeth in humans. Acta Odont. Scand. 24(3):287–306, 1966.

Andreasen, J. O., and Hjörting-Hansen, E.: Intraalveolar root fractures: radiographic and histologic study of 50 cases. J. Oral Surg. 25:414–426, September 1967.

Andreasen, J. O., and Kristerson, L.: The effect of extra-alveolar root filling with calcium hydroxide on periodontal healing after replantation of permanent incisors in monkeys. J.O.E. 8(7):349–354, 1981.

Andreasen, J. O., and Kristerson, L.: Repair process in the cervical region of replanted and transplanted teeth in monkeys. Int. J. Oral Surg. 10:128–136, 1981.

Andreasen, J. O., and Kristerson, L.: The effect of limited drying or removal of the periodontal ligament upon periodontal healing after replantation of mature permanent incisors in monkeys. Acta Odont. Scand. 39(1):1–13, 1981.

Andreasen, J. O., Reinholdt, J., Riis, I., et al.: Periodontal and pulpal healing of monkey incisors preserved in tissue culture before replantation. Int. J. Oral Surg. 7:104–112, 1978.

Arens, D. E.: Apexification, pulp capping and pulpotomy. *In* Clark, J. W. (ed.): Clinical Dentistry. Hagerstown, Md., Harper & Row, 1977.

Atrizadeh, F., Kennedy, J., and Zander, H.: Ankylosis of teeth following thermal injury. J. Periodont. 6:159–167, 1971.

Auslander, W. P., and Weinberg, G.: Anatomic repair of internal perforations with indium foil and silver amalgam: Outline of a method. N.Y. J. Dent. 39:454, December 1969.

Austin, L. T.: A review of forty cases of retained fractured roots of anterior teeth. J.A.D.A. 17:1930–1932, 1930.

Avny, W. Y., Heiman, G. R., Madonia, J. V., et al.: Autoradiographic studies of the intracanal diffusion of aqueous and camphorated parachlorophenol in endodontics. Oral Surg. 36:80–89, 1973.

Barbakow, F. H., Austin, J. C., and Cleaton-Jones, P. E.: Experimental replantation of root-canal-filled and untreated teeth in the vervet monkey. J.O.E. 3(3):89–93, 1977.

Barbakow, F. H., Austin, J. C., and Cleaton-Jones, P. E.: Histologic response of replanted teeth pretreated with acidulated sodium fluoride. Oral Surg. 45:621–628, 1978.

Barbakow, F. H., Cleaton-Jones, P. E., Austin, J. C., et al.: Changes in tooth mobility after experimental replantation. J.O.E. 4(9):265–272, 1978.

Barbakow, F. H., Cleaton-Jones, P. E., Austin, J. C., et al.: Effect of thyrocalcitonin, acidulated sodium fluoride, and neutral sodium fluoride on the mobility of experimentally replanted teeth. J.O.E. 6(11):823–828, 1980.

Barbakow, F. H., Cleaton-Jones, P. E., Austin, J. C., et al.: Healing of replanted teeth following topical treatment with fluoride solutions and systemic administration of thyrocalcitonin: a histometric analysis. J.O.E. 7(7):302–308, 1981.

Barker, B. C. W., and Mayne, J. R.: Some unusual cases of apexification subsequent to trauma. Oral Surg. 39:144–150, 1975.

Barry, G. N.: Replanted teeth still functioning after 42 years. Report of a case. J.A.D.A. 92:412, February 1976.

Baume, L. J., Holz, J., and Risk, L. B.: Radicular pulpotomy for category III pulps. Part II. Instrumentation and technique. J. Prost. Dent. 25:525–531, 1971.

Baume, L. J., Holz, J., and Risk, L. B.: Radicular pulpotomy for category III Pulps. Part III. Histologic evaluation. J. Prost. Dent. 25:649–657, 1971.

Bell, T.: The Anatomy, Physiology and Diseases of Teeth. Philadelphia, Carey and Lee Publishing, 1830.

Bender, I. B., and Seltzer, S.: The effect of diseases of the periodontium on the human pulp. Conference on Biology of the Human Pulp, Memphis, September 18, 1970.

Bennett, D. T.: Traumatized anterior teeth. Br. Dent. J. 116:7, 1964.

Bergenholz, G.: Microorganisms from necrotic pulp of traumatized teeth. Odont. Revy 25:347–358, 1974.

Berning, H. P., and Lepp, K. L.: Progressive internal resorption of teeth. Die Quintessenz Zahnarztlichen Lit. 9:49, April 1958.

Bhaskar, S. N.: Nonsurgical resolution of radicular cysts. Oral Surg. 34:458, 1972.

Bhaskar, S. N., and Rappaport, H. M.: Histologic evaluation of endodontic procedures in dogs. Oral Surg. 31:526–535, 1971.

Binnie, W. H., and Mitchell, D. F.: Induced calcification in the subdermal tissues of the rat. J. Dent. Res. 52:1087–1091, September–October, 1973.

Bjorvatn, K, and Massler, M.: Effect of fluorides and root resorption in replanted rat molars. Acta Odont. Scand. 29(1):17–29, 1971.

Blaha, L.: Dentin permeability of the root canals. Rev. Fac. Odontol. Tucuman 11:25–36, 1977.

Blomlöf, L.: Storage of human, periodontal ligament cells in a combination of different media. J. Dent. Res. 60:1904–1906, November 1981.

Blomlöf, L., Otteskog, P., and Hammarström, L.: Effect of storage in media with different ion strengths and osmolalities on human periodontal ligament cells. Scand. J. Dent. Res. 89:180–187, 1981.

Bödecker, C. F., and Lefkowitz, W.: Replantation of teeth. Dent. Items Interest 57:675–692, August 1935.

Burch, J. G., and Hulen, S.: A study of the presence of accessory foramina and the topography of molar furcations. Oral Surg. 38:451, 1974.

Burke, J. H.: Reversal of external root resorption. J.O.E. 2(3):87–88, 1976.

Burke, J. H., and Cernak, R. A.: Internal resorption following foil insertion. Oral Surg. 32:938, 1971.

Burkley, M. A., and Crabb, H. S. M.: Replantation of teeth. Br. Dent. J. 108:190, 1965.

Caffesse, R. G., Nasjleti, C. E., and Castelli, W. A.: Long term results after intentional tooth reimplantation in monkeys. Oral Surg. 44:666–678, 1977.

Camp, J. H., Williams, J. J., and Webber, R. T.: Treatment of traumatized teeth. American Dental Association, 121st Annual Session, New Orleans, October 14, 1980.

Campbell, A. D., Gear, R. D., Turner, D. W., et al.: Cell mediated response to endodontic cements: research report. J.O.E. 4(5):147–150, 1978.

Carranza, F. A., Itoiz, M. E., Cabrini, R. L., et al.: A study of periodontal vascularization in different laboratory animals. J. Perio. Res. 1:120, 1966.

Casullo, D. P.: The integration of endodontics, periodontics, and restorative dentistry in general practice. Cont. Ed. Gen. Dent. 1:140–144, March 1980.

Cathey, G. M.: ADA Annual Scientific Session, Houston, 1970.

Chacker, F. M.: The endodontic-periodontic continuum. Dent. Clinic North Am. 18(2):393–414, 1974.

Chivian, N.: Intentional replantation. J. N.J. Dent. Soc. 38(6):247, 1967.

Clark, K. B., and Hayes, P. A.: A study of the comparative effects of >>rigid>>and>> semirigid>>fixation on the healing of fractures of the mandible in dogs. J. Bone Joint Surg. 45A:731–741, 1963.

Coccia, C. T.: A clinical investigation of root resorption rates in reimplanted young permanent incisors — a five year study. J.O.E. 6(1):413–420, 1980.

Cohen, S., and Burns, R. C.: Pathways of the Pulp, 2nd Ed, St. Louis, C. V. Mosby Co., 1980.

Cohen-Scali, J. A.: Ocalexic penetration in secondary root canals and dentinal tubules. Rev. Odontost. (Paris) 6(2):95–101, 1977.

Coolidge, E. D.: The reaction of cementum in the presence of injury and infection. J.A.D.A. 18:499, March 1931.

Cox, C. F., Heys, D. R., Heys, R. J., et al: A clinical and histological profile of life: A new pulp capping agent. Midwestern Dental Meeting (printed art), Chicago, February 15, 1980.

Cunningham, G. J., and Penick, E. C.: Use of a roentgenographic contrast medium in the differential diagnosis of periapical lesions. Oral Surg. 26:96–102, 1966.

Cutright, D. E., and Bhaskar, S. N.: A new method of demonstrating microvasculature. Oral Surg. 24:422, 1967.

Cvek, M.: Treatment of non-vital permanent incisors with calcium hydroxide. II. Effect on external root resorption in luxated teeth compared with effect of root filling with gutta percha. Odont. Revy 24(4):343–354, 1973.

Cvek, M.: Clinical procedures promoting apical closure and arrest of external root resorption in non-vital permanent incisors. *In* Grossman, L. I. (ed.): Transactions of the 5th International Conference on Endodontics. Philadelphia University of Pennsylvania Press, 1973.

Cvek, M., Granath, L. E., and Hellender, L.: Treatment of non-vital permanent incisors with calcium hydroxide III. Odont. Revy 25:43–56, 1974.

Dargent, P.: A study of root resorption. Acta Odont. 117:47–61, March 1977.

Davis, M. S., Joseph, S. W., and Bucher, J. F.: Periapical and intracanal healing following incomplete root canal fillings in dogs. Oral Surg. 31:662–675, 1971.

Deeb, E., Prietto, P. P., and McKenna, R. C.: Replantation of luxated teeth in humans. J. South. Cal. Dent. Ass. 28:194–205, April 1965.

Degering, C. I.: Radiography of dental fractures. Oral Surg. 30:213–219, 1970.

Diem, C. R., Bowers, G. M., Ferrigno, P. D., et al.: Regeneration of the attachment apparatus on pulpless teeth denuded of cementum in the rhesus monkey. J. Periodontol. 45(1):18–22, 1974.

Dimashkieh, M. R.: The problem of the open apex. A new approach. J. Br. Endo. Soc. 10(1): 9–16, 1977.

Dylewski, J. J.: Apical closure of non-vital teeth. Oral Surg. 32:82–89, 1971.

Emmersten, E., and Andreasen, J. O.: Replantation of extracted molars: A radiographic histologic study. Acta Odont. Scan. 24:327, November 1966.

Epstein, L. I.: Traumatic injuries to anterior teeth in children. Oral Surg. 15:334–344, 1962.

Erausquin, J., and Devoto, F.: Alveolodental ankylosis induced by root canal treatment in rat molars. Oral Surg. 30:105–110, 1970.

Erausquin, J., and Muruzabal, M.: Tissue reaction to root canal cements in the rat molar. Oral Surg. 26:360–373, 1968.

Erausquin, J., and Muruzabal, M.: Tissue reaction to root canal fillings with absorbable pastes. Oral Surg. 28:567–578, 1969.

Feldman, G., Solomon, C., and Notaro, P. J.: Endodontic management of traumatized teeth. Oral Surg. 21:100–112, 1966.

Fish, E. W.: Surgical Pathology of the Mouth. London, Sir Isaac Pitman and Sons, 1952.

Fisher, F. J.: The effect of a calcium hydroxide/water paste on micro-organisms in carious dentine. Br. Dent. J. 133:19–21, 1972.

Flanagan, V. D., and Myers, H. I.: Delayed reimplantation of second molars in the Syrian hamster. Oral Surg. 11:1179–1188, 1958.

Flath, J.: Klinische Beobachtungen bei der echten Transplantation von retinierten Zahnen. Otsch. Stomat. 13:561–574, 1963.

Forsberg, A., and Hugglund, G.: Differential diagnosis of radicular cyst and granuloma. Dent. Radiogr. Photogr. 33:84–88, 1960.

Frank, A. L.: Resorption, perforations and fractures. Dent. Clin. North Am. 18(2):465–487, 1974.

Frank, A. L.: External-internal progressive resorption and its nonsurgical correction. J.O.E. 7(10):473–476, 1981.

Frank, A. L., and Weine, F. S.: Nonsurgical therapy for the perforative defect of internal resorption. J.A.D.A. 87:863–868, October 1973.

Frost, H. M.: Tetracycline-based histological analysis of bone remodelling. Calc. Tissue Res. 3:211–237, 1969.

Fudenberg, H. H., Stites, D. P., Caldwell, J. L., et al.: Basic and Clinical Immunology. Los Altos, Cal., Lange Medical Publishers, 1976.

Gartner, A. H., Mack, T., Somerlott, R. G., et al.: Differential diagnosis of internal and external root resorption. J.O.E. 2(11):329–334, 1976.

Goldberg, F., and Gurfinkel, J.: Analysis of the use of dycal with gutta percha points as an endodontic filling technique. Oral Surg. 47:78–82, 1979.

Grant, D., and Bernick, S.: Ankylosis and the postulated osteodepressive effect of the periodontal ligament. Abstract No. 251 of IADR Program, 1972.

Groper, J. N., and Bernick, S.: Histological study of the periodontium following replantation of teeth in the dog. J. Dent. Child. 37:24–35, 1970.

Grossman, L. I.: Intentional replantation of teeth. J.A.D.A. 72:1111–1118, 1966.

Grossman, L. I.: Endodontic Practice, 9th Ed. Philadelphia, Lea and Febiger, 1978.

Grossman, L. I., and Ship, I.: Survival rate of replanted teeth. Oral Surg. 29:899–906, 1970.

Guerini, V.: History of Dentistry. Philadelphia, Lea and Febiger, 1909.

Gurney, B. F.: Modern methods in bacteriologic control. Dent. Clin. North Am. 7:321–339, 1963.

Hammer, H.: Der histologische Vorgang bei der Zahn-replantation. Dtsch. Zahn. Mund. Kieferheilkd. 1:115–136, 1934.

Hammer, H.: Der histologische Vorgang bei der Zahn-replantation nach Vernichtung der Wurzelhaut. Dtsch. Zahn. Mund. Kieferheilkd. 4:179–187, 1937.

Hammer, H.: Replantation and implantation of teeth. Int. Dent. J. 5:439–475, 1955.

Hamner, J. E., Reed, O. M., and Stanley, H. R.: Reimplantation of teeth in the baboon. J.A.D.A. 81:662–670, 1970.

Hardy, L. B., O'Neal, R. B., and del Rio, C. E.: Effect of polylactic acid on replanted teeth in dogs. Oral Surg. 51:86–92, 1981.

Hargeaves, J. A., and Craig, J. W.: The Management of Traumatized Anterior Teeth of Children. London, E & S Livingston, 1970.

Harrington, G. W.: The period-endo question: differential diagnosis. Dent. Clin. North Am. 23(4):673–690, 1979.

Harrington, G. W., and Natkin, E.: External resorption associated with bleaching of pulpless teeth. J.O.E. 5(11):345–348, 1979.

Harris, C. A.: A Dictionary of Dental Science, Bibliography and Medical Terminology. Philadelphia, Lindsay and Blakiston, 1849.

Harris, W. E.: A simplified method of treatment for endodontic perforations. J.O.E. 2(5):126–134, 1976.

Hasselgren, G., Larsson, A., and Rundquist, L.: Pulpal status after autogenous transplantation of fully developed maxillary canines. Oral Surg. 44:106–112, 1977.

Healy, H. J.: Endodontics: Selection of case treatment procedures. J.A.D.A. 53:434, 1956.

Heithersay, G. S.: Periapical repair following conservative endodontic therapy. Aust. Dent. J. 15:511–518, 1970.

Heithersay, G. S.: Combined endodontic treatment of transverse root fractures in the region of the alveolar crest. Oral Surg. 36:404, 1973.

Heithersay, G. S.: Replantation of avulsed teeth. A review. Aust. Dent. J. 20:63–72, 1975.

Heithersay, G. S.: Calcium hydroxide in the treatment of pulpless teeth with associated pathology. J. Br. Endo. Soc. 8(2):74–93, 1975.

Heithersay, G. S.: Clinical and histological observations of the use of calcium hydroxide in endodontic therapy. Thirty-fourth Annual Meeting of the American Association of Endodontists, April 16, 1977.

Henry, J. L., and Weinmann, J. P.: The pattern of resorption and repair of human cementum. J.A.D.A. 42:270–290, 1951.

Herbert, W. E.: Three successful cases of replacement of teeth immediately following dislocation. Br. Dent. J. 94:182–183, 1953.

Holland, R., and de Souza, V.: Clinical and biological considerations of endodontic treatment. III. Filling of the root canals. Rev. Assoc. Paul Cir. Dent. 31(5):324–330, 1977.

Holland, R., and Nery, R. S.: Periapical tissue reactions of deciduous teeth to some root canal filling materials. Rev. Fac. Odontol. Aracatuba. 5(½):163–177, 1976.

Holland, R., de Mello, W., Nery, M. J., et al.: Reaction of human periapical tissue to pulp extirpation and immediate root canal filling with calcium hydroxide. J.O.E. 3(2):63–67, 1977.

Holland, R., de Souza, V., Nery, M. J., et al.: Tissue reactions following apical plugging of the root canal with infected dentin chips. Oral Surg. 49:366–369, 1980.

Hovinga, J.: Replantatie en transplantatie van tanden. Amsterdam, Oosterbaan & Le Cointre N.V.–Goes, 1968.

Hovinga, J.: Autotransplantation of maxillary canines: a long-term evaluation. J. Oral Surg. 27:701–708, 1969.

Hoyer: Pathological tooth resorption and its clinical importance. Stomatol. D.D.R. 27(1):46–49, 1977.

Hudson, J. R.: Studies on the effect of fluoride on bone resorption. J. Dent. Res. 40:724–725, 1961.

Hurst, R. V.: Regeneration of periodontal and transseptal fibres after autografts in Rhesus monkeys. A qualitative approach. J. Dent. Res. 51:1183–1192, 1972.

Ingber, J. S., Rose, L. F., and Coslet, J. G.: The biologic width — a concept in periodontics and restorative dentistry. Alpha Omegan 70(3):62–65, 1977.

Ingle, J. I., and Beveridge, E. E.: Endodontics, 2nd Ed., Philadelphia, Lea and Febiger, 1976.

Jonck, L. M.: An investigation into certain aspects of transplantation and reimplantation of teeth in men. Br. J. Oral. Surg. 4:137–146, November 1966.

Jones, P. A., Taintor, J. F., and Adams, A. B.: Comparative dental material cytotoxity measured by depression of rat incisor pulp respiration. J.O.E. 5(2):48–55, 1979.

Kaqueler, J. C., and Massler, M.: Healing following tooth replantation. J. Dent. Child. 36:303–314, 1969.

Kawahara, H. A., Yamagami, A., and Nakamura, M.: Biologic testing of dental materials by means of tissue culture. Int. Dent. J. 18(2):443–467, 1968.

Kemp, W. B., Grossman, L. I., and Philips, J.: Evaluation of 71 replanted teeth. J.O.E. 3(1):30–35, 1977.

Kennedy, G. D. C., McLundie, A. C., and Day, R. M.: Calcium hydroxide — Its role in a simplified endodontic technique. Dent. Oral. Top. Mag. 84:51–57, 1967.

Knight, M. K., Gans, B. J., and Calandra, J. C.: Effect of root canal therapy on replanted teeth of dogs. Oral Surg. 18:227–242, 1964.

Krakow, A. A.: Implants, replants, and transplants related to endodontics. In Clark, J. W. (ed.): Clinical Dentistry. Hagerstown, Md., Harper & Row, 1977.

Kronfeld, R.: Histopathology of the Teeth and Their Surrounding Structures. Philadelphia, Lea and Febiger, 1933.

Kronfeld, R.: The biology of cementum. J.A.D.A. 25:1451, September 1938.

Kuttler, Y.: A precision and biologic root canal filling technic. J.A.D.A. 56:38–50, 1958.

Langeland, K., Rodriques, H., and Dowden, W.: Periodontal disease, bacteria and pulpal histopathology. Oral Surg. 37:257–270, 1974.

Lantz, B., and Person, P. A.: Periodontal tissue reactions after root perforation in dog teeth. A histologic study. Odont. Tisk. 75:209–220, 1967.

Laws, A. J.: Calcium hydroxide as a possible root canal filling material. N.Z. Dent. T. 58:199, October 1962.

Lenstrup, K., and Skieller, V.: Replantation of accidentally avulsed teeth. Tandlaegebladet 61:570, 1957.

Lenstrup, K., and Skieller, V.: A follow-up study of teeth replanted after accidental loss. Acta Odont. Scand. 17:503–509, 1959.

Lepp, F. H.: Progressive intradental resorption. Oral Surg. 27:184, 1968.

Likins, R. C., Pakis, G., and McClure, F. J.: Effect of fluoride and tetracycline on alveolar bone resorption in the rat. J. Dent. Res. 42:1532, 1963.

Lindén, L. A.: Microscopic observations of fluid flow through cementum and dentin. In vitro study on human teeth. Odontol. Revy 19:367–381, 1968.

Lindhal, B., and Martensson, K.: Replantation of a tooth. Odontol. Revy 11:325, 1960.

Line, S. E., Polson, A. M., and Zander, H. A.: Relationship between periodontal injury, selective cell repopulation and ankylosis. J. Periodontol. 45:725–730, 1974.

Littman, S. H.: Evaluation of root canal debridement by use of a radiopaque medium. J.O.E. 3(4):135–138, 1977.

Löe, H., and Waerhaug, J.: Experimental replantation of teeth in dogs and monkeys. Arch. Oral. Biol. 3(4):176–184, 1961.

Lowman, J. V., Burke, R. S., and Pelleu, G. B.: Patent accessory canals: incidence in molar furcation region. Oral Surg. 36:580, 1973.

Makkes, D. C., Thoden van Velzen, S. K., and van den Hooff, A.: The response of the living organism to dead and fixed dead enclosed homologous tissue. Oral Surg. 46:296–306, 1978.

Makkes, D. C., Thoden van Velzen, S. K., and Wesselink, P. R.: The response of the living organism to dead and fixed dead tissue. J.O.E. 4:17–21, 1978.

Martensson, G.: Dental injuries following radical surgery on the maxillary sinus, with special reference to changes in sensitivity after Caldwell-Luc operations. Acta Otolaryng. 84(Suppl.):1–74, 1950.

Massler, M.: Therapy conducive to healing of the human pulp. Oral Surg. 34:122–130, 1972.

Massler, M.: Tooth replantation. Dent. Clin. North Am. 18(2):445–452, 1974.

Massler, M., and Malone, A. J.: Root resorption in human permanent teeth. A roentgenographic study. Am. J. Ortho. 40:619, August 1954.

Massler, M., and Perreault, J. G.: Root resorption in the permanent teeth of young adults. J. Dent. Child. 21:158, 1954.

Matsumiya, S., and Kitamura, M.: Histo-pathological and histo-bacteriological studies of the relation between the condition of sterilization of the interior of the root canal and the healing process of periapical tissue in experimentally infected root canal treatment. Bull. Tokyo Dent. Coll. 1:1–19, October 1960.

Matsumiya, S., Konde, S., Takada, Y., et al.: Histopathological study of healing process after infected root canal treatment. I Congresse della Societa Italiana di Odontomatologia o Chirurgia Maxillo-Facciale.

Maynard, J. G., and Wilson, R. D. K.: Physiologic dimension of the periodontum significant to the restorative dentist. J. Periodontol. 50(4):170–174, 1979.

McDonald, R. E., Zawawi, H. A. M., and Mitchell, D. F.: Rat connective tissue reaction to implants of pulp capping materials. J. Dent. Res. 38:738, 1959.

McWalter, G. M., El Kafrawy, A. H., and Mitchell, D. F.: Pulp capping in monkeys with a calcium hydroxide compound, an antibiotic, and a polycarboxylate cement. Oral Surg. 36:90–100, 1973.

Melcher, A. H.: Repair of wounds in the periodontium of the rat. Influence of periodontal ligament on osteogenesis. Arch. Oral Biol. 15:1183–1204, 1970.

Melcher, A. H.: On the repair potential of periodontal tissues. J. Periodontol. 47:256–260, 1976.

Messing, J.: Reimplantation of teeth. Dent. Pract. Dent. Rec. 18(7):241–248, 1968.

Meyer-Bardowicks, J.: Tooth re-implantation with maintenance of pulp vitality. Quint. Int. 8:27–30, August 1979.

Michanowicz, A. E., Michanowicz, J. P., and Abou-Rass, M.: Cementogenic repair of root fractures. J.A.D.A. 82:569, March 1971.

Miller, H. M.: Replanting human teeth. Dent Surv. 29:1439–1442, 1953.

Mitchell, D. F., and Amos, E. R.: Reaction of connective tissues of rats to implanted dental materials. 35th General Meeting, I.A.D.R., Atlantic City, No. 153 Preprinted Abstract, March 1957.

Mitchell, D. F., and Shankwalker, G. B.: Osteogenic potential of calcium hydroxide and other materials in soft tissue and bone wounds. J. Dent. Res. 37(6):1157–1163, 1958.

Monsour, F. N. T.: The reimplantation of displaced teeth. Aust. Dent. J. 15(5):361–364, 1970.

Monsour, F. N. T.: Pulpal changes following the reimplantation of teeth in dogs. A histological study. Aust. Dent. J. 16(4):227–231, 1971.

Moriya, H., et al.: Clinico-radiographic study on root canal filling with Neodyne for root canal filling. Shikwa Gakuho 77(5):773–784, 1977.

Morris, M. L.: A new hypothesis of periodontal homeostasis. J. Periodontol. 51:49, 1980.

Morris, M. L., Moreinis, A., Patel, R., et al.: Factors affecting healing after experimentally delayed tooth transplantation. J.O.E. 7(2):80–84, 1981.

Morse, D. R.: Clinical Endodontology. Springfield, Ill., Charles C Thomas, 1974.

Morse, D. R., Patnik, J. W., and Schacterle, G. R.: Electrophoretic differentiation of radicular cysts and granulomas. Oral Surg. 35:249–264, 1973.

Morse, D. R., Wolfson, E., and Schacterle, G. R.: Nonsurgical repair of electrophoretically diagnosed radicular cysts. J.O.E. 1(5):158–163, 1975.

Moss, J. P.: The indications for the transplantation of maxillary canines in the light of 100 cases. Br. J. Oral Surg. 12:268–274, 1975.

Mullaney, T. P., Camp, J., Cohen, S., et al.: Endodontic Symposium for the Family Practitioner. AAE and University of Texas at San Antonio Dental School, San Antonio, November 1979.

Mummery, J. H.: The pathology of pink spots on teeth. Br. Dent. J. 41:300, 1920.

Myers, H. I., et al.: Replantation of teeth in the hamster. Oral Surg. 7:1116–1129, 1954.

Myers, H. I., and Flanagan, V. D.: A comparison of results obtained from transplantation and replantation experiments using Syrian hamster teeth. Anat. Rec. 130:497, 1958.

Nasjleti, C. E., Caffesse, R. G., Castelli, W. A., et al.: Healing after tooth replantation in monkeys. A radioautographic study. Oral Surg. 39:361–375, 1975.

Nasjleti, C. E., Caffesse, R. G., and Castelli, W. A.: Replantation and autotransplantation of mature teeth without endodontics in monkeys. J. Dent. Res. 54:650–658, 1978.

Natiella, J. R., Armitage, J. E., and Greene, G. W.: The replantation and transplantation of teeth. Oral Surg. 29:397–419, 1970.

Neaverth, E. J., and Goerig, A. C.: Technique and rationale for splinting. J.A.D.A. 100:56–63, January 1980.

Ohman, A.: Healing and sensitivity to pain in young replanted human teeth. An experimental clinical and histologic study. Odontol. Tidskr. 73:166–227, 1965.

Oliet, S.: Apexogenesis associated with replantation. Dent Clin. North Am. 18:457–564, 1974.

Omnell, K.: Study of a root fracture. Br. Dent. J. 95:181, 1953.

Oswald, R. J., Harrington, G. W., and Van Hassel, H. J.: Replantation. 1. The role of the socket. J.O.E. 6(3):479–484, 1980.

Oswald, R. J., Harrington, G. W., and Van Hassel, H. J.: A postreplantation evaluation of air-dried and saliva-stored avulsed teeth. J.O.E. 6(5):546–551, 1980.

Pashley, D. H.: The influence of dentin permeability and pulpal blood flow on pulpal solute concentrations. J.O.E. 5(12):355–361, 1979.

Pearson, J. K., and Nicolazzo, M. R.: Immediate replantation and stabilization of avulsed teeth. Dent. Surg. 50(9):66, 1974.

Penick, E. C.: The endodontic management of root resorption. Oral Surg. 16:344, 1963.

Phillips, J. R.: Apical root resorption under orthodontic therapy. Angle Orthod. 25:1, 1955.

Pindborg, J. J.: Clinical, radiographic, and histological aspects of intraalveolar fractures of upper central incisors. Acta Odont. Scand. 13:44, June 1955.

Prichard, J.: The infrabony technique as a predictable procedure. J. Periodont. 28:202, July 1957.

Pritchard, G. B.: A specimen showing pink spot. R.´Soc. Med. Trans. 24:1600, 1931.

Pulver, W. H., Traubman, J. A., and Smith, D. J.: Immune components in normal and inflamed human dental pulp. Arch. Oral. Biol. 22(2):103–111, 1977.

Rabinowitch, B. Z.: Internal resorption. Oral Surg. 33:263, 1972.

Raisz, L. G., Nuki, K., Alander, C. B., et al.: Interactions between bacterial endotoxin and other stimulators of bone resorption in organ culture. J. Perio. Res. 16:1–7, 1981.

Rasmussen, P., and Mjör, I. A.: Calcium hydroxide as an ectopic bone inductor in rats. Scand. J. Dent. Res. 79:24–30, 1971.

Ravin, J. J., and Helbo, M.: Replantation of akcidentelt eksarticulerede taender. Tandlaegebladet 70:805–815, 1966.

Ronning, O., and Koski, K.: The fate of inorganic implants in the subcutaneous tissue of the rat. Plast. Reconstr. Surg. 37:121–124, 1966.

Rothschild, D. L., Goodman, A. A., and Blakey, K. R.: A histologic study of replanted and transplanted endodontically and nonendodontically treated teeth in dogs. Oral Surg. 28:871–876, 1969.

Rowe, D. J., and Bradley, L. S.: Quantitative analyses of osteoclasts, bone loss and inflammation in human periodontal disease. J. Perio. Res. 16:13–19, 1981.

Rubach, W. C., and Mitchell, D. F.: Periodontal disease, accessory canals and pulp pathosis. J. Periodont. 26:34, 1965.

Salinas, G.: Canal treatment of deciduous teeth with the biocalex method. Rev. Ital. Stomatol. 46(7/8):4–11, 1977.

Scott, J. N., and Zelikow, R.: Replantation — a clinical philosophy, J.A.D.A. 101:17–19, July 1980.

Seltzer, S.: Endodontology, New York, McGraw-Hill, 1971.

Seltzer, S.: Biologic aspects of endodontics. Temple University Continuing Education Course, Philadelphia, March 6–10, 1978.

Seltzer, S., and Bender, I. B.: Inflammation in the odontoblastic layer of the dental pulp. J.A.D.A. 59:720, 1959.

Seltzer, S., and Bender, I. B.: The Dental Pulp, 2nd Ed., Philadelphia, J. B. Lippincott Co., 1975.

Seltzer, S., Bender, I. B., and Ziontz, M.: The interrelationship of pulp and periodontal disease. Oral Surg. 16:1474, 1963.

Seltzer, S., Soltanoff, W., and Bender, I. B.: Epithelial proliferation in periapical lesions. Oral Surg. 27:111–121, 1969.

Seltzer, S., Bender, B., Nazimov, H., et al.: Pulpitis-induced interradicular periodontal changes in experimental animals. J. Periodont. 38:124–129, March 1967.

Seltzer, S., Soltanoff, W., Sinai, I., et al.: Biological aspects of endodontics. III. Periapical tissue reaction to root canal instrumentation. Oral Surg. 26:534–546, 1968.

Shafer, W. G., Hine, M. K., and Levy, B. M.: A Textbook of Oral Pathology, 3rd Ed. Philadelphia, W. B. Saunders Co., 1974.

Sharp, R. E.: The relationship of the pulp and the periodontium. Periodont. Abstr. 25(3):130–142, 1977.

Sherman, P.: Intentional replantation of teeth in dogs and monkeys. J. Dent. Res. 47:1066–1071, 1968.

Shovelton, D. S.: Presence and distribution of microorganisms within nonvital teeth. Br. Dent. J. 117:101, August 1964.

Shulman, L. B., Gedalia, I., and Feingold, R. M.: Fluoride concentration in root surfaces and alveolar bone of fluoride-immersed monkey incisors three weeks after replantation. J. Dent. Res. 52:1314, November 1973.

Shulman, L. B., Kalis, P., and Goldhaber, P.: Fluoride inhibition of tooth-replant root resorption in Cebus monkeys. J. Oral Ther. Pharmacol. 4:331–337, May 1968.

Sibley, L. C.: Management of root fracture. Oral Surg. 13:1475–1483, 1960.

Simon, J. H. S.: Incidence of periapical cysts in relation to the root canal. J.O.E. 6(11):845–848, 1980.

Simon, J. H. S., Glick, D. H., and Frank, A. L.: The relationship of endodontic-periodontic lesions. J. Periodont. 43:202, April, 1972.

Simon, J. H. S., Jensen, J. L., and Kimura, J. T.: Histologic observations of endodontically treated replanted roots. J.O.E. 1(5):178–180, 1975.

Simon, J. H. S., Kelly, W. H., Gordon, D. G., et al.: Extrusion of endodontically treated teeth. J.A.D.A. 97:17–23, July 1978.

Sinai, I. H.: Endodontic perforations. Their prognosis and treatment. J.A.D.A. 95:90–95, July 1977.

Sinai, I. H., and Soltanoff, W.: The transmission of pathologic changes between the pulp and the periodontal structures. Oral Surg. 36:558, 1973.

Singh, K. K., and Dudani, I. C.: Autogenous transplantation of developing mandibular third molars. J. Indian Dent. Assoc. 42:199–212, 1970.

Siskin, M.: The Biology of the Human Dental Pulp. St. Louis, C. V. Mosby Co., 1973.

Skoglund, A.: Vascular changes in replanted and autotransplanted apicoectomized mature teeth of dogs. Int. J. Oral Surg. 10(2):100–110, 1981.

Skoglund, A.: Pulpal changes in replanted and autotransplanted apicoectomized mature teeth of dogs. Int. J. Oral Surg. 10(2):111–121, 1981.

Skoglund, A., and Tronstad, L.: Pulpal changes in replanted and autotransplanted immature teeth in dogs. J.O.E. 7(7):309–316, 1981.

Skoglund, A., Tronstad, L., and Wallenius, K.: A micro-angiographic study of vascular changes in replanted and autotransplanted teeth of young dogs. Oral Surg. 45:17–28, 1978.

Söder, P. O., Otteskog, P., Andreasen, J. O., et al.: Effect of drying on viability of periodontal membrane. Scand. J. Dent. Res. 85(3):164–168, 1977.

Spangberg, L.: Biologic effect of root canal filling materials. Effect in vitro of water soluble components of root canal filling materials on Hela cells. Odontol. Revy 20:132, 1969.

Spangberg, L., and Langeland, K.: Biologic effects of dentinal materials. Toxicity of root canal filling materials on Hela cells in vitro. Oral Surg. 35:402, 1973.

Speer, M. L., Madonia, J. V., and Heuer, M. A.: Quantitative evaluation of the immunocompetence of the dental pulp. J.O.E. 3(11):418–423, 1977.

Stahl, S. S.: Pathogenesis of the inflammatory lesion in pulp and periodontal tissue. Periodontics 4:190, 1966.

Stanley, H. R.: Human Pulp Response to Operative Dental Procedures. Gainesville, Fla., Storter Printing Co. 1976.

Stanley, H.: Personal Communication, January 1981.

Stanley, H. R., and Lundy, T.: Dycal therapy for pulp exposures. Oral Surg. 34:818–827, 1972.

Stanley, H, R., Weisman, M. I., Michanowicz, A. E., et al.: Ischemic infarction of the pulp: Sequental degenerative changes of the pulp after traumatic injury. J.O.E. 4(11):325–335, 1978.

Stevens, O. O.: Mouth protectors: evaluation of twelve types — second year. J. Dent. Child. 32:137–143, 1965.

Stevens, R. M.: Tooth replantation. U.S. Navy Med. 71:21–26, July 1980.

Stewart, G. G.: Calcium hydroxide-induced root healing. J.A.D.A. 90:793–800, April 1975.

Stewart, G. G.: The recognition and treatment of vertical root fractures. AAE 37th Annual Session, Los Angeles, April 17, 1980.

Stone, S., Ramfjord, S. P., and Waldron, J.: Scaling and gingival curettage: A radioautographic study. J. Periodontol. 37:416, 1966.

Strindberg, L. Z.: Dependence of the results of pulp canal therapy on certain factors: an analytic study based on radiographic and clinical follow-up examinations. Dent. Abstr. 2:176, 1956.

Stuart, W. W., Crowley, L. V., Turner, D. W., et al.: Humoral response to endodontic cements. J.O.E. 5(7):214–217, 1979.

Sugiyama, F.: Clinical evaluation of calcium hydroxide as a root canal filling material. Shikwa Gakuho 49:145, 1944.

Sweeney, E. J., Moore, D. J., and Dooner, J. J.: Retentive strength of acid-etched anterior fixed partial dentures: an in vitro comparison of attachment techniques. J.A.D.A. 100:198–202, February 1980.

Taylor, G. N., Madonia, J. V., Wood, N. K., et al.: In vivo autoradiographic study of relative penetrating abilities of aqueous 2% parachlorophenol and camphorated 35% parachloropheral. J.O.E. 2(3):81–86, 1976.

Torneck, C. D.: Reaction of rat connective tissue to polyethylene tube implants. Oral Surg. 24:674–683, 1967.

Torneck, C. D.: Controversies in the rationale of treatment. The 36th Annual Session of the American Association of Endodontists, Atlanta, April 29, 1979.

Torneck, C. D., Smith, J. S., and Grindall, P.: Biologic effects of endodontic procedures on developing incisor teeth. IV. Effect of debridement procedures and calcium hydroxide camphorated parachlorophenol paste in the treatment of experimentally induced pulp and periapical disease. Oral Surg. 35:541–554, 1973.

Toto, P. D., and Restarski, J. S.: The histogenesis of pulpal osontoclasts. Oral Surg. 16:172, 1963.

Tronstad, L.: Reaction of the exposed pulp to Dycal treatment. Oral Surg. 38:945–953, 1974.

Tronstad, L.: Scientific Session: American Association of Endodontists, 33rd Annual Meeting, Hollywood, Fla., April 1976.

Tronstad, L.: Tissue reactions following apical plugging of the root canal with dentin chips in monkey teeth subjected to pulpectomy. Oral Surg. 45:297–304, 1978.

Tronstad, L., Andreasen, J. O., Hasselgren, G., et al.: pH changes in dental tissues after root canal filling with calcium hydroxide. J.O.E. 7(1):17, 1981.

Vaes, G.: Lysosomes and the cellular physiology of bone resorption. Dingle, J.-I., and Fell, H. B., (eds.): In Lysosomes in Biology and Pathology, Vol. I. Amsterdam, North-Holland Publishing Co., 1969.

Van Hassel, H. J., Oswald, R. J., and Harrington, G. W.: Replantation 2. The role of the periodontal ligament. J.O.E. 6(4):506–508, 1980.

Van Mullem, P. J., Simon, M., Lamers, A. C., et al.: Hard tissue resorption and deposition after endodontic instrumentation. Oral Surg. 49:544–548, 1980.

Vertucci, F. J., and Williams, R. G.: Furcations canals in the human mandibular first molar. Oral Surg. 38:308, 1974.

Waerhaug, J.: Effect of c-avitaminosis on the supporting structures of teeth. J. Periodont. 29:87–97, 1958.

Waldron, J. M.: Personal communication. November 1981.

Walsh, J. S., Kafrawy, A., and Roche, J. R.: The effect of apical modification on the vitality of replanted permanent monkey teeth. J. Dent. Child. 45:146–150, 1978.

Warner, G., Orban, B., Hine, M. K., et al.: Internal resorption of teeth: Interpretation of histologic findings. J.A.D.A. 34:468, April 1947.

Webber, R. T.: The expanded role of calcium hydroxide. American Association of Endodontists, Annual Session, Philadelphia, May 1981.

Webber, R. T., del Rio, C. E., Brady, J. M., et al.: Sealing quality of a temporary filling material. Oral Surg. 46:123–130, 1978.

Webber, R. T., Schwiebert, K. A., and Cathey, G. M.: A technique for placement of calcium hydroxide in the root canal system. J.A.D.A. 103:417–421, September 1981.

Weine, F. S.: Replantations. Ill. Dent. J. 42:657–662, October 1973.

Weine, F. S.: Endodontic Therapy, 2nd Ed., St. Louis, C. V. Mosby Co., 1976.

Weiss, M. B., and Bjorvatan, K.: Pulp capping in deciduous and newly erupted permanent teeth of monkeys. Oral Surg. 29:769–775, 1970.

West, N. M.: A possible impediment to biologic root-end closure. J.O.E. 6(11):842–844, 1980.

Wilkinson, F. C.: Pathology of replanted teeth. Aust. J. Dent. 30:269, 1926.

Witech Laboratory: Calciobiotic root canal sealer with calcium hydroxide. Manufacturer's advertisement distributed March 1981, Erie, Pa.

Woehrle, R. R.: Cementum regeneration in replanted teeth with differing pulp treatment. J. Dent. Res. 55:235–238, 1976.

Worth, G.: Postgraduate lecture. USAIDR, Walter Reed Army Hospital, Winter, 1973.

Wuehrmann, A. H., and Mason-Hing, L. R.: Dental Radiology, 3rd Ed. St. Louis, C. V. Mosby Co., 1973.

Yoshiki, S., and Mori, M.: Enzyme histochemistry of tissue reaction to calcium hydroxide. Bull. Tokyo Dent. Col. 2:32–39, 1961.

Zadik, D., Chosack, A., and Eidelman, E.: The prognosis of traumatized permanent anterior teeth with fracture of the enamel and dentin. Oral Surg. 47:173–175, 1979.

Zander, H. A., and Law, P. B.: Pulp management in fractures of young permanent teeth. JADA 31:195, 1944.

8

Root Canal Fillings with Silver Points: The Rigid Core Techniques

MICHAEL A. HEUER, D.D.S., M.S.

HISTORICAL BACKGROUND

Metals of various types and forms have had a long history of use as filling materials in the root canals of human teeth. As early as 1757, gold and lead were suggested as materials to fill root canals prior to the re-implantation or transplantation of teeth, a dental surgical practice common to the period. In the nineteenth century, particularly before the use of gutta percha became widespread following its introduction in the post–Civil War period, gold foil and gold wire were commonly used as root canal filling materials. As late as 1930, Grove reported modifications of gold wire for use as root canal fillings and recommended the pre-fabrication of gold points for better adaptation to the technique. In the quarter century preceding 1930, methods utilizing tin foil, lead wire or points, copper amalgam, or gold-tin alloys for root canal therapy each had proponents. Of all the metals advocated, only silver points have gained any acceptance by endodontic practitioners. There are several reasons for this development.

One of the principal reasons for selecting silver as the metal of choice relates to what is known as its oligodynamic effect (i.e., the toxic effect of exceedingly small quantities of pure metals in solution upon living cells). This was first noted by the Swedish scientist Arhennis, who observed that storage of contaminated water in copper vessels resulted in sterilization of the water because of the antimicrobial effect of minute amounts of copper dissolved from the vessel walls. The Swiss botanist Naegeli used the word "oligodynamic" to describe this phenomenon. In the 1920's and 1930's German dentists, principally Trebitsch, Greth, and Eckstein, were among the first to study and recommend the use of silver in endodontics, based upon this property of the metal. Grossman, following an extended visit to Germany in 1928, attempted to introduce the use of silver points in root canal therapy to his American colleagues. The concern over root canal infection and the search for disinfecting agents and sealing materials were very real in the first half of the twentieth century, as the theory of focal infection was widespread and pervasive at that time.

By a synthesis of Grove's idea of the pre-fabrication of metal points and the oligodynamic concepts of European dentists, Elmer A. Jasper of St. Louis was able to convince dental manufacturers and practitioners of the practicality of the silver point technique in endodontics. What Jasper advocated was the manufacture of silver points in sizes to match the sizes of existing root canal instruments. Once the root canal was enlarged by a particular sized root canal file, a silver point of that same size was fitted and cemented into the tooth to seal the root canal system. This step, introduced by Jasper in 1933, remains the central concept of the technique to the present time.

In the two decades following the introduction of the technique, the University of Michigan, under the leadership of Ralph F. Sommer, became a leading center for the advocacy and promulgation of this new therapy. Sommer's groups developed an extended rationale for the technique and, by adding refinements, adapted it to a wide selection of clinical endodontic cases. The apparent simplicity and adaptability of the technique had great appeal to the relatively inexperienced practitioners. The intense interest of the Michigan group, as well as their students, stimulated much basic research into root canal anatomy, instrumentation, and filling materials in a prolonged effort not only to provide a scientific basis for the technique but to standardize the armamentarium and procedure. Ironically, the net result of this research (which did eventually lead to the development of standards for root canal instruments and endodontic filling materials) was to discourage the use of silver points as a universal root canal filling material.

PHILOSOPHY OF TREATMENT

The basic premises of the philosophy were expressed in Sommer's text, *Clinical Endodontics*, which has been out of print for some years. Essentially, these are as follows: (1) The root canal system of a *mature tooth* is circular in cross section in the apical one third of the root regardless of its cross-sectional configuration in either the middle or the cervical third of the root. (2) The *mature tooth* has an apical constriction at the dentino-cemental junction of the root to which the root canal system is to be instrumented and filled. (3) The cross-sectional diameter of the root canal system of a *mature tooth* is comparable to the cross-sectional diameter of root canal files and to silver points manufactured to match the size and taper of these root canal files. (4) Enlargement of a mature root canal system by a root canal file selected to *remove irregularities* from the cross-sectional circular configuration of the *apical one third* of the root will result in a root canal preparation that conforms to the size and taper of a pre-fabricated silver cone. (5) Precise fitting and cementing of the pre-fabricated silver cone into the root canal preparation in the *apical one third* of the root result in a hermetic seal of the root canal system. (6) Sealing the apical one third of the root canal system with a silver cone cemented into the root *will not* obturate the middle or cervical thirds of the root canal system. Therefore, accessory points of gutta percha must be laterally condensed around the central core of silver to fill and seal these areas of the root.

These premises developed during a period of time in which the use of gutta percha softened or dissolved in chloroform or in eucalyptol, with or without the utilization of heated instruments, constituted the major alternative for filling root canals. Today, the rationale for the use of silver points is as valid as it was four decades ago. Why, then, have silver points and the silver point filling technique fallen into such disrepute among endodontic practitioners?

USE OF SILVER POINTS TODAY

The relative ease of the clinical procedure and the improved radiographic esthetics of completed cases when compared with other types of root canal fillings give a false sense of security to an inexperienced clinician. What could be simpler than placing a radiopaque wire through a tooth and producing a picture of that dense "filling" from apex to crown? The success of silver point root canal fillings (or any type of root canal filling for that matter) depends upon the ability to *seal* the root canal space *laterally*, not upon the ability to reach the apex of the root. In order to seal a root canal, a silver point must fit the preparation as precisely as possible in the apical portion of the root, and even if fitted well, it relies upon root canal sealer cement to effect a lateral seal of the space. The technique in practice is neither simple nor predictable as to the efficacy of the apical seal, based on radiographic interpretation. With increasing numbers of such endodontic procedures being completed, this dichotomy between theory and practice became increasingly apparent, and it was soon recognized that silver points and silver point techniques were not a universal solution to filling root canals.

The first problem that became obvious was the discrepancy between the size and taper of the root canal files and the size and taper of silver points available commercially. This led to the concept of standardization of instruments and filling materials by a concerted action on the part of practitioners, dental organizations, and dental manufacturers and is an ongoing process even today. Although standardized instruments and filling materials have brought improvements in the design and fabrication of products, they have not completely resolved the problems associated with fitting pre-fabricated points into preparations made with matching instruments. The most significant design feature to facilitate this process was the introduction of a standardized taper to both instruments and points, regardless of their nominal size.

As time went by, the increasing utilization of cast gold or pre-fabricated posts and/or cores for strength and retention purposes when restoring endodontically treated teeth made the use of silver point root canal fillings as described by Sommers less practical. The use of a silver point with auxiliary cones of gutta percha laterally condensed around it to obturate the root canal of an anterior tooth does not make for easy resolution of a restorative problem if a post in the root canal is required. Either the root canal filling will need to be removed and redone (this time using all gutta percha or a silver point sectioned so as not to extend incisally beyond the apical portion of the root) or an attempt (usually unsuccessful) will have to be made to drill out a post preparation of sufficient depth without perforating the root wall or dislodging the silver master core. The needs of restorative dentistry added emphasis to the trend toward all gutta percha root canal fillings or modifications of silver point fillings by the use of apical seals only.

Questions as to the validity of the concept that root canal anatomy lends itself to precision preparations of the root canal system were soon raised. Investigations by several authors created doubts as to whether preparations of a root canal in the apical one third of the root were indeed circular in cross section, as postulated. Evidence suggested that in most instances they were not. In addition, the central axis of the root canal preparation seldom corresponded to the central axis of the natural root canal that preceded it, and preparations to the sizes suggested by advocates of silver points were by and large inadequate to thoroughly debride the walls of a root canal. In spite of standardized instruments, the techniques for using these instruments by clinicians were far from standardized. The practical result is that a standardized preparation of the root canal is probably more fiction than fact. Clinicians who use root canal instruments primarily in a linear or filing mode will never be able to produce a preparation that is circular in cross section, whereas clinicians who use root canal instruments primarily in a rotary or reaming mode most likely can produce a circular preparation, but only in those instances in which the root canals are straight or access to the area of the preparation is uninhibited.

If a proper preparation cannot be attained, how can an acceptable seal be effected? Evidence from dye and radioisotope penetration studies suggests it cannot. These studies make it abundantly clear that the efficacy of a root canal seal by means of a solid core such as a silver point depends primarily on the concurrent use of a proper root canal sealer cement. A silver point without root canal sealer cement is beyond any reasonable doubt the most ineffective root canal filling available. Although silver cones with sealer cement are certainly superior to gutta percha cones used without solvents, root canal sealer cements, or mechanical compaction, they are definitely inferior to gutta percha cones used with root canal sealer or mechanical compaction as far as sealing the apex of a tooth is concerned. When silver cones with sealer cement are compared with gutta percha cones dissolved in or used with gutta percha solvents or when they are compared with gutta percha cones compacted without either solvents or sealer cements, there is considerable doubt as to which system is superior.

In spite of abundant evidence of abuses of silver point root canal filling techniques leading to clinical failures, investigations of the clinical efficacy of silver point root canal fillings compared with gutta percha root fillings fail to reveal any significant differences in clinical success. This is somewhat surprising in light of the claims made for a high incidence of lateral root canals in human teeth, as evidenced by radiographs taken after root canal systems have been obturated by gutta percha techniques designed to fill lateral canals. Collaborating evidence from anatomic studies of high incidences of lateral root canal systems of the natural dentition has not been presented. One might therefore suspect that the acutely flared preparations necessary for these condensation techniques may be producing some artifactual minute perforations of the root canal wall during either preparation or condensation. Lateral root canals that are demonstrated radiographically by evidence of the loss of alveolar lamina dura laterally have been sealed by any number of root filling techniques in clinical practice. However, there can be no doubt that those techniques in which the middle and cervical areas of the root canal wall can be subjected to extrusion pressures during root canal filling will be the most successful. Silver point techniques that are capable of providing such forces only in the apical third of the root, if at all, are predictably less successful in these cases.

The coup de grâce to use of silver points as the filling material of choice for endodontics resulted from investigations of the corrosion and cytotoxicity of silver. The corrosive behavior of silver points has been investigated by standard potentiostatic techniques. Silver was found to corrode spontaneously in sulfide media (Na_2S or Na_2SO_4) at -450 mv with respect to a standard calomel electrode and to corrode in chloride media (0.9% NaCl or Ringer's solution) at 100 mv. The corrosion films formed were noncontinuous and nonpassivating and allowed corrosion to continue at high current densities. In human serum, two separate, slightly passivating regions of corrosion were noted at approximately 200 mv and 400 mv. The first region was felt to be due to the formation of AgCl and the second to the formation of either Ag_2CO_3 or Ag_2O.

Histologic studies of pure silver implants in connective tissue over several decades show variable fibrous encapsulation, tissue discoloration, macrophages, and dark silver particles in tissue reactions that range from very mild to mild to fairly well tolerated to well tolerated. Only when pure silver was implanted in dog femur (definite tissue reaction) or cat brain (severe reaction) were adverse tissue effects noted. Tissue or cell cultures of HeLa cells or fibroblasts showed no cytotoxicity caused by pure silver.

In 1971, clinical cases were reported by three authors in which partial or complete in vivo destruction of a silver point used to fill a root canal was observed. In one patient, the apical 2 mm of a silver point located totally within the root structure disintegrated over a period of 35 months; in another patient, focal argyria appeared in the mucoperiosteum following silver point root canal filling 4 years earlier; and in the third patient, that portion of a silver point extending into the apical tissues separated from that portion retained in the tooth 8 years postoperatively. All of these, as well as other reported clinical cases, revealed black corroded silver cones on surgical examination.

The following year Seltzer published a study of 25 silver cones retrieved from 13 teeth that had been diagnosed as endodontic failures owing to the development of pain and/or swelling. Five silver points from three successful asymptomatic cases were also examined. Silver points from both successful and unsuccessful cases showed some degree of corrosion; however, gross amounts of corrosion were exhibited in unsuccessful cases. Tissue cultures revealed these points to be cytotoxic, whereas new, unused, or uncorroded silver points showed no cellular inhibition. X-ray diffraction showed that the corrosion products consisted of silver salts, principally sulfide, sulfate, carbonate, and silver amine sulfate amide hydrate. Seltzer concluded that the corrosion products of silver were the cytotoxic factors and not the metallic silver itself.

The fact that silver points corrode and that this corrosion is at least in part responsible for endodontic clinical failure when silver points are used to seal the root canal has since been substantiated by other investigators. Since it is also known that silver does not corrode in the presence of eugenol or zinc oxide–eugenol root canal sealer cements, it is reasonable to assume that the corrosion of silver points clinically can be lessened by ensuring that these points are seated entirely within the confines of the root canal, surrounded and protected by a sealer cement. This, in fact, seems to be the situation in clinically successful cases. However, if, as Seltzer surmises, the corrosion products of silver are cytotoxic, what is not clear is why when silver is implanted in connective tissue (when its exposed surface area and corrosion potential are greatest) do we not see the histologic evidence of cytotoxicity? The answer in all probability relates to the effectiveness of the apical seal as well as to the metal itself. Perhaps the necessary corrosion reactions leading to cytotoxic silver salts exist only in the absence of an apical seal and in the presence of degraded serum proteins.

In summary, the choice of silver as a material for use in active biologic systems is not tenable in current medical or dental practice. However, a half century of root canal treatment in which silver point root canal fillings were done successfully by thousands of dentists in tens, if not hundreds, of thousands of teeth cannot be condemned out of hand. The advent of endodontics as a special area of dental practice and the introduction of endodontics into significantly more dental practices than at any other time owe a debt in part to the advocates of the silver point technique, who championed the cause of conservative endodontics by means of a system within the capability of the vast majority of dental practitioners. The influence of the philosophy of silver points will long be felt, owing to the progress made in the standardization of instruments, materials, and techniques in endodontics, as well as to resurgent interest in the technical and mechanical aspects of endodontic practice. In today's spectrum of endodontic know-how, silver point root canal fillings still hold a place of respect, albeit limited, in the wide range of options available to the thoughtful practitioner.

Materials and Instruments

Silver used in endodontics is manufactured into tapering points or cones designed to match the sizes of root canals prepared by standardized instruments. The surface texture and shape of silver points vary considerably from manufacturer to manufacturer. The tips of the points vary from well-defined machined conical tapers to irregular nondescript pointed ends. The surface texture varies from smooth amorphous undulations to sharply defined grooves perpendicular to the long axis of the point proper, as if the metal were spun on a lathe. The nominal sizes of silver points are given in Table 8–1. Preciseness of shape affects the accuracy of fit, and surface texture affects both the adherence of sealer cement and the corrosive potential.

Despite the manufacturing differences, the chemical compositions of commercial brands of silver points used in endodontics have been found to be similar, and potentiostatic investigations failed to show any significant differences in their corrosion behavior. The silver content of these filling points ranges from 99.8 to 99.9 per cent, with nickel and copper being the elements in next highest concentration. Nickel and copper have not been detected in the corrosive fibers studied. The hardness values for silver points average 112 Knoop hardness number, which corresponds to a range of Knoop values expected for cold-worked samples of commercial grade silver (99.9 per cent). This is comparable to a mean Knoop hardness number of 62 for human dentin and 120 for Class I inlay soft gold casting alloy. The microstructure of endodontic silver points is indicative of cold-drawn wire, with an etched surface similar to that of 99.9 per cent silver that has been cold rolled. The tensile strength values of 307 MPa (44,491 psi) to 450 MPa (65,194 psi) determined for silver points fall into the range of values to be

TABLE 8–1 Nominal Sizes of Silver Points*

Size Designation	Projected Diameter at Tip (mm)	Diameter D 1 mm from Tip (mm)	Diameter D_3 3 mm from Tip (mm)	Diameter D_2 16 mm from Tip (mm)
10	—	—	—	—
15	—	—	—	—
20	0.20	0.22	0.26	0.52
25	0.25	0.27	0.31	0.57
30	0.30	0.32	0.36	0.62
35	0.35	0.37	0.41	0.67
40	0.40	0.42	0.46	0.72
45	0.45	0.47	0.51	0.77
50	0.50	0.52	0.56	0.82
55	0.55	0.57	0.61	0.87
60	0.60	0.62	0.66	0.92
70	0.70	0.72	0.76	1.02
80	0.80	0.82	0.86	1.12
90	0.90	0.92	0.96	1.22
100	1.00	1.02	1.06	1.32

All dimensions measured to an accuracy of 0.005 mm.
Tolerance ± 0.02 mm.
Taper proportion 0.02 mm per 1 mm of uniform taper.
Overall length not less than 30 mm ± 2.0 mm.

expected for cold-worked silver. The mechanical data available indicate the degree of cold working associated with silver points, probably in the range of 20 to 50 per cent. No definitive values for percentage of elongation, proportional limits, or modules of elasticity have been determined for endodontic silver points. As previously noted, the corrosion behavior of silver points has been investigated by standard potentiostatic techniques as well as observed in scanning electron microscope studies.

It is absolutely essential that a root canal sealer cement be used in conjunction with silver points; hence, the selection of that cement assumes some importance. Root canal sealer cements are of three broad generic types: (1) those based upon zinc oxide–eugenol formulations; (2) those that do not contain eugenol, including several polymeric systems; and (3) those that contain active ingredients for which therapeutic claims are made. The therapeutic sealers have little place as sealer cements to be used in conjunction with silver points, as the paraformaldehyde or iodoform contained in them adds nothing to the desired physical properties of the cement and their contribution to asepsis in the root canal environment is dubious. Of the non-eugenol–containing sealer cements only Diaket, an organic polyketone, and AH26, an epoxy type resin system adapted to endodontics, have found much favor. Chloropercha or eucapercha root canal sealer cements, usually solutions of gutta percha and rosin, have little use when silver points are to be sealed into a root canal system. Silastic and Hydron, when employed as endodontic filling materials, are used without any core materials such as silver points or gutta percha.

With the exception of Diaket or AH26, the root canal sealer cements most suitable for cementing a silver point into a root canal are based upon zinc oxide–eugenol formulations. Principally these are derived from three basic formulations — those of Rickert, Grossman, and, to a lesser degree, Wach. The essential ingredients of all three are the powder zinc oxide, rosins, and radiopaque agents and the liquid eugenol with or without resins added. Rickert (Kerr) root canal sealer uses oleoresins and precipitated silver in the powder, whereas the powder component of the Grossman (Procosol) and Wach sealers contains bismuth or barium salts. Wach's sealer powder contains no resin. The liquid component of Rickert's sealer contains Canada balsam (as does Wach's sealer) in addition to eugenol, whereas Grossman's sealer liquid consists of eugenol alone. Trace amounts of eucalyptol and beechwood creosote are also contained in the Wach sealer liquid, the former ingredient acting as a solvent for gutta percha when used with gutta percha root canal fillings. All three formulas at one time or another contained traces of ingredients intended to lend antiseptic qualities to the material, but these have been deleted by and large with the passage of time.

Zinc oxide–eugenol sealing cements may not be optimal materials for use in endodontics. Zinc oxide–eugenol sets by a combination of chemical and physical processes, yielding a hardened mass of zinc oxide embedded in a matrix of long, sheath-like crystals of zinc eugenolate ($[C_{10}H_{11}O_2]_2Zn$). Excess eugenol is invariably present and is absorbed by both the zinc oxide and the eugenolate. Hardening of the mixture is due to the zinc-eugenolate formation; the unreacted eugenol remains trapped and tends to weaken the mass. Free eugenol usually remains after setting of zinc oxide–eugenol cements, including root canal sealers, and reacts with fresh dentin by increasing its microhardness (probably because of protein precipitation) in direct proportion to the amount available. More important are the high degree of cytotoxicity of eugenol and the antigenic potential of tissues affected by it. Free eugenol comes in contact with apical tissues in decreasing amounts from the time of insertion of the freshly mixed unset sealer cement until the material ultimately disintegrates in tissue serum. Silver points have not been demonstrated to interact chemically with zinc oxide–eugenol sealer cements, but the relatively unstable nature of these materials in biologic systems prejudices the long-term effectiveness of a silver point root canal filling, which depends upon stable materials for surface protection from corrosion as well as continuity of apical seal. Although at present no better substitutes for the zinc oxide–eugenol endodontic sealer cements have been developed, these facts fuel the continuing search for them.

The setting time of root canal sealer cements ranges from less than 15 minutes to none at all. As might be expected, higher temperature and humidity decrease the time of setting. Setting times of less than 30 minutes may prevent manipulation of the cement when sealing the root canal, whereas sealer cements that do not set at all most likely will remain chemically active (hence more cytotoxic) and will not possess desirable sealing properties.

The flow rate of the sealer cement is important, as it is one measure of the cement's viscosity. This property affects not only the ability of the sealer to penetrate the recesses or irregularities of the root canal preparation but also its handling characteristics both within and without the root canal system. Based on scientific evidence, the flow rates of Rickert's sealer and AH26 are comparable with Grossman's sealer; the flow rate for Diaket is somewhat less. In some studies Diaket exhibits a viscosity unsuitable for most endodontic procedures.

The film thickness of root canal sealer cements is another important factor, as it in part determines the luting potential of the cement. The allowable film thickness for fine grain (Type I) zinc phosphate cements used in restorative dentistry is 25 μm. The film thickness of Rickert's sealer approaches this and that of Diaket exceeds it, whereas Grossman's sealer has a film thickness somewhat less than 25 μm.

The solubility of root canal sealers in aqueous solutions is a critical factor, as it relates to the stability of these cements in tissue fluids. Whereas the Rickert sealer shows water absorption increases of less than 1 per cent, some forms of Grossman sealer show increases of greater than 2.5 per cent. Volume changes measured at 7, 30, and 90 day intervals show that stability is reached after 30 days and a 3 per cent decrease in volume of the Rickert sealer occurs, whereas some forms of Grossman's sealer show continuous decreases in volume from 1.25 per cent at 7 days to 2 per cent at 30 days and 3.25 per cent at 90 days. Kerr's Tubliseal, a two-paste zinc oxide–eugenol system, shows the same continuous decrease in volume, ranging from 1.5 to 5 per cent. Measurements of volume changes from sealer cements that fail to set were unobtainable.

All the sealer cements under consideration here have demonstrated properties of radiopacity nearly twice that of the gutta percha cones usually used in endodontic practice and as such can be detected on clinical radiographs.

For use as a cementing agent with silver points, the ideal root canal sealer must set within a reasonable time period of not less than 30 minutes at room temperature (perhaps less at body temperature and increased humidity), have shear rate sensitivity, behave like a pseudoplastic material, have flow characteristics suitable to clinical conditions, have a film thickness suitable for luting a metal to dentin, be relatively insoluble in aqueous solutions, demonstrate volume stability once set, and be radiopaque. Based on these criteria, the Rickert formula of Kerr appears to be most suitable. AH26 would appear to be an acceptable alternative, but data relating to physical properties have not been reported.

The major criticisms of Rickert's material have been its tendency to stain tooth structure if left in contact with dentin and the rapidity of its setting time. By understanding the nature of the material, i.e., precipitated silver causing the stains and Canada balsam contributing to rapid setting times, the criticisms are easily overcome by reasonable precautions in mixing and removal from visible dentinal surfaces.

A suggested inventory of materials and supplies for an operator wishing to practice silver point root canal filling techniques is given in Table 8–2.

TABLE 8–2 Materials and Supplies for Root Canal Filling

Silver points in standardized sizes 20 through 60
Root canal sealer cement
Gutta percha accessory filling points — size A fine
Baseplate gutta percha (pink) in 4 $\times$ 4 $\times$ 1 mm squares
Zinc oxyphosphate cement — extra fine white
IRM temporary cement
Chloroform USP
Alcohol — 95% ethanol
Rubber dam — 4 $\times$ 4 or 5 $\times$ 5 inch pre-cut squares
Cotton pellets — #3
Cotton rolls — 2½ inch
Cotton gauze — 2 $\times$ 2 inch
Cotton Q-tips
Local anesthetic as necessary

TABLE 8–3 **Instruments for Root Canal Filling**

BASIC (10 instruments)

Mouth mirror, front surface #5
Explorer, DE #5
Explorer, endodontic DE #DG16
Periodontal probe, DE Goldman-Fox/Williams
Excavator, endodontic DE #33
Plastic instrument, Woodson #2
Plastic instrument, Woodson #3
Cotton pliers, college non-pinch with serrated extra fine tips
Cotton pliers, endodontic self-locking with serrated tips
Ruler, endodontic 6 inch stainless steel

FILLING SUPPLEMENT (10 instruments plus cement slab)

Root canal pluggers, Luks #1, 2, 3, and 4
Root canal spreaders, #D11 and D12
Plastic instrument, Mortenson #2
Hemostat, Halsted-Mosquito, curved 4¾ inch*
Scissors, crown and collar, curved 5 inch
Cement spatula, #22
Cement slab, 2 × 2 × ½ inch tempered glass

*May substitute either Steiglitz forceps or silver point pliers.

When filling root canals with silver points, the dental practitioner will need an appropriate selection of instruments in order to perform effectively and efficiently. A suggested inventory of instruments for silver point root canal fillings is given in Table 8–3.

Some comments concerning this selection are in order. The basic armamentarium listed is applicable to and used for all endodontic procedures, including the filling of the root canal. It has been carefully selected so as to be suitable for the diagnosis and evaluation of a suspected endodontic problem, the preliminary coronal access preparation and exploration of the root canal system, the preparation of the root canal, the placement of intraradicular or intracoronal dressing, and the placement of temporary restorations following treatment.

It is assumed that in addition to the basic instrument supply suggested for endodontics several other items would be readily available for use in the dental office. Necessary for every endodontic treatment appointment, including that scheduled for filling the root canal, would be a small alcohol or other type burner, glass slabs or treated paper, mixing pads suitable for cements of various types, a straight 5 inch utility scissors, and the rubber dam instruments including punch, clamp forceps, clamps (#9, 2A, 12A, and 13A Ivory) and rubber dam frame (Ostby or Young). A selection of burs to meet most, if not all, the requirements of endodontic treatment need not be extensive. Experience has shown that friction grip (FG) burs of surgical length sizes 2, 4, and 6 (round) and 558 (cross-cut fissure) plus regular length 701 (tapered fissure) and 1557 (round bur end-straight fissure) burs are all that are required. A 770S safe-ended diamond stone, also friction grip, is a valuable addition to this basic selection.

In clinical practice, an autoclave bag contains the following sterilized instruments and supplies: root canal files sizes 10 through 60 (11 instruments), a 3 ml irrigation syringe with a 23 gauge needle (disposable), two cotton rolls, six 2 × 2 inch gauze pads, and two cotton Q-tips. The working blades of the instruments are inserted into one of the cotton rolls, with sizes 10 to 35 having their handles protruding from one end and sizes 40 to 60 having their handles protruding from the other. In this way the color code identification is clearly visible, and instruments having the same color code are readily distinguishable from one another.

The supplementary armamentarium contains those instruments essential for the filling of the root canal. This selection is easily adaptable to either the silver point or the laterally condensed gutta percha techniques. The two essential instruments for silver point filling procedures are the small hemostat and the crown and collar scissors. Either a Steiglitz forceps or a specially designed silver point pliers can be substituted for the small hemostat. It should be noted that in this instrument selection the Luks pattern root canal pluggers sizes 1 through 4 correspond in size to endodontic files #35, 55, 85, and 100, respectively. The D11 and D12 root canal spreaders have tip sizes that correspond to endodontic filling points of approximately size 25, but the taper of these instruments is larger than either instruments or filling points in the standardized system.

Root Canal Preparation

A radicular preparation of a tooth has two main objectives. The first is to cleanse and sanitize the root canal system by removing any soft tissue debris and bacterial contamination. The second is to shape the root canal(s) to receive a root canal filling.

The principal parts or regions of a root canal preparation are shown in Figure 8–1. In the usual sequence of root canal instrumentation the apical constriction that occurs at or near the dentino-cemental junction is located and verified by radiograph to determine the working length or *extension* of the preparation. The apical constriction will in turn be either maintained or very minimally enlarged so as to function as the apical *resistance form* of the preparation. The *retention form* or apical collar is developed immediately coronal to the resistance form in the apical one third of the preparation. This precise conical portion of the preparation is the most crucial area for success or failure if solid core root canal fillings are to be used, as this is the portion of the root into which they must fit. Occlusal to the retention form and flaring outward through the coronal access cavity preparation is the *convenience form* or flare of the root canal preparation.

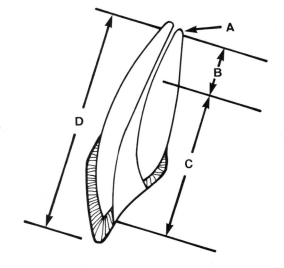

Figure 8–1 Principal parts of a root canal preparation. *A,* Resistance form. *B,* Retention form. *C,* Convenience form. *D,* Extension.

TABLE 8–4   Classification of Root Canal Systems and Preparations

CLASS I	*Root Canal: Uncomplicated* mature system with a straight or slightly curved root canal and an apical constriction
	Preparation: Uncomplicated preparation with resistance and retention form. Varying degrees of apical-occlusal flare to a straight or slightly curved preparation of size 40 to 60
CLASS II	*Type A* *Root Canal: Complicated* mature system with severely curved, dilacerated, or bifurcated root canals and apical constrictions
	Preparation: Complicated with resistance and retention form in a minimally flared preparation of less than size 50 in diameter
	Type B *Root Canal: Complicated* mature system with ancillary, lateral, or accessory root canals and apical constrictions
	Preparation: Complicated with resistance and retention form in a maximally flared preparation of more than size 40 in diameter
CLASS III	*Type A* *Root Canal: Immature* root canal with flaring of apical foramen and no apical constriction present
	Preparation: Complicated with no resistance or retention form and little flare beyond natural anatomy; apical size 100 or more in diameter
	Type B *Root Canal: Mature* root canal with loss of root apex and/or apical constriction by iatrogenesis or pathosis
	Preparation: Uncomplicated with no resistance form, but with retention form; varying degrees of apical-occlusal flare and preparations of any size from 40 to 100
CLASS IV	*Root Canal:* Primary teeth subject to or undergoing resorption

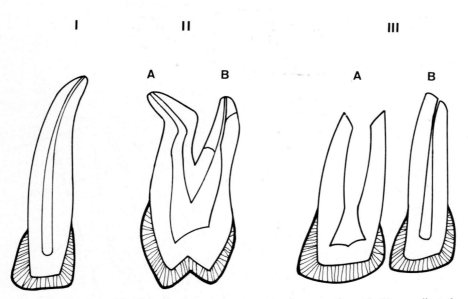

Figure 8–2 Classification of root canal systems and preparations. I, Uncomplicated mature tooth with straight root canal. II*A*, Complicated mature tooth with curved root canal. II*B*, Complicated mature tooth with lateral root canal. III*A*, Immature root canal. III*B*, Mature root canal with loss of apex.

Root canal systems or root canal preparations can be classified according to their complexity, the severity of curvature present, the presence of lateral or accessory root canals, and the presence or absence of an apical constriction or resistance form. Such a classification schema is shown in Table 8–4 and Figure 8–2. Classification of the root canal system predetermines in part the type of instrumentation technique likely to be most suitable for cleansing and shaping of the root, the type of filling material to select in order to seal the prepared root canal, and the type of filling technique to be used with the material selected. Root canal filling materials and techniques ought to be selected based upon the type of case presenting rather than selecting those cases that are treatable based upon the limitations of one's particular root canal material or technique.

Keeping the foregoing principles in mind, the preparation of a root canal system for any filling technique is a rather universal procedure. Once the extension (working length) has been established and confirmed, the preparation of the retention form begins by introducing the smallest root canal file to the working length and rotating it from one quarter to one half turn clockwise to engage the root canal wall. The instrument is then retracted from the root canal, wiped clean by twisting counterclockwise between alcohol-dampened gauze, and re-introduced to the working length. This process is repeated at the working length until the instrument size in use can be rotated 360 degrees without resistance, and only then should the next largest sized standardized instrument be used in the root canal. During instrumentation the root canal should be kept flooded with sodium hypochlorite irrigating solution, which is refreshed when instrument sizes are changed or even sooner. Instruments should not be precurved prior to introduction into the root canal system nor should filing actions of the instruments in an apical-occlusal direction be employed, as it is the rotary cutting action of the root canal files that creates the conical shape of the apical collar and maintains its circular cross section. The sequence of quarter to half turns and retraction is repeated with the next sized instrument until free rotation is achieved. A progression of larger and larger root canal files, each penetrating to the working length, is used in this fashion until the walls of the root canal are stripped of their predentinal surface and smoothly rounded into a conical apical collar that extends occlusally from the apical resistance form for not less than 2 to 3 mm.

Based upon the root canal anatomy and the potential preparation classification, the type of filling material and technique to be used to seal the root canal must now be considered.

The first determinant will be the presence or absence of an apical constriction. In any root canal preparation it is important not to pack the apical region with dentinal filings or tissue debris during instrumentation, but rather maintain a patent hollow tube between the apical soft tissues and the oral cavity at all times. The presence of an apical resistance form in the final preparation is essential if plastic or paste root canal fillings are to be used. However, this is not such a critical feature of the preparation utilizing solid core root canal fillings such as silver cones.

The second determinant is the shape of the apical collar or retention form of the preparation. The length of the apical collar in an apical-occlusal direction need not be great for use with gutta percha filling techniques. In lateral condensation techniques utilizing gutta percha master cores, apical collar length should not be less than 1 to 2 mm or more than 3 to 4 mm. In more plastic gutta percha techniques or paste fillings an apical collar may not

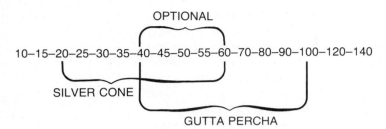

Figure 8–3 Apical diameter of preparation and selection of root canal filling core material.

be necessary at all. The apical collar or retention form is the critical feature of preparations designed for root canal fillings using solid cores of silver. When a silver core filling technique is under consideration, the length of the apical collar should not be less than 4 to 5 mm, or, better yet, it should extend over the entire length of the apical one third of the root.

The size or diameter of the retention form or apical collar also has a bearing upon the selection of a root canal filling material, as can be seen in Figure 8–3. When the diameter of the apical collar is much less than the diameter of a #40 root canal file, the ability to adapt a master cone of gutta percha accurately is impaired, whereas when the diameter of an apical collar is in excess of the diameter of a #60 root canal file, the usefulness of a fitted silver cone is questionable. In sizes smaller than 20 or larger than 100, master cores of gutta percha or silver are not practical in most cases.

The third determinant is the flare of the convenience form from the apical collar to the occlusal coronal access preparation. Solid core or silver cone techniques require very little, if any, flare to the convenience form beyond that inherent in the natural root canal system. Gutta percha techniques require much flare to the convenience form in order that the spreaders or pluggers used to compact the material can reach unimpeded into the apical region of the root.

Once the basic retention form has been established as previously described, in which the bulk of the pulp canal contents has been removed and a definitive apical amputation of the pulp has been accomplished, the actual root canal preparation for root canal filling can be initiated. A wide root canal system flaring buccal-lingual in an oval pattern, as seen in ribbon-shaped roots, or in all directions, as seen in conical roots, lends itself to a short, wide apical collar and a flaring convenience form. A narrow or bifurcated root canal system that assumes a circular cross-section shape in the middle third of the root lends itself to long, narrow apical collars with little flare to the convenience form. Sharp curves to a root canal, particularly in root canals with constricted diameters, preclude wide flaring preparations. Consequences of the presence of lateral or accessory root canals are lessened if the thickness of lateral root dentin in the region of their location can be reduced and access to them obtained. Root canals that can be instrumented only with precurved instruments or root canal files used in an apical-occlusal filing motion are less likely to produce apical collars that are conical in form or circular in diameter than are uncurved root canal instruments rotated in the root canal.

If one has determined that a silver point filling is suitable, then the previously described technique of instrumentation for establishment of the apical collar is continued with larger and larger instruments until the proper apical-occlusal length of the apical collar (retention form) is attained or until the uncurved instruments can no longer negotiate the root canal system. The walls of the root canal occlusal to the apical collar are lightly honed on each surface to remove surface debris and irregularities but without making any aggressive attempt to increase the flare of the convenience form. A recommended pattern of instrumentation for honing is as follows: Insert a root canal file one size larger than that preparing the apical collar to a level slightly apical to the occlusal termination of the retention form and, maintaining pressure against the buccal wall of the root canal, retract it quickly from the tooth. Repeat this process, gradually moving the location of the instrument from distal to mesial on the buccal wall. Follow honing of the buccal wall by irrigating the root canal system and inserting the file to the working length of the root, followed in turn by rotation and withdrawal, as in preparing the apical collar. Repeat the honing process on the mesial wall of the root canal moving from buccal to lingual, irrigate, and re-prepare. The procedure is repeated on the lingual and distal walls of the root canal, as described, enclosing the circle.

If a gutta percha filling has been selected, a technique of recapitulation or serial filing of the root canal is necessary. This technique entails the insertion of successively larger sized instruments to points in the root canal short of the apical collar, followed by reinsertion of the instrument preparing the apical collar itself to the full working length of the root canal after each successive instrument is used. The net effect, dependent in part upon the apical-occlusal distance used between each successively larger sized instrument, is to increase significantly the flare of the root canal from the occlusal termination of the retention form to the occlusal coronal access cavity preparation (much as the sequence of tubes one inside another increases the diameter of a telescope). If the flare obtained is insufficient, engine-driven reamers or drills are used in the cervical portion of the root to increase it even further. Serial filing techniques or engine-driven reamers are contraindicated in most filling techniques in which silver cones would be used. The exception may be in those instances in which laterally condensed gutta percha around a central core of silver would be used for sealing the middle and/or cervical thirds of a root canal. Even in these cases, however, much less aggressive use of flaring techniques is required.

It is with these factors in mind that the preparation for root canal filling is concluded and the selection of the root canal filling core material is predetermined. A comparison of a preparation for gutta percha and that for a silver cone is shown in Figure 8–4.

GUTTA PERCHA   **SILVER POINT**

CHARACTERISTIC

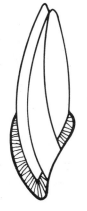

Figure 8–4 Comparison of preparations for gutta percha and silver point root canal fillings.

RESISTANCE FORM

yes   no

RETENTION FORM

no   yes

CONVENIENCE FORM

flare   natural

APICAL DIAMETER

40–100   20–60

CLASSIFICATIONS

I, IIB, III   I, IIA, IIIB

TECHNIQUE

Recapitulation   Rotation

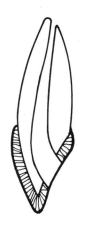

Filling the Root Canal

The root canal system of a tooth is ready for filling when the following criteria have been met: The root canal has been cleansed and prepared according to the preceding description. The tooth is comfortable; i.e., there is little, if any, sensitivity to either chewing or percussion, and sensitivity to palpation of the mucoperiosteum in the apical region and spontaneous pain are absent. The root canal is dry, without hemorrhage, exudate, or purulent material. If bacteriologic cultures have been taken, these are demonstrably negative. A single-sitting root canal procedure precludes the evaluation of many of these criteria prior to root canal filling, just as prolonged or overzealous treatment may preclude the attainment of them.

Assuming the tooth in question is ready for root canal filling, has been isolated by means of the rubber dam, and has had both the temporary restorations that seal the coronal access cavity preparation and the intraradicular dressings removed, the procedure for filling a single rooted tooth with a silver point root canal filling would proceed as follows:

The root canal should be dried with a paper point. This serves two purposes, as it enables the clinician to detect any exudate in the root canal (which will invariably be present if the recommended instrumentation procedure has been followed) and will dry out the system so as to preclude the extrusion of exudate or residual intracanal medicaments into the apical tissues.

A root canal instrument (K file) of the size used to prepare the apical collar is then introduced into the dry root canal to the working length of the tooth. Using this instrument (or one standardized size larger) without irrigation to re-prepare the retention form in the root provides a check on the working length and size and a fresh, dry dentinal surface prior to root canal filling.

Select a silver point of the same size as the working instrument used to fit into the root canal. With experience, the silver point can be cut to a length equal to the working length of the root canal file. Neophytes, however, should use the entire 30 mm long points for trial fitting. Using the hemostat or point forceps, grasp the silver point at a distance from its tip equal to the working length of the root canal file and insert the silver point into the root canal. The point should be firmly seated, so much so that additional pressure in an apical direction cannot force the point beyond the established working length or through the apex of the tooth. Additional apical pressure results only in a buckling of the unsupported portion of the point, which is to be avoided. The point should fit so well that it cannot be easily removed from the root canal — certainly not without the use of the hemostat. Silver points that can be placed and/or removed with cotton forceps *do not* properly fit the root canal preparations they were intended for.

The first thing the clinician will note is that the silver point does not extend to the exact length into the tooth that the root canal file did. This is to be expected, as the silver point will not extend into the very apical portion of the preparation, which was cut by the pointed tip of the root canal instrument. Therefore, a good fit would be short of the extension of the root canal file by at least the length of the tip of that file. What is required is that the point be wedged into the shape of the apical collar retention form with as much wall contact as possible circumferentially and not be caught by the acutely tapered conical shape of the instrument tip or the apical constriction

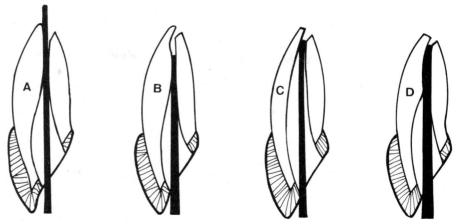

Figure 8–5 Fitting the silver point. *A*, Overextended. *B*, Underextended. *C*, Lack of frictional retention. *D*, Correct fit.

of the resistance form without any other wall contact. For this reason it may be desirable in some cases to eliminate the apical constriction and/or resistance form during root canal preparation to insure that the point is being held firmly by the retention form alone.

If the silver point has not been cut to the working length of the root canal file prior to fitting, then once seated it should be cut off with the crown and collar scissors level with the occlusal reference plane of the tooth. In any event at this time it is important that the point be fitted well into the root canal and extend from a position just short of the apical termination of the preparation to a position level with the reference plane on the occlusal surface from which the working length or extension was determined. You should *not* attempt to mark the occlusal extension of the silver point by bending it or using markers or placing notches in it. Cut it off level with the occlusal plane and then take a radiograph of the tooth so as to verify the accuracy of placement.

Three major problems may be encountered when fitting the silver point into the root canal or when viewing the radiographic verification of its fit. These are depicted in Figure 8–5.

Suppose the point does not seat to the working length of the root canal file responsible for the preparation? If the silver point had been cut to the working length prior to fitting, this problem would be evident before any radiograph was taken, but in any event the radiograph would reveal a situation not unlike that shown in Figure 8–5*B*. When faced with this problem, the first action should be to reconfirm the working length with a root canal file to eliminate the possibility of measurement error or an unforeseen obstruction of the preparation. If the working length is found to be correct, the problem is most likely due to an attempt to fit a silver point whose diameter is at the high range of the allowable tolerance into a preparation made by a root canal file at the low range of the allowable tolerance. The maximum discrepancy attributable to this cause amounts to 0.04 mm, which translates to an apical-occlusal extension of 2.0 mm, as the tapers are identical. Fortunately, the principle of mechanics involved in the cutting of materials always produces a hole of greater diameter than the diameter of the instrument that cuts it, so that the underextension of a silver point attributable to this cause will be less than 2.0 mm. To correct the problem, two options are available, the first of which is preferred. This is to select a silver point of a smaller size and then, using the crown and collar scissors, cut off a portion of its apical end. For each millimeter of the apical end of a silver point removed in this fashion, the diameter of the tip remaining will increase by 0.02 mm. Thus, a size 25 silver point can be converted to a size 28 by the removal of 1.5 mm of its apical end. After cutting, the tip of this resized silver point should be rounded by stroking with a fine cuttlefish disc held between the fingers, so as to remove any sharp edges or flashes produced by the scissors. The disc need not be engine driven, as the silver is very soft and easily abraded. The resized point is then fitted into the root canal — hopefully to the proper extension. An alternative solution to the problem of underextension, suitable only for extreme cases, is to recut the preparation using a larger sized root canal file and then repeat the fitting procedure.

Suppose the point does not seat at the working length or extends beyond the confines of the root canal? If the silver point had been precut to length prior to placement, this problem would also be detectable before taking a radiograph and most certainly would be revealed on the film, as depicted in Figure 8–5A. Overextension of the silver point is easily corrected. That portion of the tip of the silver point that extends beyond the tooth is cut off with the crown and collar scissors, the cut tip is rounded off with a cuttlefish disc as described previously, and the point is reinserted into the root canal. Pressure in an apical direction upon the refitted point should not result in any extension of the point into the root canal beyond the established occlusal reference plane. It is extremely important to have the occlusal end of the silver point cut flush with the occlusal reference plane of the tooth when the initial trial fit of the point is attempted so that this reference point remains constant during adjustments to the apical extension. If the refitted point drops deeper into the preparation than did the initial overextended point, the retention form of the preparation is not restraining the point. When this happens, the refitted point should be discarded after recording its length and noting the amount of overextension removed previously. A fresh silver point of a size larger than the diameter of the tip of the refitted point is selected. For example, if 3 mm of overextension had been removed, this equals 4×0.02 mm of taper or an apical diameter that is now 0.08 mm greater than that of the original point. Hence the new point would have to be at least two sizes larger than the original one was (a size 25 point having 3 mm of its apex removed equals a size 33 point; therefore, a size 35 point is selected to replace it under these circumstances). The fresh silver point should fit the root canal preparation slightly short of what might be expected in more normal circumstances. This is due to the lack of any resistance form in the root canal preparation to prevent the root canal sealer cement from extruding out of the tooth and to the high probability of the architecture of the apex of such teeth being that of two truncated cones joined by their apices. The objectives are to confine the root canal filling to the root canal preparation proper, represented by the truncated cone of the preparation, and to prevent any extension of either sealer or core material into the apical foramen, represented by the short, angulated, truncated cone at the apex. In effect, a Class IIIB preparation is what is being dealt with in most of these cases.

If the point seats to the working length but does not resist removal with the hemostat, it is said to have no frictional retention or "tugback." The problem is evident during manipulation of the point but *is not* revealed on a radiograph. This situation is depicted in Figure 8–5C, in which the only portion of the silver point in contact with tooth structure is at the very apex. This is due to one of two factors. Either the root canal system has a large natural flare and the retention form is not large enough to take this into account, or the root canal has been overprepared by recapitulation or serial filing and the apical collar has been lost. This problem is invariably encountered when attempts are made to fit silver points into root canal preparations designed for gutta percha root canal fillings. To correct the situation, either re-prepare the root canal for silver (if this enlargement of the apical third of the root is technically feasible) or use gutta percha as the core material of choice. In rare selected cases a compromise composite root canal filling consisting of a central core of silver fitting into a short complex apical collar surrounded by laterally condensed gutta percha cones may be considered. Under no circumstances should a single point of silver be cemented into such a preparation, as the success of treatment is overwhelmingly dependent upon sealer cement closing the lateral voids that are present.

The ideal fit of a silver point into a prepared root canal is depicted in Figure 8–5D. In this instance the point extends to a level just short of the working length of the instruments used to prepare the root canal and makes contact with as much of the surface of the apical collar as possible, preferably the entire apical third of the root or certainly not less than the terminal 4 to 5 mm of the preparation. The point cannot be forced apically through the tooth, as the converging walls of the retention form of the preparation restrain it, and cannot be withdrawn from the tooth without the forceful use of the seating hemostat or forceps. The entire procedure is analogous to the trial seating of an inlay or onlay restoration in operative dentistry. Just as the cementation and finishing of the restoration occur after trial seating, so the cementation and finishing of a silver point root canal filling are done after trial fitting, as described. This step of trial fitting is crucial to the success of silver point root canal fillings, for the fit of the fillings determines their ability to cement. By contrast, the fitting of master cones of gutta percha, although important, is not nearly as critical to success or failure, as the gutta percha is molded during the root canal filling procedure by the use of spreaders or pluggers. Remember, no one trial seats an amalgam restoration in operative dentistry, as the material adapts to the walls of the cavity preparation during condensation.

The fitted silver point could simply be cemented into place using a root canal sealer and thereby sealing the root canal system, and this has been recommended by some authors. This approach, however, does not take into account the need for coronal restoration of the tooth following filling of the root canal and is not recommended in practice. The following technique is one that is adaptable to a wide variety of clinical conditions and has proved to be effective and efficient in experienced hands. This technique is illustrated in Figure 8–6.

First, determine the level in the pulp chamber or the prepared root canal at which the central core of silver will terminate after the root canal filling is completed. If post placement in the root following root canal filling is planned, the degree to which the post will extend into the root canal will also have to be determined at this time. Internal posts should be considered in most single-rooted teeth, in the most accessible root of bi-rooted teeth, and

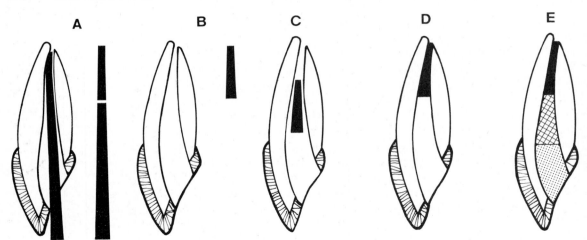

Figure 8–6 Cementing the silver point and filling the root canal. *A*, Filling and sectioning the point. *B*, Coating the preparation and apical portion of the point with sealer cement. *C*, Placing the apical portion of the point in the tooth. *D*, Seating the apical portion of the point to place. *E*, Finished root canal filling.

in the distal root of mandibular molars or the palatal root of maxillary molars. In the inaccessible roots of bicuspids, the mesial roots of mandibular molars, or the buccal roots of maxillary molars (i.e., in those roots of the posterior teeth in which silver cones are likely to be used in current practice) the occlusal termination of the silver core is usually in the area of the pulpal floor orifices to the root canals. In any event once the occlusal level of the silver core after root canal filling has been determined, the silver is cut in two pieces. This provides an apical segment that will be cemented into the root and an occlusal segment that will ultimately be discarded. The two segments laid end to end equal in length the undivided silver point that has been pre-fitted into the tooth (Fig. 8–6*A*).

The root canal preparation should be dry, as noted previously. Preferably the operator should be able to pass a sterile paper point through the canal to the apical soft tissue beyond, and subsequent examination would show a dry paper point with a minute spot of red blood at the very tip of its apex. This assures the operator that the canal is clean, free of exudate, and patent from apical tissues to occlusal access cavity preparation.

The root canal sealer cement should be mixed on a glass slab to a heavy, tacky consistency. When the flat blade of the cement spatula is pressed into the freshly mixed cement and then raised vertically, the cement should cling to the spatula and slab, forming a thick, viscous thread between the two for a distance of 1 cm or more. It is important to have the cement at this consistency rather than too thin, which would result in an uneven seal, or too thick, which would impede placement into the root canal preparation. In cases in which the root canal preparation exceeds size 35, the cement can be transferred to the preparation by means of a paper point, but in smaller sized preparations a root canal instrument may be necessary. In these cases a root canal file one size smaller than that which prepared the canal is used. The objective is to coat the walls of the retention form of the root canal preparation with a film of root canal sealer cement. In doing this the convenience form is also coated with sealer. Paper points coated with sealer cement are wiped against the root canal walls. When using the root canal file, however, the instrument is rotated counterclockwise during withdrawal, depositing material in the process. Some authors recommend the use of engine-driven lentula spirals for this step, but in most instances these spiral devices are unnecessary. The apical portion of the pre-fitted silver point should also be coated with sealer cement. The location of sealer cement on the surface of the root canal preparation and on the apical portion of the pre-fitted silver point is shown in Figure 8–6B.

With the hemostat or point forceps, place the cement-coated apical portion of the pre-fitted silver point into the root canal preparation, positioning it as far apically as possible (Fig. 8–6C). Then, gripping the occlusal portion of the pre-fitted silver point at its occlusal end, place the point into the tooth so that its apical end butts against the occlusal end of the apical portion resting in the root canal. Using apical pressure and the occlusal portion of the pre-fitted section of the silver point as a ramrod, seat the apical portion of the pre-fitted point to place in the retention form or apical collar of the root canal preparation. A root canal plugger with a marker set at a length equal to that of the occlusal portion of the pre-fitted silver point can be substituted for the hemostat–occlusal portion ramrod described above. In most molar teeth the Mortonson plastic instrument will extend from the occlusal plane of the coronal access cavity preparation to the pulpal floor of the tooth and can be used not only to determine the occlusal level for termination of the silver root canal filling but also as a substitute instrument for the final seating of the silver points during cementation. If the silver points have been pre-fitted accurately prior to cementation, there is little danger of pushing the apical portion of the pre-fitted point through the apex of the tooth during cementation (Fig. 8–6D). Of more concern is that the point has indeed seated to the level achieved during fitting. Therefore, once the point has been seated, its position should be checked radiographically. On rare occasions the point, rather than seating, has buckled within the root canal (a danger in preparations with overly flared convenience forms) or the seating instrument has slipped off the occlusal tip of the point when apical pressure was applied. A buckled point can be straightened by passing a smooth explorer alongside, as the silver is soft and malleable. An unseated point can be seated by re-application of the seating instrument. Removing excess sealer cement from the root canal orifice assists in this procedure when it becomes necessary.

Once the silver point is cemented into the apical portion of the root and its position verified radiographically, excess sealer cement in the pulp chamber of the tooth and the orifice to the root canal should be removed by wiping the cavity preparation with cotton pellets dampened with chloroform. In a tooth or root in which a dowel preparation is to be made, several options are open to the operator. He or she can (1) prepare the dowel or post room at this time; (2) wipe the sealer cement from the unfilled middle and/or cervical portions of the root and leave the space empty for the restorative dentist to prepare the post room, as is sometimes done in patient referral situations; or (3) fill the unfilled middle and/or cervical portions of the root with gutta percha. In most instances this last option is preferred. A section of a standardized gutta percha cone approximately equal in diameter to the diameter of the root canal preparation at the level where the silver point terminates is placed within the unfilled preparation and compacted vertically by means of warm root canal pluggers. This process is repeated until the anatomic level of the pulp chamber is reached. In posterior teeth in which

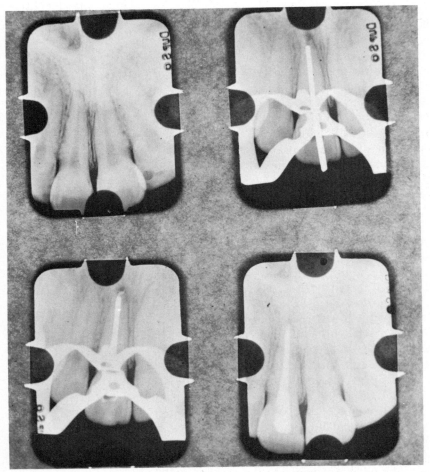

Figure 8–7 Silver point canal filling. *Top left,* Pretreatment. *Top right,* Trial fit of silver point. *Lower left,* Seating of apical portion of silver point. *Lower right,* Finished root canal filling.

the silver point root canal fillings are terminated at the pulpal floor orifices to the root canals, it is wise to compact gutta percha across the entire floor of the pulp chamber to a thickness of approximately 1 mm. This provides a level base for the bases or temporary restorations to follow and a visible indicator (pink) of the location of the floor of the pulp chamber for any operator who may have to re-enter the tooth. Once the gutta percha base has been compacted to place, the remaining coronal portion of the access cavity preparation can be closed with a good grade of zinc oxyphosphate cement. This can either extend through to the occlusal surface, becoming a temporary restoration as well as an internal base to be part of the preparation of the tooth for subsequent restoration, or it can be restricted to the internal portion of the tooth, where it will be used as a base and the surface portion of the tooth then temporarily restored with a suitable material such as IRM cement (Fig. 8–6*E*).

Examples of the technique of filling a root canal with a single silver cone, as described above, are shown in three clinical cases in which the preoperative films, working length determinations, trial fitting of the silver cone, cementation of the silver cone, and finishing of the root canal filling can be seen (Figs. 8–7 to 8–9).

Use of the technique as described avoids the necessity of having to cut off the occlusal extensions of silver points in the pulp chamber of a tooth once the points have been cemented into the roots. Even though when the pulp chamber floor is cleaned of excess sealer, gutta percha is compacted around the protruding points and an oxyphosphate cement base is placed *before* they are cut off, it is still difficult to cut these extensions precisely without dislodging the root canal filling. Only under the extenuating circumstances in which very fine silver points must be used in very constricted openings should this alternative technique be considered. A small diamond stone is used to cut off the extensions, as it has less tendency to entangle or dislodge them than does a bur.

It has often been recommended that silver points should be "notched" or partially cut just before cementation and then work-hardened by twisting back and forth so as to break at the notches after sealing in the roots. This technique of removing excess silver has been used by many practitioners; however, it does not work well when the silver points are less than size 35, since such small points are too fragile for manipulation. Unless the notching is cut completely around the circumference of the silver point, the ability to strain-harden and break is much reduced. This creates clinical problems such as the hazard of withdrawing the apical portion from its apical seat when removing the occlusal portion. Only in a few teeth with limited access and large preparations has this alternative technique been found to have merit.

Precisely machined silver points in which the apical portion is threaded into an occlusal portion are commercially available. This system does not

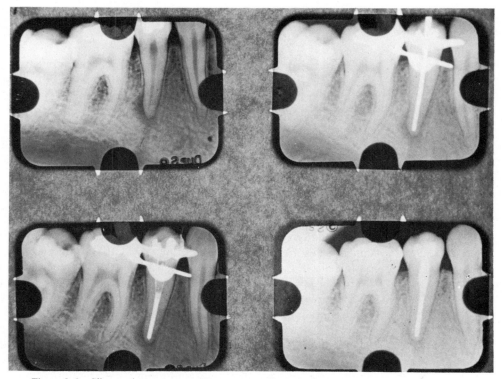

Figure 8–8 Silver point root canal filling. *Top left,* Pretreatment. *Top right,* Trial fit of silver point. *Lower left,* Seating of apical portion of silver point. *Lower right,* Finished root canal filling.

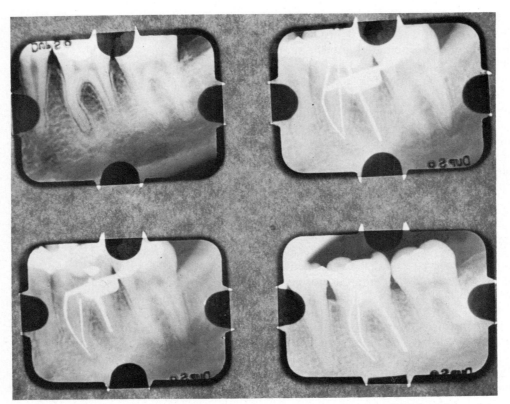

Figure 8–9 Silver point root canal filling. *Top left,* Pretreatment. *Top right,* Trial fit of silver points. *Lower left,* Seating of apical portion of silver point. *Lower right,* Finished root canal filling.

allow apical adjustments to be made in the silver point during trial fitting, nor is it available in the small sizes normally associated with silver point root canal fillings; hence, its use in practice is very limited. The idea, of course, is to cement the point to place and then unscrew and discard the occlusal portion. By contrast, the proposed technique recommended in this chapter uses readily available materials with simple instrumentation in an effective and efficient manner.

SUMMARY AND EVALUATION

The filling of root canals with silver points under the circumstances described is a viable technique in modern endodontic practice. Although its popularity in the United States has waned in recent years, it is undergoing a revival in Scandinavia. In Sweden, studies conducted as to the effectiveness of the carry-over of high quality endodontic care from the dental schools to clinical practice have revealed that teaching of the Ostby type gutta percha techniques leaves something to be desired. However, teaching of "standardized techniques," which in many particulars resemble the technique and philosophy described in this chapter, results in a demonstrably higher level and more consistent quality of endodontic care in clinical practice. This was the American experience after World War II and, as previously noted, was one of the leading factors in the dispersion of high quality endodontic care among the dental profession in North America.

That silver point, or rigid core, techniques are abused in practice cannot be denied. Figure 8–10 shows an example of the consequences of several of these abuses combined in a single clinical case. The patient presented with a history of repeated swellings and discharges from a black, stained area of the mucosa over the root of her maxillary left central incisor despite two root canal fillings and a surgical procedure (Fig. 8–10A). A periapical radiograph of the region dramatically shows the root canal fillings, loss of root apex, and apical pathosis (Fig. 8–10B). Several major abuses of silver point technique are apparent. The silver point does not seal the apex of the tooth. When the

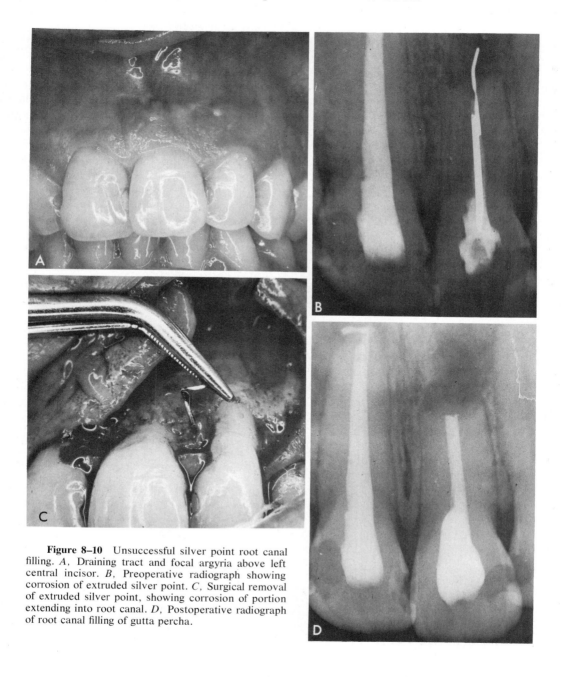

Figure 8–10 Unsuccessful silver point root canal filling. *A,* Draining tract and focal argyria above left central incisor. *B,* Preoperative radiograph showing corrosion of extruded silver point. *C,* Surgical removal of extruded silver point, showing corrosion of portion extending into root canal. *D,* Postoperative radiograph of root canal filling of gutta percha.

tooth was intact and the apical resistance and retention forms of the root canal preparation were present, the silver point was highly unlikely to have fit either. This is evident when one compares the size of the root canals of the adjacent incisors with the size of the silver point in the apex of the tooth in question. The basic principles of root canal preparation and fitting of the silver point were undoubtedly never seriously taken into consideration. Addition of a second silver point to the middle and cervical portions of the root did not alleviate this underlying problem. On the contrary, it added a second problem by precluding the possibility of restoring the tooth with a core and crown. (Fortunate in this instance!) Surgical removal of the root apex further complicated the case, as any possibility of the fit of the silver core into an apical retention form or collar was eliminated. Apicoectomies after silver point procedures without retrograde filling *increase* the possibility of recurrent failure. As far as apical surgery is concerned, the probability of improving the apical seal of a root canal without retrograde filling is nil following the silver point procedure when the critical retention form is affected. However, in the condensed gutta percha technique the apical seal may be improved, as the failures that occur in these cases are due to a lack of apical compaction, whereas the seal is effective higher in the root. The probable location of effective seal in the silver point technique is at the apex and seldom, if ever, in the midsection of the root — the reverse of the probable situation in the condensed gutta percha technique.

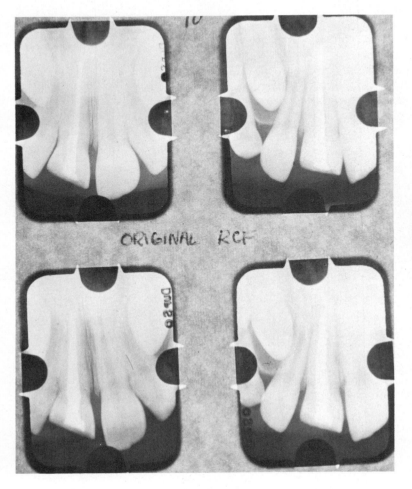

Figure 8–11 Unsuccessful root canal filling. *Top left* and *right,* Pretreatment with silver point and laterally condensed gutta percha to coronal surface. *Lower left* and *right,* Post-treatment with laterally condensed gutta percha in root and cement in coronal portion.

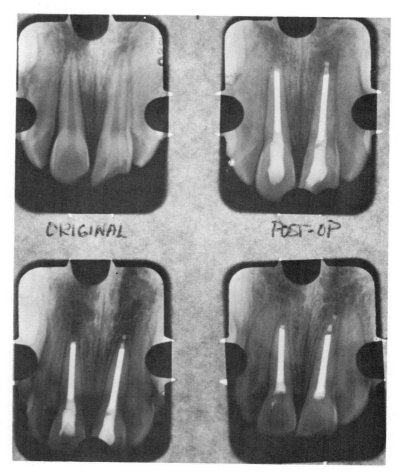

Figure 8–12 Unsuccessful (?) root canal fillings. *Top left*, Pretreatment nonvital teeth with apical areas. *Top right*, Root canal fillings. *Lower left* and *right*, One and 2 year reexaminations with repair of apical areas.

ORIGINAL

POST-OP

Surgical removal of the silver point in this case revealed that the black corrosion seen on the point itself was on that portion of the point that extended into the unsealed root canal (Fig. 8–10*C*). The clean portion in the tissue was responsible for the deposition of silver salts into the cells of the apical granuloma and overlying mucoperiostium. The questions of toxic corrosion products and their relationship to unsealed root canals raised in this case remain unresolved. The refilling of the root canal with condensed gutta percha, a material and technique more suitable to the requirements of a Class IIIB case, is shown in Figure 8–10*D*.

An unsuccessful root canal filling that did not cause clinical symptoms is shown in Figure 8–11. The principal problem in this case is that the central core of silver and the surrounding gutta percha accessory points extend to the coronal surface of the tooth. This does not allow for proper coronal restoration and results in discoloration of the coronal tooth structure. To attempt to cut the silver point down into the tooth to a depth sufficient to eliminate the root canal filling material from the crown, let alone to a depth suitable for an internal core, would undoubtedly result in dislodgment of the point, if not perforation of the root. From an endodontic viewpoint, the technical procedure and clinical result are excellent. From a dental viewpoint, the case is a disaster that requires re-treatment (as was done). In current practice, this root canal probably would not be prepared for nor filled with a silver point.

Similar questions of success or failure can be raised in regard to the

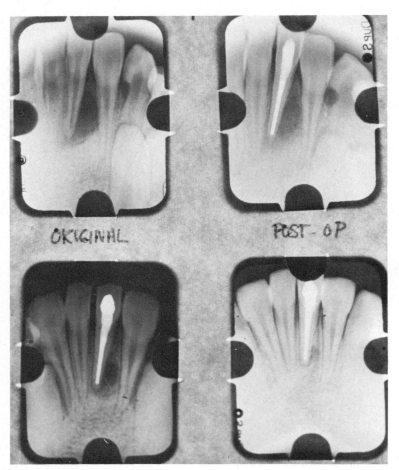

ORIGINAL   POST-OP

Figure 8–13 Unsuccessful (?) root canal filling. *Top left,* Pretreatment nonvital tooth with apical area. *Top right,* Root canal filling. *Lower left* ·and *right,* One and 2 year reexaminations with repair of apical areas.

cases illustrated in Figures 8–12 and 8–13. Both cases show excellent clinical results, with repair and resolution of apical lesions associated with nonvital teeth. Although the silver points do not extend into the coronal area of the tooth and coronal restoration was feasible, their extension into the cervical portion of the root precludes the future construction of post-cores and crowns, should this be necessary. The ability to precisely control the position of the silver point filling in the root canal is dramatically shown in these cases in which the lateral or vertical condensation of gutta percha so often leads to extrusions of filling materials beyond the apex. Are these cases successful? In a limited sense, yes; in the broadest sense, no.

Two examples of successful silver point root canal fillings are shown in Figures 8–14 and 8–15. Figure 8–14 clearly shows the positioning of the silver points within the roots, the gutta percha over them, and the coronal zinc oxyphosphate cement seal, as recommended in the text. Figure 8–15 shows the more usual root canal configurations to which silver point root canal fillings are readily adaptable. Provision for internal coring of the coronal restoration has been provided and utilized in the construction of the retainer for the fixed prosthesis. Evidence of apical repair is also seen in the 14 month evaluation period. Such short-term success with silver point root canal fillings is conceded by even the most ardent opponents of this technique.

The more typical recall and re-examination sequence in endodontic practices has been that of 3 months, 1 year, and 2 years, as shown in Figure 8–16. This case also demonstrates the technique of sealing the apical portion of the root with silver and a subsequent core and restoration of the crown. In practice, the clinician is ill advised to leave the root canal space occlusal to the silver point that seals the apex void of root canal filling material. A better practice is to seal this area with vertically compacted gutta percha, as recommended, and then, if a core is desired, remove this at a later time. The hazard of not sealing lateral canals in this region of the root is always present, and unfilled root spaces, such as that seen in this case between the gold core of the occlusal restoration and the silver point in the apex, are to be avoided.

A major criticism of silver point root canal filling techniques has been leveled at their supposed inability to seal lateral root canals. If the root canal preparations are adequate and the root canal fillings precise, silver points do seal lateral root canals, as shown in Figures 8–17 and 8–18. In these cases, as the tapered silver point was driven to position within a root canal preparation of the same taper, the sealer cement present between the point and the wall of the preparation was compressed and forced laterally. In Figure 8–17, this occurred on the distal aspect of the apical third of the root, whereas in

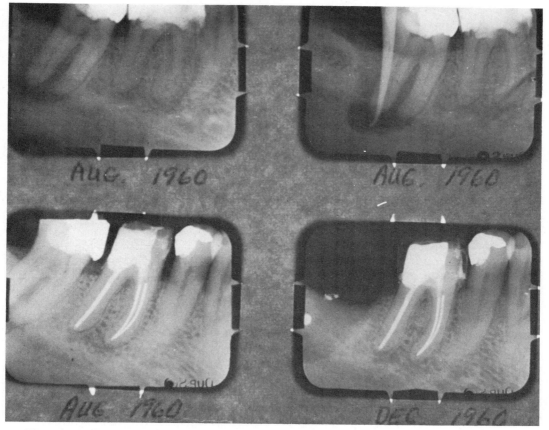

Figure 8–14 Successful root canal filling. *Top left* and *right,* Pretreatment with inoperable second molar and pulpotomy in operable first molar. *Lower left,* Root canal filling. *Lower right,* Re-examination after 3 months.

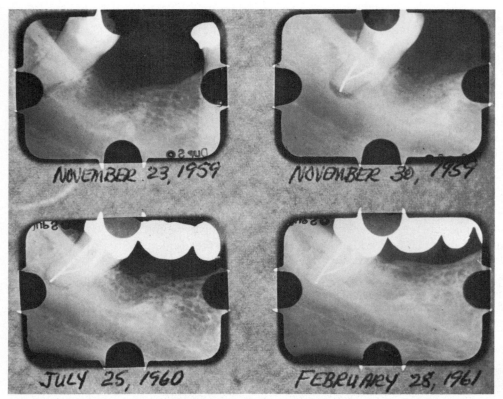

Figure 8–15 Successful root canal filling. *Top left,* Pretreatment nonvital tooth with apical area. *Top right,* Root canal filling. *Lower left* and *right,* Re-examination after 7 and 14 months.

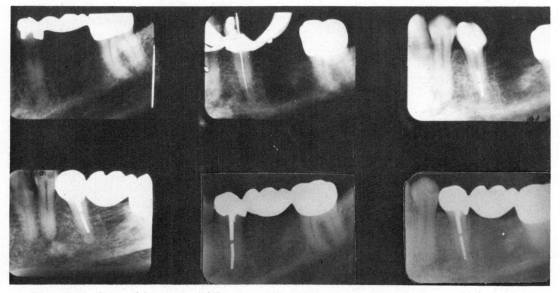

Figure 8–16 Successful root canal filling. *Top,* Pretreatment, length determination, and root canal filling. *Lower,* Re-examination at 3 months, 1 year, and 2 years, showing core and restoration.

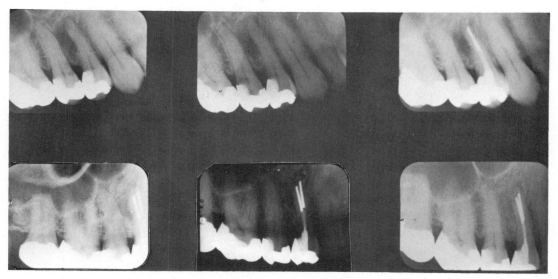

Figure 8–17 Successful root canal filling with lateral canal obturation. *Top,* Pretreatment nonvital tooth with lateral root area and root, filling with lateral and apical canal seal. *Lower,* Re-examination at 3 months, 1 year, and 2 years, showing repair of lesion.

Figure 8–18 this took place on the distal aspect of the medial roots of a molar. These cases demonstrate the necessity of having retention forms prepared for silver points that not only are adequate in size (diameter) but also extend well toward the occlusal or incisal of the tooth.

There is ample proof of the longevity of properly executed silver point root canal fillings. Figure 8–19 illustrates a case in the author's experience in which the buccal roots were sealed with silver points terminating at the floor of the pulp chamber and the palatal root was sealed with gutta percha over the apical silver point. With today's fashions in endodontics, the palatal root

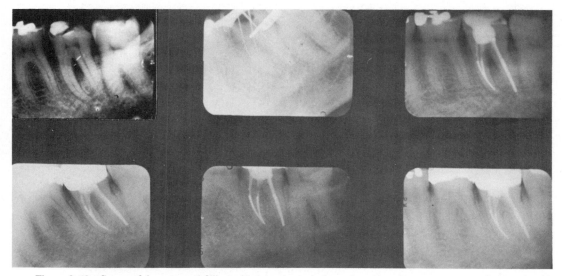

Figure 8–18 Successful root canal filling with lateral canal obturation. *Top,* Pretreatment nonvital tooth with bifurcation involvement. *Lower,* Re-examination at 3 months, 1 year, and 2 years, showing repair of bifurcation lesion.

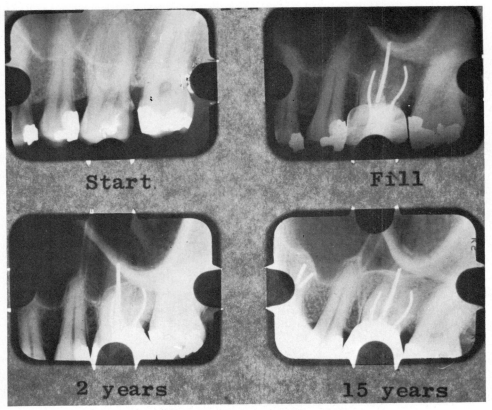

Figure 8–19   Successful root canal filling of 15 years.

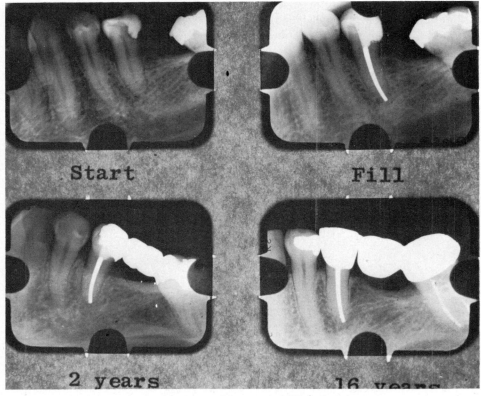

Figure 8–20   Successful root canal filling of 16 years.

would undoubtedly be sealed with all gutta percha and the buccal roots with either gutta percha or silver, as shown. Two cases of 16 years' duration are shown. In one case (Fig. 8–20), sufficient core room was not provided, but this has not prevented the successful use of this bicuspid tooth as an abutment for a fixed prosthesis. In the other case (Fig. 8–21), adequate core room was provided but was never used, and although the radiographic esthetics of this case leave something to be desired, its clinical success is undeniable. Many seemingly routine cases at the time of treatment have exhibited long-term success, as exemplified by the case shown in Figure 8–22.

A critical and objective assessment of the silver point root canal filling technique permits a prognostication for its future. The use of rigid core filling points of pure silver is likely to be discontinued, particularly if a suitable substitute for the metal is developed. This substitute would have to possess the essential physical properties associated with silver points, i.e., radiopacity, flexibility and/or rigidity, and workability with enhanced biocompatibility. Radiopaque plastic points of precision sizes seem to be the best alternatives, but as yet are not available commercially. If these plastic points were able to combine chemically with the sealer material used in cementing them into the root canal system, one of the present root canal filling interfaces could be eliminated. At present, with silver point techniques as well as with most gutta percha techniques, one interface exists between the wall of the root canal filling and the sealer cement and a second interface between the sealer cement and the master core. An advantage of paste or single-system root canal fillings such as Hydron is the elimination of

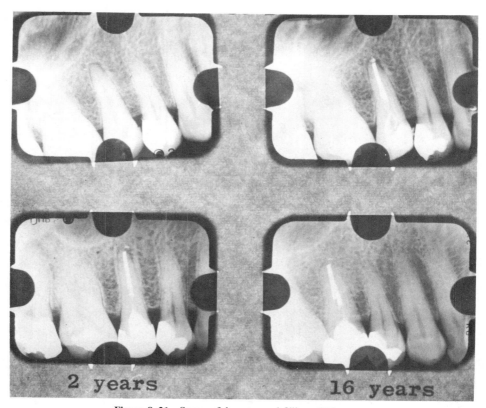

Figure 8–21 Successful root canal filling of 16 years.

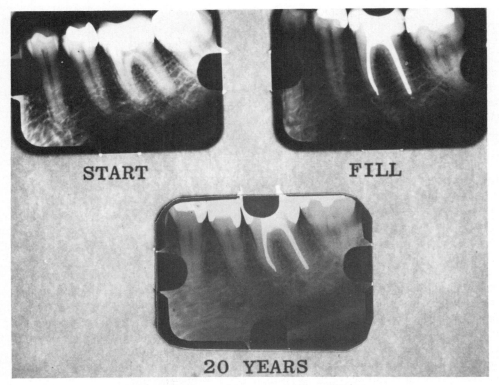

Figure 8–22 Successful root canal filling of 20 years.

one of these interfaces. The attractiveness of a root canal filling technique that provides consistency of result due to preciseness of control by the operator will do much to continue the concept and practice of rigid core filling techniques in endodontics.

REFERENCES

1. Auerbach, M. B.: Filling the root canals of molar teeth with silver wire. J.A.D.A. 46:270, March 1953.
2. Beal, F. H.: Endodontic sealing properties of cavit, chloro-rosin, gutta percha, N2 and silver cones using radioisotopes. MS Thesis, Loma Linda University, May 1972.
3. Besner, E.: The use of silver points in root canals should be discouraged. Va. Dent. J. 50:34, August 1973.
4. Brady, J. M., and del Rio, C. E.: Corrosion of endodontic silver cones in humans: A SEM and X-ray microprobe study. J. Endod. 1:205, June 1975.
5. Campbell, E., Meirowsky, A., and Hyde, G.: Studies on the use of metals in surgery: Comparative fibroblast culture. Ann. Surg. 114:472, September 1941.
6. Cassidy, R. E.: The chilled silver point as a root canal filling material. Oral Surg. 28:235, August 1969.
7. Clark, D. M.: Radioisotope determination of apical seal of silver after ultrasonics. Oral Surg. 43:771, May 1977.
8. Cohen, S., and Burns, R. C. (eds.): Pathways of the Pulp, 2nd Ed. St. Louis, The C. V. Mosby Co., 1980, pp. 173–180.
9. Council on Dental Materials, Instruments and Equipment: Dentists' Desk Reference: Materials, Instruments and Equipment, 1st Ed. Chicago, American Dental Association, 1981, pp. 166–177.
10. Craig, R. G. (ed.): Dental Materials: A Problem Oriented Approach, 1st Ed. St. Louis, The C. V. Mosby Co., 1978, pp. 231–260.

11. Dixon, C. A., and Rickert, U. G.: Tissue tolerance to foreign materials. J.A.D.A. 20:1458, August 1933.
12. Dubrow, H.: Silver points, gutta percha and their role in root canal fillings. J.A.D.A. 93:976, November 1976 (see Letters, J.A.D.A. March 1977).
13. Feldman, G., and Nyborg, H.: Tissue reactions to root filling materials. II. A comparison of implants of silver and root filling material AH26 in rabbits' jaws. Odont. Rev. 15:33, No. 1, 1964.
14. Feldman, G., Nyborg, H., and Conrado, C. A.: Tissue reactions to root filling materials. III. A comparison between implants of the root filling material N2 and silver in the jaws of rabbits. Odont. Rev. 18:387, No. 4, 1967.
15. Grossman, L. I.: Filling root canals with silver points. Dental Cosmos 78:679, July, 1936.
16. Grossman, L. I.: Endodontic Practice, 10th Ed. Philadelphia, Lea & Febiger, 1981, pp. 303–308.
17. Gutmann, J. L.: Can root canal filling with silver points provide an effective root canal seal? A perspective. J. D.C. Dent. Soc. 54:35, Winter 1979.
18. Harris, W. E.: Disintegration of a silver point: Report of a case. J.A.D.A. 83:868, October 1971.
19. Harrison, J. W., and Todd, M. J.: The effect of root resection on the sealing property of root canal obturations. Oral Surg. 50:264, September 1980.
20. Healy, H. J., and Weine, F. S.: The use of measurement of control handles with silver points for endodontic fillings. Fortn. Rev. Chic. Dent. Soc. 52:9, July 1966.
21. Hunter, H. A.: Effects of gutta percha, silver points and Rickert's root sealer on bone healing. J. Can. Dent. Assoc. 23:385, July 1957.
22. Ingle, J. I.: Root canal obturation. J.A.D.A. 53:47, July 1956.
23. Ingle, J. I.: A standardized endodontic technique using newly designed instruments and filling materials. Oral Surg. 14:83, January 1961.
24. Ingle, J. I., and Beveridge, E. E.: Endodontics, 2nd Ed. Philadelphia, Lea & Febiger, 1976, pp. 240–245.
25. Jarrett, J. H., and Narang, R.: Metallic pigmentation from endodontic silver cones. S.C. Dent. J. 38:17, Spring 1980.
26. Jasper, E. A.: Root canal therapy in modern dentistry. Dental Cosmos 75:823, September 1933.
27. Jasper, E. A.: Adaptation and tissue tolerance of silver root canal fillings. J. Dent. Res. 20:355, August 1941.
28. Jasper, E. A.: Essentials in endodontic practice. Oral Surg. 2:1199, September 1949.
29. Kawahara, H., Yamagami, A., and Nakamura, M.: Biological testing of dental materials by means of tissue cultures. Int. Dent. J. 18:443, January 1968.
30. Kesel, R. G.: Critique of methods of filling root canals. *In* Grossman, L. I. (ed.): Transactions of the Second International Conference on Endodontics. Philadelphia, University of Pennsylvania Press, 1958, p. 158.
31. Kirchoff, D. A.: Localized argyria after a surgical endodontic procedure: Report of a case. Oral Surg. 32:613, October 1971.
32. Luks, S.: Gutta percha versus silver points in the practice of endodontics. N.Y. Dent. J. 31:341, October 1965.
33. Marshall, F. S., and Massler, M.: The sealing of pulpless teeth evaluated with radioisotopes. J. Dent. Med. 16:172, October 1961.
34. Messing, J. J.: Precision apical silver point cones. J. Br. Endo. Soc. 3:22, April–June 1969.
35. Moodnik, R. M., Levey, M. H., Besen, M. A., and Borden, B. G.: Retrograde amalgam filling: A SEM study. J. Endod. 1:28, January 1975.
36. Mullaney, T. P.: Silver point break-off technique for endodontic therapy. J. Can. Dent. Assoc. 33:253, May 1967.
37. Nagai, K., and Imazeki, T.: Correlational study between metallographical findings of metals and their tissue reactions in the vital body. J. Nihon U. School Dent. 2:66, December 1959.
38. Natkin, E., Van Hassel, H. J., and Steiner, J. C.: The comparative merits of silver cones and gutta percha in the treatment of fine canals of molar teeth. J. Br. Endo. Soc. 3:59, October–December 1969.
39. Neagley, R. L.: The effect of dowel preparation on the apical seal of endodontically treated teeth. Oral Surg. 28:739, November 1969.
40. Nicholls, E.: Sectional root filling with silver points. Dent. Pract. Dent. Rec. 8:241, April 1958.
41. Randell, S.: Fracture of a silver point root canal filling after eight years. Ill. State Dent. J. 40:29, January 1971.
42. Ritchie, G. M., Weine, F. S., and Smulson, M. H.: Modification for successful use of silver points in endodontics. J. Acad. Gen. Dent. 20:35, March 1972.
43. Seidler, B.: The technic and rationale of filling root canals. N.Y. J. Dent. 24:376, November 1954.

44. Seidler, B.: Root canal filling — an evaluation and method. J.A.D.A. 53:567, November 1956.
45. Seltzer, S., Green, D. B., Weiner, N., and DeRenzis, F.: A scanning electron microscope examination of silver cones removed from endodontically treated teeth. Oral Surg. 33:589, April 1972.
46. Short, L. C.: Use of silver points in root canal obturation. J. Miss. Dent. Assoc. 29:10, November 1973.
47. Siskin, M.: The obturation of the root canal. Dent. Clin. North Am. 1:855, November 1957.
48. Soltanoff, W., and Parris, L.: Controlled silver points filling technique for endodontically involved teeth. J.A.D.A. 65:301, September 1962.
49. Sommer, R. F., Ostrander, F. D., and Crowley, M. C.: Clinical Endodontics, 3rd Ed. Philadelphia, W. B. Saunders Co., 1966, pp. 216–218, pp. 256–274.
50. Spangberg, L.: Biological effects of root canal filling materials. Odont. Rev. 20:133, Nos. 2, 3, 4, 1969.
51. Spangberg, L.: Biological effects of root canal filling materials. Odont. Tedskr. 77:121, April 1969.
52. Strean, L. P.: Oligodynamic action of silver in root canal antisepsis: Preliminary report. Dent. Cosmos 78:241, March 1936.
53. Tainter, J. F., and Ross, P. N.: Opinions and practices of American Board of Endodontics Diplomates. Dent. J. 44:321, July–August 1979.
54. Tayler, R. L.: Physical and chemical properties of selected endodontic silver points. MS Thesis, Northwestern University, June 1975.
55. Venable, C. S., Stock, W. G., and Beach, A.: The effects on bone of the presence of metals based upon electrolysis. Ann. Surg. 105:917, June 1937.
56. Wais, F. T.: Variations in the diametric measurements of root canal files and corresponding sizes of silver root canal points. MS Thesis, University of Michigan, May 1954.
57. Walker, R. T.: The use of amalgam in conventional root canal therapy. J. Br. Endo. Soc. 12:99, July 1979.
58. Weine, F. S.: Endodontic Therapy, 2nd Ed. St. Louis, The C. V. Mosby Co., 1976, pp. 263–286.
59. Weine, F. S., Healy, H. J., and Lippert, J. L.: Use of silver points with improved digital control. J.A.D.A. 83:125, July 1971.
60. Weisman, R. V., et al.: Corrosion of silver and titanium points. J. Br. Endo. Soc. 9:81, July 1976.
61. Wright, J. J. N.: Root canal filling technique using newly designed instruments and silver points. Roy. Can. Dent. Corp. Quart. 3:2, January 1963.
62. Zielke, D. R., Brady, J. M., and del Rio, C. E.: Corrosion of silver points in bone: A SEM and microprobe analysis. J. Endod. 1:356, November 1975.
63. Zwener, O.: Effect of dowel preparation on the apical seal of endodontically treated teeth. J. Endod. 8:687, August 1980.

9

New Directions

INTRODUCTION

MELVIN GOLDMAN, D.D.S.

For the most part, endodontic texts have favored the word "obturate" when describing the filling of the root canal. Obturate connotes total obliteration of a space and this is, of course, the ultimate goal of all endodontic therapy. However, the passing years have produced much research that demonstrates the difficulty of attaining the ultimate goal. Gutierrez and Garcia,[1] Davis et al.,[2] Brayton et al.,[3] Goldman,[4] Wollard et al.,[5] and Larder et al.[6] have published research findings clearly delineating the highly complex anatomy of the root canal space (Figs. 9–1 and 9–2) and the lack of ability of semisolid or solid materials to completely fill or

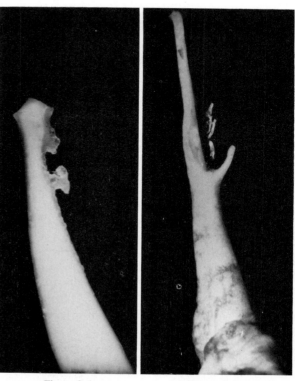

Figure 9–1 Silicone model of prepared canal of upper central incisor. (From Davis, S. R. et al.: Oral Surg. 34:642, 1972.)

Figure 9–2 Silicone model of prepared canal of upper cuspid. (From Davis, S. R. et al.: Oral Surg. 34:642, 1972.)

Figure 9–1   **Figure 9–2**

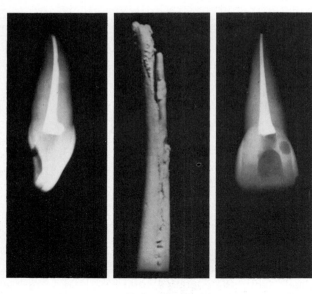

Figure 9–3 Note that the radiographs may indicate a well-condensed gutta percha filling. However, when the tooth structure is dissolved away, the resulting model is far from well condensed. (From Brayton, S. M. et al.: Oral Surg. 35:226, 1973.)

''obturate'' this space (Figs. 9–3 and 9–4). Their work corroborates the work of Hess[7] and emphasizes the need for new directions in endodontic therapy.

One new direction is obviously pointed toward materials for filling that are capable of flowing into irregular spaces, cul-de-sacs, fins, and so forth, for the above-mentioned research clearly indicates that these are present in the vast majority of teeth. A second direction should be toward the redesign of endodontic instruments, for papers by Mizrachi et al.,[8] Walton,[9] Moodnik et al.,[10] and others have shown that our present instruments cannot possibly clean the root canal space as thoroughly as we once believed could be done. A third direction must be toward better irrigants and irrigation techniques, for papers by McComb and Smith,[11] McComb et al.,[12] Baker et al.,[13] and Goldman et al.[14] have shown that our present techniques and materials are not producing the clean canals that we assumed were resulting from our efforts.

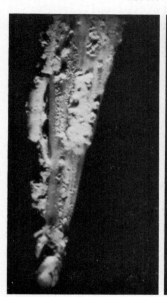
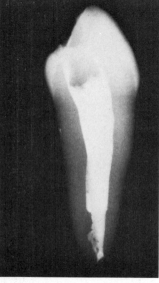

Figure 9–4 Lower bicuspid displaying a lack of correlation between the radiograph and the model similar to that shown in Figure 9–3. (From Brayton, S. M. et al.: Oral Surg. 35:226, 1973.)

Clearly, therefore, if we accept that the goals of therapy are to have a root canal space as clean as possible and filled in all its irregularities, new directions for endodontics are in order. In the following pages we will discuss several aspects of this premise and perhaps establish some signposts toward the endodontics of tomorrow.

Since the preceding discussion applies to endodontic therapy, let us begin by discussing each aspect in general and then describing a new filling technique and material that have recently become available.

INSTRUMENTS AND INSTRUMENTATION

The purpose of instrumentation is threefold: (1) to completely remove all pulp tissue and its remnants; (2) to remove all necrotic debris and/or bacteria; and (3) to smooth, shape, and enlarge the canal space to conveniently accept a filling. A search of the literature reveals that there is a dearth of information about the origin of root canal instruments and instrument design. Broaches to remove pulp tissue are simply barbed shafts that engage soft tissue and require no further discussion except to emphasize that they must always be used so as not to bind in the canal and must never be forced or curved.

K-type files and reamers are twisted, tapered pieces of steel made from either triangular or square blanks and have not been changed for many years. The one vast improvement was provided by Ingle,[15] when he proposed and devised a means of standardizing the diameter, taper, and working length of all endodontic instruments. The various manufacturers have complied with the profession's request for standardization and manufacturing tolerances, and this has somewhat eased the burden of the practitioner. Hedstrom files have become popular in the recent past, and many feel that they are superior to K-type files. Unfortunately, when double-blind studies have been carried out, they have uniformly failed to demonstrate that one kind of file is superior to another.[8, 10] In fact, these studies have shown that neither K-type nor Hedstrom files adequately fulfill the requirement of thoroughly removing all material from the root canal space. Scanning electron microscopy by Moodnik et al.,[10] McComb and Smith,[11] McComb et al.,[12] Mizrachi et al.[8] and Goldman et al.[14] all demonstrate that (1) many areas of the canal wall are untouched by the instruments, (2) debris may be left behind, and (3) a "smeared layer" is found on many areas of the wall of the canal space. The nature of this "smeared layer" has been the subject of investigation, and more will be reported on this later in the chapter (Figs. 9–5 and 9–6).

Another facet of canal preparation must be considered with the advent of mechanical preparation aids. Many claims have been made by both proponents of this technique and the manufacturers. Among the advantages claimed are faster preparation of the canal space, elimination of the rubber dam, and more thorough preparation. Unfortunately these are merely claims and again, when subjected to the scrutiny of double-blind research studies, are not capable of being substantiated. Harty and Stock,[16] O'Connell and Brayton,[17] Weine et al.,[18] and others have shown that mechanical preparation of the canal space is not faster, is not better, and has no significant advantages over our present system of hand-held instruments, unless one considers that the use of a rubber dam is a significant disadvantage.

However, our present methods do leave much to be desired, for

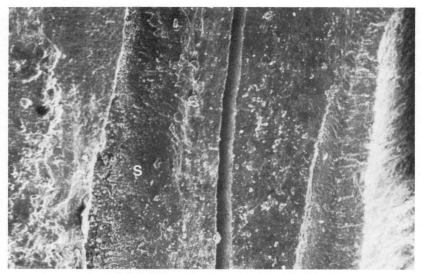

Figure 9–5 Scanning electron microscope photograph of canal wall showing ''smeared layer.'' Note that dentinal tubules cannot be seen. Area (S) is magnified in Figure 9–6. (Original magnified 60×.) (From Goldman, L. B. et al.: Oral Surg. 48:79, 1979.)

certainly the canal space is not as clean as it should or could be. It is obvious that there is a great need for redesigned instruments. Hopefully these will be forthcoming in the not too distant future.

IRRIGANTS AND IRRIGATION TECHNIQUES

Several factors become apparent when one considers the highly irregular root canal space. The most obvious is that since our present instruments

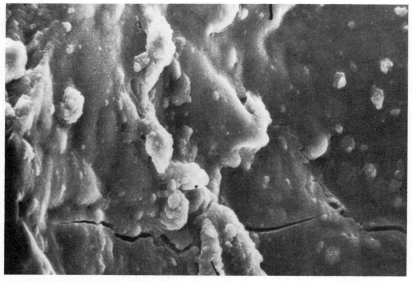

Figure 9–6 Enlargement of area S in Figure 9–5. Note that dentinal tubules are not seen. (Original magnified 2000×.) (From Goldman, L. B. et al.: Oral Surg. 48:79, 1979.)

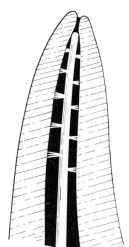

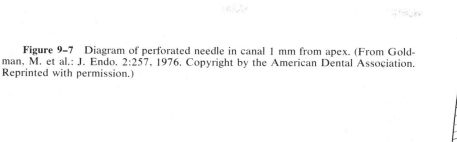

Figure 9–7 Diagram of perforated needle in canal 1 mm from apex. (From Goldman, M. et al.: J. Endo. 2:257, 1976. Copyright by the American Dental Association. Reprinted with permission.)

and instrumentation techniques do not reach many areas of the root canal space, we must reach and cleanse those areas in another manner. Thus, the importance of irrigation and irrigation solutions is tremendously enhanced. Again, the scrutiny of double-blind research studies indicates that we are sorely lacking in our ability to thoroughly cleanse the canal space. McComb and Smith,[11] McComb et al.,[12] Mizrachi et al.,[8] and others have demonstrated that our irrigation techniques are not accomplishing their purpose. That is, the canal space, *especially in the apical portion,* is not being thoroughly cleaned by either instrumentation or irrigation. Goldman et al.[19] have described a new type of perforated irrigation needle and demonstrated that the conventional needle used in the recommended nonbinding manner did not succeed in spraying the irrigating solution throughout the length of the canal space. The perforated needle (Fig. 9–7), which is sealed at its apical end and has perforations along the side, can be placed to within 1 mm of the apex and any irrigating solution can be sprayed directly on the walls of the canal space along almost its entire length. Mizrachi et al.,[8] McComb and Smith,[11] and McComb et al.[12] also emphasized the salutary effects of large volumes of irrigating solutions. Goldman et al.[14] recently published a scanning electron microscopic (SEM) study using a 20 ml final flush of NaOCl and showed a significantly cleaner canal when using the perforated needle than when using the conventional needle.

The "smeared layer" that was referred to earlier is also under investigation. Its presence was reported by several investigators,[10, 11, 12] who also reported that an EDTA solution was able to remove it. Goldman et al.[20] investigated the efficacy of several irrigating solutions and in the course of these investigations discovered that the smeared layer was present *only on that portion of the wall that had been instrumented* (Fig. 9–8). The smeared layer was not removed by prolonged soaking in 5% NaOCl, but was removed by a 17% solution of EDTA (Fig. 9–9). This would indicate that this layer is caused by instruments in contact with the wall and is probably composed of a slurry of dentin filings, for it is removed by a chelating agent and is not affected by an organic tissue solvent such as 5% NaOCl. Recently, Wayman et al.[21] also showed that a smeared layer was present and that it was removed by solutions of citric acid in various strengths and was not affected by the NaOCl. This would seem to corroborate Goldman and associates' findings as to the nature of the smeared layer.

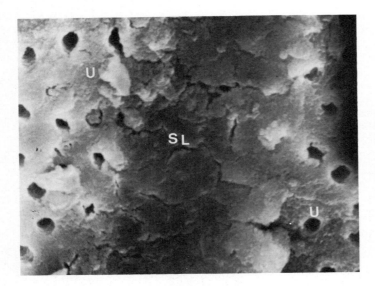

Figure 9–8 Scanning electron microscope photograph of prepared canal soaked in 5% NaOCl for several hours. The dark area in the center is a groove made by the file. The smeared layer is SL. On either side (U) is a portion of the canal wall that is not instrumented and is very clean, with clearly patent dentinal tubules. (Original magnified 2000×.) (From Goldman, L. B. et al.: Oral Surg. 52:197, 1981.)

Of course, the question arises now as to whether it is necessary to remove the smeared layer. Goldman et al.,[20] Moodnik et al.,[10] McComb and Smith,[11] and McComb et al.[12] have all determined that the layer is not adherent to the surface of the wall. Goldman et al.[20] have determined that the smeared layer is about 1 micron thick. However, it does block the dentinal tubules, and all indications are that any layer that is interposed at the interface of the filling and the wall cannot be beneficial. In addition, other studies by Benkel et al.[22] have shown that a filling material such as poly-HEMA (to be discussed) is able to penetrate the dentinal tubules (Fig. 9–10). All intracanal drugs that are used in endodontics operate by vaporizing throughout the canal. If the dentinal tubules are blocked, they may contain bacteria, which then could not be reached by either the bactericidal vapors of the intracanal drugs or the irrigating solutions.

Therefore, it would seem that the smeared layer cannot serve any useful purpose but rather, on the one hand, could hinder effective bactericidal

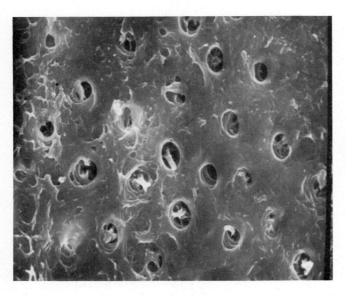

Figure 9–9 A section of instrumented canal wall flushed with EDTA. The section is very clean with no evidence of a "smeared layer." (From Goldman, L. B. et al.: Oral Surg. 52:197, 1981.)

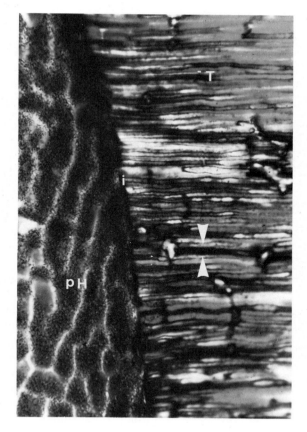

Figure 9–10 High power photomicrograph of area of canal wall demonstrating poly-HEMA in the tubules (pH = poly-HEMA, T = tubules, i = interface between filling and dentin; arrows point to material in tubule). (Original magnified 480×.) (From Goldman, M. et al.: J. Endo. 2:196, 1976. Copyright by the American Dental Association. Reprinted with permission.)

action and, on the other hand, could block more effective sealing by a filling material.

Thus, in the past several years a better understanding of the root canal space has led to important strides being taken to develop a more efficient means of delivering any irrigation solution and also to developing more efficient irrigation solutions or a combination of same.[20, 21]

FILLING MATERIALS AND TECHNIQUES

As with irrigation and irrigation solutions, some important innovations have appeared recently that seem to point toward new directions. These take into account the highly irregular root canal space and attempt to provide a means of more completely filling this space. One that has been available for some time is the endodontic pressure syringe, which is used with a zinc oxide–eugenol (ZOE) paste. The second is the use of thermoplasticized gutta percha with a special syringe. These two previously available materials are used with innovative techniques to better suit the needs that have become apparent.

The third is a new material, a hydrophilic plastic called poly-HEMA, which has recently been introduced and which seems to have many advantages. The following is a description of this material and the technique of its use.

Poly-hydroxy-ethylmethacrylate (Poly-HEMA)

Physical and Chemical Properties.   Poly-HEMA is a hydrophilic plastic that was developed for use as a biocompatible implant material. Wichterle and Lim[23] first described the material and pointed out that its hydrophilic property allowed for the free interchange of low molecular weight solutes in and out of the material. The chemical composition and the safety data have been exhaustively studied and need not be repeated here.[24-28] Suffice it to say that the material has a long history of nontoxicity and superior biocompatibility when used as an implant. The adaptation and use of poly-HEMA as a root canal filling material have been reported,[22, 29-31] and it seems to have many qualities that make it useful for this purpose. A delivery system for its use has been developed, which makes the material simple and easy to deliver into a root canal space. The superior biocompatibility of poly-HEMA makes it ideal for a filling material, since even if there is an inadvertent slight overfill into the periapical tissues (which, of course, is not recommended), the material will be well tolerated and seems to exert no toxic effect. Kronman et al.[32] have reported that poly-HEMA will not support bacterial growth, and Goldman et al.[33] have reported that it is not penetrable by highly motile *Proteus* bacteria. These factors, along with the histologic evidence of penetration of dentinal tubules (see Fig. 9–10), as reported by Benkel et al.,[22] seem to indicate a superior seal.

When the paste and powder are mixed, they form a gel. When the gel is forced through the delivery system by the pressure of the syringe, it becomes a liquid because of its thixotropic nature. Thixotropy is the property of a gel whereby it becomes a liquid when subjected to pressure and returns to a gel state when the pressure is released. This provides a material that is ubiquitous and flows freely into all the irregularities. Once the pressure is released, the material returns to its gel state and then proceeds to complete polymerization and cross-linking. The working time in the canal is 6 to 8 minutes, which allows for working radiographs of the fill to be seen and correction of the fill if necessary. Polymerization is complete in 15 to 17 minutes. The peak exotherm (in the small quantities in the root canal) is 37° C. The free monomer (which is soluble) is 0.17 per cent of the total weight.

Before polymerization and cross-linking are complete, the material is completely soluble, and on occasion an overfill into the periapex will seem to have disappeared in follow-up radiographs taken some time later. However, the solubility is available only *before* polymerization, and depending on the amount of fluid available in the periapical tissue, some of the excess may be dissolved away in the first 6 to 8 minutes. Once polymerization and cross-linking have been completed (after 15 minutes), there is no known solvent for the material, and it has not been seen to be broken down by the body, according to any histologic studies to date.

Instrumentation.   The preparation of the canal space to receive the poly-HEMA filling does not differ substantially from the techniques of preparation for any of the other filling regimens. Canals should be thoroughly debrided and filed and shaped. Whether one prepares to the apical opening or just short of it is not of great importance and depends only upon the habits of the clinician. The use of K-type files, Hedstrom files, or mechanical aids is also not of significance, depending, again, only upon the expertise of the clinician. It is recommended that the coronal one third of the canal be carefully flared to facilitate the insertion of the delivery tip. This flaring can be done with hand instruments or with a #3 or #4 Gates-Glidden bur. Probably it is better to prepare the entire canal one or two sizes larger than one is accustomed to. There are two reasons for this. (1) Research studies showing the irregularity of the root canal space indicate that we probably should prepare our canals larger than we are accustomed to, in order to render them as clean as possible. (2) The material is made radiopaque by the addition of 35% barium sulfate ($BaSO_4$). The radiopacity is not as evident as with gutta percha or silver cones, and thus a slightly larger canal enhances the radiographic appearance. Barium sulfate has a toxicity rating of zero.[34]

After preparation is completed, the canal should be thoroughly washed with irrigating solution, the proper intracanal dressing placed, and the canal sealed, but one must be aware of certain precautions concerning irrigants and intracanal medication. Tests done on the polymerization of the materials showed that alcohol, EDTA, and R-C Prep have minimal effects on polymerization. Lidocaine (Xylocaine), water, NaOCl, and H_2O_2 have borderline effects, since they affected the polymerization slightly when present at the 10 per cent level. However, if the canal is thoroughly dried by paper points, there is no problem. Surprisingly, saline inhibited polymerization at very low levels, as did providone-iodine solution and formocresol. Therefore, the last three materials should not be used when poly-HEMA is to be the filling material.

Delivery System and Filling Technique. The criteria for determining when the canal space is ready to be filled with poly-HEMA are the same as those generally accepted by the profession for filling with other materials. That is, the tooth must be comfortable and must not display percussion or palpation sensitivity or any other clinical symptoms, and there must be no sinus tract. The use of the rubber dam is mandatory and cannot be eliminated.

Before the filling technique is outlined, the specially designed armamentarium must be described.

DELIVERY SYSTEM. The delivery system has two components: a syringe and a delivery tip. The syringe consists of a cylindrical barrel that houses a plunger and is machined to very close tolerances. The plunger has threads placed at its proximal end below a crossbar, which is used to turn the plunger (Figs. 9–11 and 9–12). The delivery tips are available in four different sizes — #24, the largest, corresponds to a #60 file; #26 corresponds to a #50; #28 corresponds to a #40; and #30, the smallest, corresponds to a #30

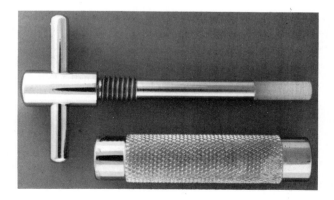

Figure 9–11 Delivery syringe for poly-HEMA.

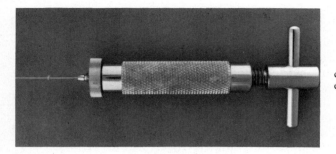

Figure 9–12 Delivery syringe assembled with delivery tip ready for use. (From Goldman, L. B. et al.: Quint. 2:101, February 1979.)

file. The tip is 1¾ inches long, with a blunted distal end. The proximal end of the tip is attached to a hub and a reservoir. The latter has a volume of 0.5 ml (Fig. 9–13).

Recently a newer model of the delivery system has been marketed. This is a one-handed syringe that uses a permanent stainless steel reservoir to which a disposable dental needle with a metal hub is attached (Fig. 9–14). There is also a new mixing capsule being marketed. The paste and powder are placed into the capsule, the small plastic pellet is placed inside, and the mix is placed in any amalgamator (Fig. 9–15).

In order to have complete polymerization, the root canal filling material is supplied in preweighed containers of paste and powder. The specific ratios are 2.55 gm of paste to be mixed with 0.45 gm of powder. The powder is supplied in small plastic capsules. Mixing directions are included with each kit and are quite simple.

Filling Technique. The technique that has been developed to utilize poly-HEMA as the sole root canal filling material is not difficult. However, as with any technique, there are certain steps that must be followed to insure complete filling of the canal space:

1. Isolate the tooth with a rubber dam and remove the temporary filling and the intervisit dressing. Probe the canal to insure the patency of the preparation, making certain that there are no ledges or other obstructions present. You may flush the canal with any appropriate irrigant. Dry the canal thoroughly with appropriately sized sterile absorbent paper points *to the apex.*

2. Select the filling tip that fits tightly to a point 1 mm short of the working length. The tip is supplied with a stylus that should be left in place so that the lumen will not be crimped if a curve is required in the tip to negotiate a curved canal (Fig. 9–16). A marker is put on the tip, which is then placed into the canal to the desired depth (Fig. 9–17). A periapical radiograph should be taken to verify the tip's position. *Note:* In multi-rooted teeth; several tips can be placed and one radiograph taken to verify (Fig. 9–18).

3. After the proper tip has been fitted and the proper length marked, it should be removed from the tooth. A sterile absorbent paper point, large enough to fit the canal 1 mm from the working length, *should be left in the canal until just prior to the introduction of the root canal filling material.*

4. Open the plastic pouch containing the paste and squeeze the entire contents of the pouch onto a clean, dry slab. Add the entire capsule of powder. Using a clean, dry stainless steel spatula, thoroughly mix the two components for *60 seconds,* using the entire surface of the slab. It is very important to thoroughly incorporate all the powder into the paste to insure a

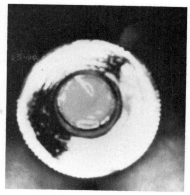

Figure 9–13 Reservoir end of delivery tip filled with material. It holds about 0.5 cc.

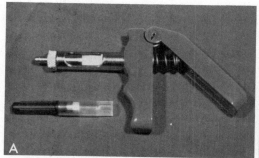

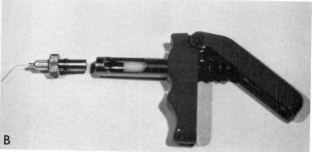

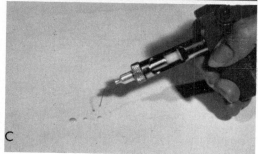

Figure 9–14 Delivery system utilizing one-handed syringe with permanent stainless steel reservoir to which a disposable dental needle with a metal hub is attached. *A*, Syringe and needle to be attached. *B*, Syringe hub and reservoir detached, ready for filling with mixed Hydron. *C*, A few drops of the material being extruded.

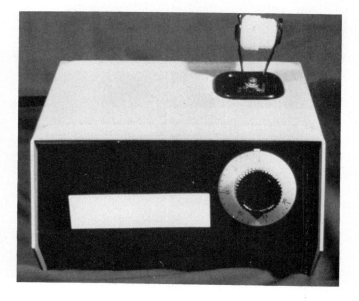

Figure 9–15 Capsule ready to be mixed (see text).

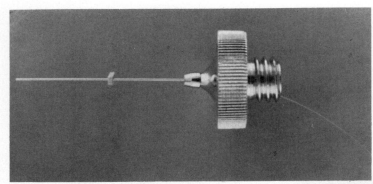

Figure 9–16 Delivery tip with stylus in place and rubber marker. (From Goldman, L. B. et al.: Quint. 2:101, February, 1979.)

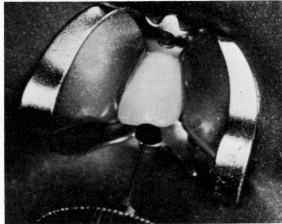

Figure 9–17 Tip placed into tooth to depth indicated by marker. (From Goldman, L. B. et al.: Quint. 2:101, February, 1979.)

Figure 9–18 Three delivery tips placed into molar, each with a different colored marker. (From Goldman, L. B. et al.: Quint. 2:101, February, 1979.)

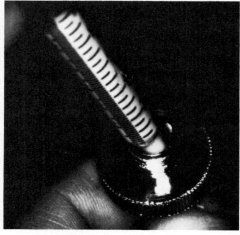

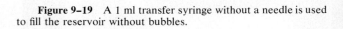

Figure 9–19 A 1 ml transfer syringe without a needle is used to fill the reservoir without bubbles.

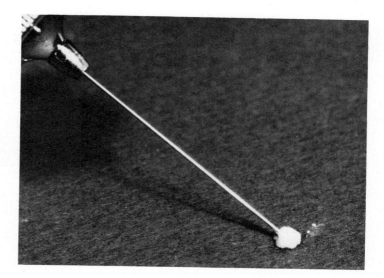

Figure 9–20 The syringe is assembled and a small amount of material is forced out to be certain that the system is patent and delivering. (From Goldman, L. B. et al.: Quint. 2:101, February, 1979.)

homogeneous mix by pressing the spatula firmly against the slab while mixing. After 20 to 30 seconds, a pale pink color develops, indicating the onset of polymerization.

5. Remove the stylus and load the mixed material into the tip receptacle using a 1 ml transfer syringe (without a needle). The syringe is then placed in the receptacle end of the delivery tip and the poly-HEMA is deposited, without entrapping air bubbles (Fig. 9–19). The barrel of the syringe is placed on the tip and tightened by turning *counterclockwise*.

6. Place and engage the plunger by turning the crossbar clockwise one or two turns or until a small amount of the material is extruded from the end of the delivery tip (Fig. 9–20). The tip is then placed in the canal to the previously determined length, so that it is slightly wedged near the apex.

7. With the tip in its most apical position, the crossbar should be turned *one or two half turns. Remember:* the volume of the root canal is only 0.02 to 0.04 ml. Gently release the tip from the bound position, withdraw about 1 mm, and keep turning the crossbar continuously until the material is seen in the pulp chamber. The tip is slowly withdrawn *while turning the plunger* to continuously deposit the paste so as to prevent the formation of voids.

8. After removal of the delivery tip, a sterile cotton pledget is used to condense the excess material into the canal. Additional pledgets should be used to remove *all* excess polymer from the pulp chamber.

9. A periapical radiograph should be taken to verify the completeness of the filling. If incomplete, the tip can be reloaded and the canal refilled by reinserting the tip through the previously deposited material. Because the working time is between 6 and 8 minutes, there should be no problem in reintroducing the tip. Once a successful filling is obtained and all excess polymer is removed from the pulp chamber, a stiff mix of a polycarboxylate cement or Cavit* may be condensed into the access cavity and pulp chamber, filling it completely. Since poly-HEMA absorbs fluid and expands slightly after setting, the temporary filling may be forced out of the tooth if this material is not removed from the pulp chamber before the temporary filling is placed.

---

*Premier Dental Supply Co., Philadelphia, Pa.

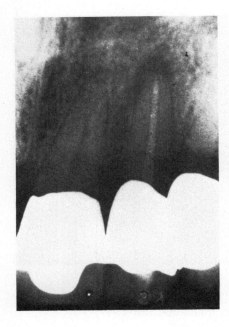

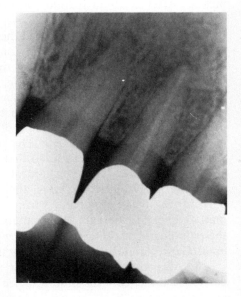

Figure 9–21   Immediate post-fill radiograph. (From Goldman, L. B. et al.: Quint. 2:101, February, 1979.)

Figure 9–22   Check radiograph more than 1 year post-fill.

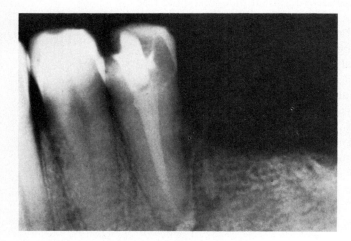

Figure 9–23   Immediate post-fill radiograph. Note that a small amount of material seems to have extruded through a sinus tract.

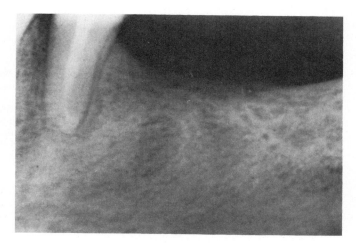

Figure 9–24 Radiograph 1 year post-fill. Note healing. Patient removed excess, which protruded through a sinus tract. Small apical overfill remains, for the material is nonresorbable and biocompatible.

10. After the rubber dam is removed, a final radiograph should be obtained (Fig. 9–21). Follow-up films are taken later (Figs. 9–22 to 9–24).

11. The delivery tip is discarded, but it is imperative to disassemble the syringe immediately and wash it thoroughly before polymerization begins.

Summary. Poly-hydroxy-ethylmethacrylate (poly-HEMA), as formulated for use as a root canal filling material, has many advantages. It seems to fulfill the 11 requirements for a root canal filling material that Grossman lists in his text.[35]

1. It is easily introduced into the root canal.

2. It is liquid or semisolid upon insertion and becomes solid afterward. Its final set consistency in the root canal space is closely akin to rubber base impression material.

3. It seals the canal laterally as well as apically (see Fig. 9–10).

4. Although it does shrink after being inserted, the hydrophilic property causes it to absorb fluid to a net expansion of about 9 per cent.

5. It is not affected by moisture.

6. It does not encourage bacterial growth.

7. It is radiopaque owing to addition of 35% $BaSO_4$ (which has a toxicity of zero).

8. It cannot stain tooth structure.

9. It does not irritate periapical tissue.

10. It is sterile in the package before insertion.

11. It is easily removed from the root canal if necessary.

REFERENCES

1. Gutierrez, J. H., and Garcia, J.: Microscopic and macroscopic investigation on results of mechanical preparation of root canals. Oral Surg. 25:108, January 1968.
2. Davis, S. R., Brayton, S. M., and Goldman, M.: The morphology of the prepared root canal utilizing injectable silicone. Oral Surg. 34:642, October 1972.
3. Brayton, S. M., Davis, S. R., and Goldman, M.: Gutta-percha root canal fillings (Part I). Oral Surg. 35:2, February 1973.
4. Goldman, M.: Evaluation of two filling methods for root canals. J. Endo. 1:2, February 1975.
5. Wollard, R. R., Brough, S. O., Maggio, J., and Selzer, S.: SEM examination of root canal filling materials. J. Endo. 2:4, April 1976.

6. Larder, T., Prescott, A., and Brayton, S. M.: Gutta-percha — a comparative study of three methods of obturation. J. Endo. 2:40, October 1976.
7. Hess, W.: The Anatomy of the Root Canals of the Teeth of the Permanent Dentition, Part I. New York, Wm. Woods & Co., 1975, pp. 1–47.
8. Mizrachi, S. J., Tucker, J. W., and Seltzer, S.: A scanning electron microscopic study of the efficacy of various endodontic instruments. J. Endo. 1:324, October 1975.
9. Walton, R.: Histologic evaluation of different methods of enlarging the pulp canal space. J. Endo. 2:10, October 1976.
10. Moodnik, R. M., Dorn, S. O., Feldman, M. J., Levey, M., and Borden, B. G.: Efficacy of biomechanical instrumentation — an SEM study. J. Endo. 2:261, September 1976.
11. McComb, D., and Smith, D. C.: A preliminary scanning electron microscopic study of root canal after endodontic procedures. J. Endo. 1:238, July 1975.
12. McComb, D., Smith, D. C., and Beagrie, G. S.: The results of in vivo endodontic chemomechanical instrumentation — a scanning electron microscopic study. J. Br. Endo. Soc. 9:11, 1976.
13. Baker, N. A., Eleazer, P. D., Averback, R. E., and Seltzer, S.: Scanning electron microscopic study of various irrigation solutions. J. Endo. 1:127, April 1975.
14. Goldman, L. B., Goldman, M., Kronman, J. H., and Lin, P. S.: Scanning electron microscopic study of a new method of irrigation during endodontic treatment. Oral Surg. 48: 79, July 1979.
15. Ingle, J. J.: A standardized endodontic technique utilizing newly designed instruments and filling materials. Oral Surg. 14:83, January 1961.
16. Harty, F. J., and Stock, G. J. R.: The giromatic system compared with hand instrumentation in endodontics. Br. Dent. J. 137:239, 1974.
17. O'Connell, D. T., and Grayton, S. M.: Evaluation of root canal preparation with two automated endodontic hand pieces. Oral Surg. 39:2, February 1975.
18. Weine, F., Kelly, R., and Bray, K.: Effect of preparation with endodontic hand pieces on original canal shape. J. Endo. 2:10, October 1976.
19. Goldman, M., Kronman, J. H., Goldman, L. B., Clausen, H., and Grady, J.: New method of irrigation during endodontic treatment. J. Endo. 2:257, September 1976.
20. Goldman, L. B., Goldman, M., Kronman, J. H., and Lin, P. S.: The efficacy of several irrigation solutions for endodontics — an SEM study. Oral Surg. 52:2, August 1981.
21. Wayman, B. E., Kapp, W. M., Pirrero, G. J., and Lazzari, E. P.: Citric and lactic acid as root canal irrigants in vivo. J. Endo. 5:9, September 1979.
22. Benkel, B. H., Rising, D. W., Goldman, L. B., Rosen, H., Goldman, M., and Kronman, J. H.: The use of a hydrophilic plastic as a root canal filling material. J. Endo. 2:7, July 1976.
23. Wichterle, O., and Lim, D.: Hydrophilic gels for biologic use. Nature 180:117, 1960.
24. Dreifus, M., Holeckova, E., and Wichterle, O.: Evaluation of hydrocolloid plastic substances on tissue cultures. Cesk. Oftal. 18:268, July 1962.
25. Barvic, M.: Reaction of the living organism to the presence of acyrlic allografts and possible carcinogenic effects of such grafts. Acta Univ. Carol. Med. 8:707, 1962.
26. Kocvara, S., Kliment, K., Kubat, J., Stol, M., Ott, Z., and Dvorak, J.: Gel-fabric prosthesis of the ureter. J. Biomed. Mat. Res. 1:325, 1967.
27. Tollar, M., Stol, M., and Kliment, L.: Surgical suture materials coated with a layer of hydrophilic hydron gel. J. Biomed. Mat. Res. 3:301, 1969.
28. Sprincl, L., Vacil, J., and Kopecek, J.: Biological tolerance of ionogenic hydrophilic gels. J. Biomed. Mat. Res. 7:123, 1973.
29. Rising, D. W., Goldman, M., and Brayton, S. M.: Histologic appraisal of three experimental root canal filling materials. J. Endo. 1:172, May 1975.
30. Kronman, J. H., Goldman, M., Lin, P. S., and Kliment, C.: Evaluation of intracytoplasmic particles in histiocytes after endodontic therapy with a hydrophilic plastic. J. Dent. Res. 56:7, July 1977.
31. Goldman, L. B., Goldman, M., Kronman, J. H., and Kliment, C.: The use of a hydrophilic plastic as a root canal filling material — delivery system and technique. Quint 2:172, February 1979.
32. Kronman, J. H., Goldman, M., Goldman, L. B., Coleman, E., and Kliment, C. K.: Microbiologic evaluation of poly-HEMA root canal filling material. Oral Surg. 48:2, August 1979.
33. Goldman, L. B., Goldman, M., Kronman, J. H., and Letourneau, J. M.: Adaptation and porosity of poly-HEMA in a model system using two microorganisms. J. Endo., 6:8, August, 1980.
34. Sax, N. I.: Dangerous Properties of Industrial Materials. New York, Van Nostrand Reinhold Corp., 1968, p. 452.
35. Grossman, L. H.: Endodontic Practice, 6th ed. Philadelphia, Lea & Febiger, 1965, p. 235.

INJECTION MOLDED GUTTA PERCHA

JAY MARLIN, D.M.D.

The root canal system is usually obturated with solid materials, such as silver cones or gutta percha in conjunction with a sealer. Gutta percha possesses flow properties, especially when heated; whereas silver does not. Although solvents can also be utilized to facilitate the flow of gutta percha, voids are frequently left when the solvents evaporate. Advantage has been taken of both heating and solvent types of flow characteristics.[1-6] Currently, the obturation techniques most commonly used involve lateral condensation, vertical condensation of warm gutta percha, or gutta percha softened by a solvent such as chloroform.

Until recently, gutta percha did not satisfy two of Grossman's requirements for an ideal root filling material.[7] Specifically, it was not a semisolid upon insertion, becoming a solid afterward, and it would on occasion shrink after being inserted, when used with a solvent. With the recently developed technique of injection molded thermoplasticized gutta percha. these shortcomings are overcome.

Injection molding involves heating the gutta percha to a plastic state and forcing it, under mechanically generated pressure, into a prepared root canal space. The formulation of gutta percha used in endodontic therapy is characterized as "low heat," meaning that it softens in the range of 93° C.[7a] The heat at which gutta percha decomposes has not been published. In the initial experiment by Yee et al.,[8] gutta percha would extrude from the experimental syringe at a glycerin bath temperature of 110° C, but consistent flow was obtained at 160° C. The present syringe (unloaded) reaches a maximum temperature of 176° C in the heating element and a maximum of 123° C at the needle tip. The high temperatures in both of these syringes are necessitated by the extremely poor conductivity of the gutta percha. Maximum temperatures are used for short periods of 2 to 3 minutes to facilitate the flow, while at the same time preventing breakdown of the gutta percha. After injection, the material is condensed as it solidifies, so that it retains the shape of the internal outline of the root canal system.

With this approach, there is excellent adaptation to the surfaces of the root canal walls and complete obturation without any evidence of shrinkage.[8-9] In an in vitro study by Yee et al.,[8] teeth were cleaned and shaped utilizing a standardized method and were then obturated with injection molded thermoplasticized gutta percha, with and without a sealer. The results were compared with results from control teeth obturated by lateral condensation with sealer, as described by Luks,[5] and by vertical condensation of warm gutta percha with a sealer, as detailed by Schilder.[6] Utilizing radiographs, visual inspection of fillings recovered after tooth decalcification, and dye penetration, it was found that the injection molded technique resulted in a sealing of the root canal space that was equal to or better than that resulting from the control techniques. Fin-like extensions, cul-de-sacs, and webs along the pulp chamber floor, many of which remained untouched during the cleaning and shaping procedures, were obturated with the injection molded technique, as were multiple foramina and accessory and lateral canals.

The technique was further evaluated by Torabinejad et al.,[9] utilizing the scanning electron microscope. These findings confirmed the earlier observations that injection molded gutta percha in conjunction with the use of sealer represents a practical approach to the obturation of the root canal space in vitro.[8] Adaptation of the injected gutta percha root canal fillings to the root canal space is equal or superior to that of fillings produced by generally accepted procedures that were tested and are known to be clinically successful.

TECHNIQUE

Practical aspects of the experimental techniques of injection molding needed technical improvement and development before the method could be clinically applied on a large scale. This author in conjunction with two engineers, Don Herskovitz and Martin Stiglitz, developed the current injection molding device (Fig. 9–25) to facilitate usage. The syringe consists of several components: a barrel, a plunger, an inherent heating element with its control mechanism, and an assortment of 18, 20, and 26 gauge needles. Canals that are not sufficiently prepared to accept a 25 gauge needle would compromise success with any technique used.

The barrel inserts into the heating element so that their cylinders are continuous. This section of the assembled syringe is insulated to protect patient and clinician from thermal injury. The needle is attached onto the free end of the heating element. The plunger pushes the gutta percha through the barrel and heating element, where it is softened so that it can be extruded through the needles. The plunger is designed to prevent backward flow of gutta percha. The needles are designed to retain the heat so as to facilitate the flow of the thermoplasticized gutta percha.

Local anesthesia, pretreatment, rubber dam application, and access are all accomplished in the usual manner. The objective of the cleaning and shaping procedure is to shape the root canal system appropriately for obturation with gutta percha. A constriction at the apical terminus of the canal is required to limit the apical flow of filling material at that point, as it would be for any gutta percha technique. After the desired shape of the root canal system has been obtained, culturing and temporization are handled in the usual manner and the patient is scheduled for the obturation procedures.

At the filling appointment, the syringe is loaded from the rear with

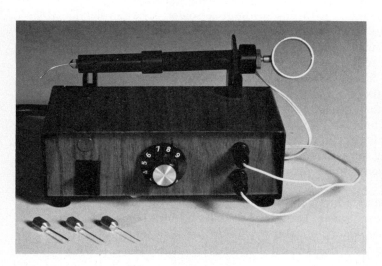

Figure 9–25 Injection molding syringe with control unit. The unit regulates the voltage to the heating element contained within the syringe, which allows extrusion of gutta percha of the correct consistency through the specially designed needles. The syringe is fully insulated to prevent thermal injury to both patient and clinician. Dental gutta percha is loaded ahead of the plunger, which is designed to prevent backward flow of the plasticized material.

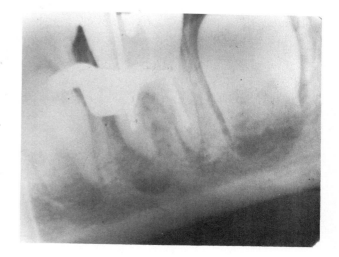

Figure 9–26 Mandibular left first molar. Needles fit in mesio-buccal and distal canals.

commercially available gutta percha cones. The control unit regulates the current to provide the appropriate heat within the syringe. A needle is selected to fit the canal to within 3 to 5 mm of the apex (Fig. 9–26), with smaller canals requiring insertion closer to the apex. A drop of sealer is wiped along the coronal half of the canal. The sealer acts as a lubricant, which facilitates both the flow and the condensation of the gutta percha. When the gutta percha is heated to the appropriate temperature, it flows freely from the needle. At this consistency it will adhere to a surface and string into a thread-like strand several inches from that surface to the tip of the needle (Fig. 9–27). At the proper temperature, the gutta percha is not uncomfortable to the touch.

The initial deposition of injected gutta percha is illustrated in Figure 9–28. A series of pluggers, which are dipped in alcohol to prevent adhesion of the gutta percha to the instrument, are used to condense the filling material to the apex. Additional gutta percha is injected to fill the body of the canal. The completed procedure is illustrated in Figure 9–29.

The usual period of time required to introduce the gutta percha and fill a

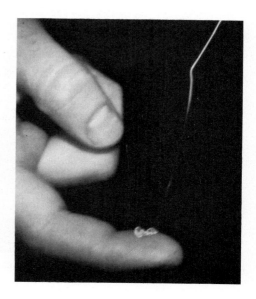

Figure 9–27 Extrusion of gutta percha of the proper consistency. Gutta percha is adherent to any surface, in this case a finger. It is noteworthy that at the correct consistency the gutta percha is not uncomfortable to the touch. At this stage, one has the ability to draw the gutta percha into an extremely fine thread.

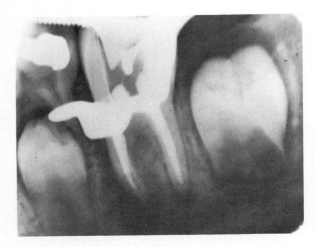

Figure 9–28 Initial deposition of injected gutta percha in all canals.

canal is 30 seconds to 1 minute. On completion of the injection process, the gutta percha retains sufficient plasticity to allow manual condensation for up to 2 to 4 minutes, depending on the diameter of the canal.

The two illustrated cases (Fig. 9–30) show that the technique can be utilized throughout the mouth. Six month to 1 year recall radiographs of 56 teeth with original periapical radiolucencies show a 96.4 per cent incidence of partial or complete resolution; of 69 teeth without any original periapical radiolucent areas, 97.2 per cent revealed no radiographic changes. All patients were clinically comfortable.[10]

SUMMARY

In summary, a new method of root canal obturation utilizing injection molded gutta percha has been described. In vitro and in vivo evaluation indicates that it is at least equivalent and possibly superior to conventional obturation approaches. Additionally, the injection molding technique offers several advantages. First, it is a simpler method for introducing sufficient gutta percha to fill the root canal system. Second, there is considerable

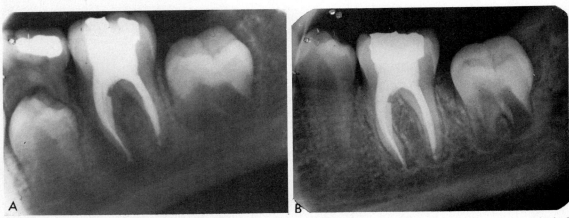

Figure 9–29 *A*, Completed case after condensation. *B*, 6 month recall. Note extent of bone fill in periapical areas.

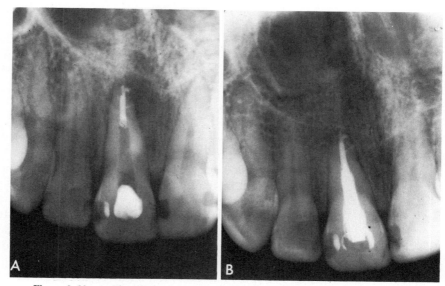

Figure 9–30 *A*, Final film of maxillary left central incisor with post space preparation. Post space can be prepared immediately after condensation. Note lateral canal into area. *B*, 6 month recall, showing complete resolution of periapical and lateral areas and post reinforcement.

conservation in chair time, which potentially can make endodontic treatment available to more patients. Finally, the technique holds the promise of being more efficient *without* sacrificing quality.

REFERENCES

1. Coolidge, E. D.: The teaching of the technique of cleaning, curetting and filling root canals. J. Nat. Dent. Assoc. 5:335, April, 1918.
2. Callahan, J. R.: Resin solution for the sealing of dental tubuli and as an adjuvant in the filling of root canals. J. Allied Dent. Soc. 9:53, March, 1974.
3. Conrad, W. K.: Materials used in root-canal technique in dental practice. Dental Cosmos 76:311, March, 1934.
4. Berg, B.: The endodontic management of multirooted teeth. Oral Surg. 3:399, March, 1953.
5. Luks, S.: Gutta percha versus silver points in the practice of endodontics. N.Y. State Dent. J. 31:341, 1965.
6. Schilder, H. Filling root canals in three dimensions. Dent. Clin. North Am. 11:723, 1967.
7. Grossman, L. I.: Endodontic Practice, 6th ed. Philadelphia, Lea & Febiger, 1965, p. 339.
7a. Gabel, A. B.: American Textbook of Operative Dentistry. Philadelphia, Lea & Febiger, 1956, pp. 612–614.
8. Yee, F. S., Marlin, J., Krakow, A. A., and Gron, P.: Three dimensional obturation of the root canal using injection-molded, thermoplasticized dental gutta percha. J. Endo. 3:168, May 1977.
9. Torabinejad, M., Skobe, Z., Trombly, P. L., Krakow, A. A., Gron, P., and Marlin, J.: Scanning electron microscopic study of root canal obturation using thermoplasticized gutta percha. J. Endo. 4:245, August 1978.
10. Marlin, J., Krakow, A. A., Desilets, R. P., and Gron, P.: Clinical use of injection-molded thermoplasticized gutta-percha for obturation of the root canal system. A preliminary report. J. Endo. 7:277, June 1981.

"ENDOSONIC ENDODONTICS," THE ULTRASONIC SYNERGISTIC SYSTEM

HOWARD MARTIN, D.M.D.
WALTER CUNNINGHAM, D.D.S., M.S.

INTRODUCTION

Ultrasonic energy is being increasingly employed in biology and medicine as an advanced method for developing controlled physical and chemical changes. Endosonic endodontics, an ultrasonic synergistic system, is an advancement in endodontic treatment that utilizes this high technology within biologic parameters. The system introduces a facile, almost completely automated technique that enables the operator to rapidly debride, shape, irrigate, disinfect, and obturate the root canal system.

This is achieved by the use of a newly designed endosonic handpiece that allows an endosonic file to be attached to an ultrasonic power source (Fig. 9–31). In addition, new advances in metallurgic bonding have allowed the development of a diamond-coated endosonic file that has been shown to be an important part of the ultrasonic debridement system. The endosonic handpiece has a flow-through component that enables a biocidal irrigant to pass along the file and into the root canal system (Fig. 9–32). The file and the irrigant are energized and activated by the ultrasonic energy transmitted through the handpiece. This energized file is able to rapidly and effectively debride the intracanal wall, while the activated irrigant is able to flush, remove, and clean the canal. In addition, the ultrasonic activation of the irrigant enhances its bactericidal qualities for greater disinfecting ability. Obturation is accomplished by using the oscillatory heating mechanism and vibrational energy of ultrasound to weld the gutta percha into a compressed, homogeneous mass that seals the canal in its various dimensions.

Ultrasound, the basis of the system, is a form of mechanical energy. The ultrasonic energy has three important components: separate effects, additive effects, and interactive effects. These three action forms of energy have been combined into one multidimensional system — endosonic endodontics, the ultrasonic synergistic system of endodontics.

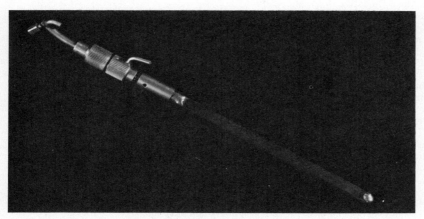

Figure 9–31   The endosonic handpiece with attached transducer (photograph by Ray Wilder).

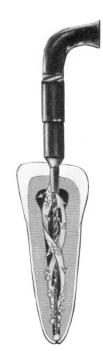

Figure 9–32 Endosonic irrigation (drawing by Phyllis Reidy).

INTRACANAL DENTIN REMOVAL

Endodontic debridement consists of the complete removal of organic debris and necrotic dentin. In the endosonic system, the endosonic file is activated by ultrasonic waves that pass through the endosonic handpiece. As the ultrasonic wave passes within the instrument, a continuous transfer of energy occurs along the entire length of the file that energizes the endosonic file into a very efficient and highly active three-dimensional state for canal preparation.[1]

A further innovation in ultrasonic mechanical debridement is the development of the endosonic diamond file. Diamond particles have excellent properties for conducting ultrasonic energy, and the structure and high elastic constants of a diamond make it one of the hardest cutting materials available. Owing to the constant irrigation and energy wave, the endosonic diamond files are disinfected and self-cleansing. This is because a germicidal irrigant, e.g., sodium hypochlorite, is continuously flowing over, around, and along the file while the constant vibratory oscillating action of the energy sound wave cleans and prevents debris from clogging the asperities of the diamond. Thus, chemo-mechanical root canal debridement is improved by utilizing a more effective intracanal dentin-removing instrument.

The significant superiority of the dentin-removing ability of the energized endosonic instruments, especially the endosonic diamonds, as compared with hand manipulation, is shown in Table 9–1.[2] Standardized canals were developed in roots and then prepared with hand instrumentation or files and diamonds powered by ultrasound. The roots were gravimetrically analyzed before and after instrumentation to determine the amount of intracanal dentin removed. The results demonstrate that the use of ultrasound as the energy source enables the operator to mechanically prepare the root canal with greater ease and effectiveness. When coupled with the

TABLE 9–1   A Comparison of Dentin-Removing Ability*

Type of File	Power Source	Mean Weight Loss (mg)
K-type	Hand	2.56 ± 0.63
Diamond (fine)	Hand	3.01 ± 0.49
Diamond (coarse)	Hand	5.54 ± 0.84
K-type	Ultrasound	4.67 ± 1.14
Diamond (fine)	Ultrasound	7.20 ± 1.05
Diamond (coarse)	Ultrasound	11.40 ± 2.18

*From Martin, H., Cunningham, W., and Norris, J.: Oral Surg. 50:566, 1980.

synergistic component of flow-through irrigation, this allows a canal preparation that enhances debridement, disinfection, and obturation. It achieves the very important goal of an exceptionally clean root canal by the multidimensional synergistic ultrasonic system of endosonic endodontics.

DEBRIDEMENT

Endodontic debridement is considered the key to successful therapy, but numerous canal cleansing studies have shown conventional or serial techniques of filing to be only partially successful. The endosonic system, however, incorporates a highly efficient intracanal dentin-removing method, coupled with an improved and activated high-volume irrigation system. The activation of the irrigant with ultrasonic energy enables the intricate canal morphology to be penetrated and flushed clean of organic debris (Figs. 9–33 and 9–34).[3, 4] The ability to clean the root canal ramifications is due to several physical actions of ultrasound. The implosion and stress-vacuum effects of cavitation dislodge, withdraw, and disperse debris into solution, allowing for easy aspiration and removal. Implosion is the shearing of fluids due to the energy of ultrasound, leading to transient voids and the immediate inward

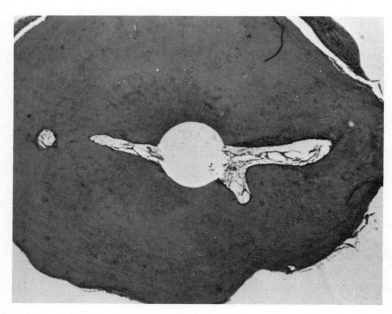

Figure 9–33 Apical portion of hand-filed canal illustrating remaining debris.

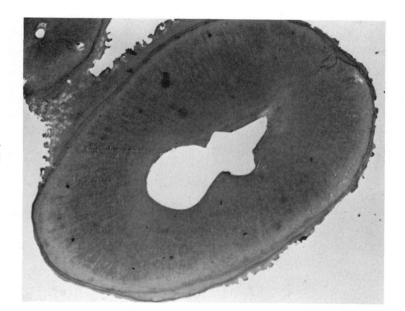

Figure 9–34 Apical portion of ultrasonically filed canal illustrating clean canal space.

collapse of these areas. The implosion effect creates severe pressure changes, localized heat gradients, shock, and rupture of the surrounding fluids and particles (e.g., bacteria) in the area. As such, a vacuum effect is also created, based upon classic principles of mechanical physics. The vacuum action causes the aspiration of debris from the canal ramifications into the main channel. This allows for easy aspiration and removal by the usual suction apparatus. The severe agitation of cavitation creates an effective scrubbing action, which also enhances the cleansing effectiveness (Fig. 9–35). The scanning electron microscope photograph illustrates the exceptionally clean wall of the canal and its dentin tubules.[4] This was accomplished by flow-through irrigation, activated by ultrasound, using 2.5% sodium hypochlorite alone. This demonstrates the improved chemical action of endosonic irrigation, which is a significant feature in the multidimensional endosonic system. Additionally, the synergistic component of

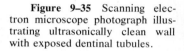

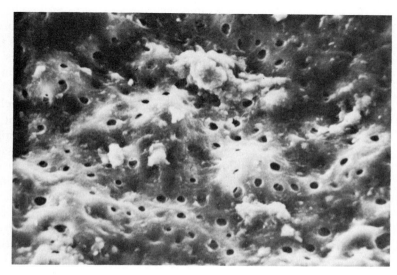

Figure 9–35 Scanning electron microscope photograph illustrating ultrasonically clean wall with exposed dentinal tubules.

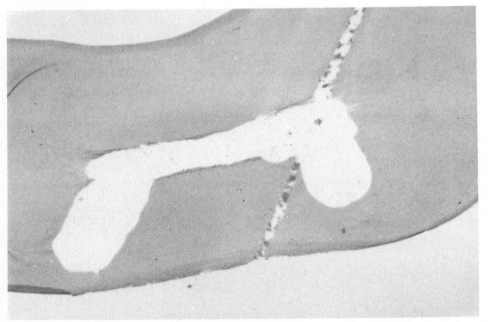

Figure 9–36 Intercanal space and mesial canals debrided and cleansed by endosonic activated irrigation with 2.5% sodium hypochlorite.

heat activation due to cavitation and hysteresis adds to and improves the ability of sodium hypochlorite irrigant to act as a solvent.[5] This allows the activated irrigant to clean the intercanal space between mesial canals in mandibular molars (Fig. 9–36) and the many aberrations of single canals. The additive components of dentin and debris removal by aspiration lead to improved morphologic access. In essence, an intracanal ultrasonic bath is created that leads to a significantly cleaner root canal in all its dimensions.

DISINFECTION

Ultrasonic debridement and continuous high volume irrigation, along with aspiration, enable the irrigant to be a more effective biocidal agent since organic detritus that depletes the solution is rapidly removed from the root canal. The endosonic file accurately guides the biocidal irrigant into the canal, and precurving allows for penetration of both irrigant and file into dilacerations. The ultrasonic energy acts as a catalytic activator for the irrigant flowing through the endosonic attachment and along the file. The energized file agitates and stirs the irrigant, thus producing a significant increase in chemical activity as well as the high pressure, disruptive effects of cavitation. The physical actions of cavitation, heating, and acoustic streaming lead to bacterial destruction by disrupting the cell membrane, by affecting bacterial nuclear material, and by altering the bacterial biochemical enzyme systems. It has been shown that the energy of ultrasound on microorganisms, by means of these physio-chemical effects, increases the irrigant's biocidal activity and significantly reduces the bacterial population (Table 9–2).[6] A more severe test included the killing of the spore *Bacillus subtilis*, in a neutral saline solution within the canal, by endosonics versus

TABLE 9–2   Bactericidal Effect of Ultrasonics with Medicament and Horse Serum Protein**

Time (min)	STAPHYLOCOCCUS AUREUS		STREPTOCOCCUS FAECALIS	
	NaOCl	Acid Pentanedial	NaOCl	Acid Pentanedial
0.0	2,400,000	3,300,000	2,600,000	3,700,000
2.0	6,000	40,000	0	940
4.0	4,800	12,000	0	0
6.0	0	0	0	0

*From Martin, H.: Oral Surg. 42:92, 1976.

hand manipulation. The results showed that hand treatment reduced spores by 62 per cent, whereas endosonics killed 86 per cent of the spores, indicating significant superiority for disinfection by endosonics.[7] In addition, the warming of sodium hypochlorite irrigant improves its ability to kill organisms known to be a part of the endodontic microbial flora.[8] The inherent energy loss within the ultrasonic generator, due to hysteresis, is utilized to warm the irrigant as it flows through the endosonic handpiece. By reduction of concentration and concurrent warming, the biocidal activity of NaOCl may be maintained while the irritation potential is reduced.

Therefore, this ultrasonic synergistic system makes use of these separate effects of ultrasound — physio-mechanical, chemical, and thermal — in an additive and synergistic manner to significantly improve root canal disinfection.

OBTURATION

Ultrasonic obturation of the root canal is achieved by utilizing an endosonic plugger to weld and compact gutta percha by means of thermo-acoustic and mechanical vibratory actions. Ultrasonic vibrations generate heat, which can be used to weld gutta percha cones into a homogeneous mass. Simultaneously, the softened gutta percha is being condensed by the vibratory motions of the endosonic plugger.

These actions effectively force the filling material laterally into the morphologic ramifications of the root canal system, thereby creating a solidly condensed, three-dimensional obturation.

Technique.   The technique used in ultrasonic obturation is both simple and controllable. Once proper access has been obtained, the canal orifice is located and length is determined in the classic manner.

The endosonic file is then utilized, as illustrated in Figure 9–37, for the rapid and efficient debridement and shaping of the root canal. Smaller sized files, e.g., #10, #15, and #20, are generally used in posterior canals. This allows for easier penetration as well as maintenance of the apical matrix and canal form. Each ultrasonically activated file accomplishes the dentin removal of files two to three times its own size. The middle and cervical portions of the canal are prepared with the endosonic diamond file for greater bulk-dentin removal and to prepare the proper tapered funnel. Simultaneously, the high-volume irrigant and aspiration cleanse the root canal space of debris and microorganisms.

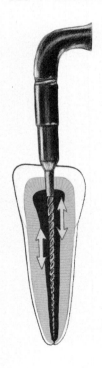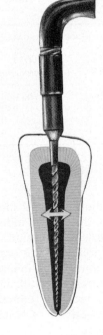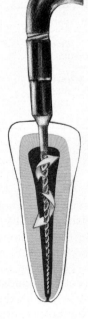

Figure 9–37 Endosonic file manipulation for canal preparation (drawing by Phyllis Reidy).

When canal preparation has been completed, the canal is dried in the standard manner with appropriately sized absorbent points. The endosonic plugger is then used with gutta percha and sealer to warm and compact the filling material into the complex anatomy of the root canal space. This ultrasonic technique combines the features of both the warm and lateral condensation methods into one simple procedure.

CLINICAL FEATURES OF ENDOSONIC ENDODONTICS

Endodontic treatment has been shown to cause or create inflammatory reactions in the periapical area with the subsequent clinical manifestation of pain. The noxious agents are bacteria, chemical and mechanical irritation, and necrotic material. In a comparative clinical study of conventional and endosonic procedures,[9] the elicitation of postoperative pain was less frequent with endosonics. This result may be linked to the reduced intrusion of canal contents into the periapical tissues. In vitro quantitative testing demonstrated that endosonics produced less extrusion of canal debris than did the conventional technique.[10]

REFERENCES

1. Martin, H., Cunningham, W., Norris, J., and Cotton, W.: Ultrasonic versus hand filing of dentin: A quantitative study. Oral Surg. 49:79, 1980.
2. Martin, H., Cunningham, W., and Norris, J.: A quantitative comparison of the ability of diamond and K-type files to remove dentin. Oral Surg. 50:566, 1980.
3. Cunningham, W., Martin, H., and Forrest, W.: Evaluation of root canal debridement by the ultrasonic synergistic system. Oral Surg. 53:401, 1982.

4. Cunningham, W., and Martin, H.: A scanning electron microscope evaluation of root canal debridement with the endosonic ultrasonic synergistic system. Oral Surg. 53:527, May, 1982.
5. Cunningham, W., and Balekjian, A.: Effect of temperature on collagen-dissolving ability of sodium hypochlorite endodontic irrigant. Oral Surg. 49:175, 1980.
6. Martin, H.: Ultrasonic disinfection of the root canal. Oral Surg. 42:92, 1976.
7. Cunningham, W., Martin, H., Pelleu, G., and Stoops, D.: A comparison of anti-microbial effectiveness of endosonic and hand root canal therapy. Oral Surg. 54:238, Aug., 1982.
8. Cunningham, W., and Joseph, S.: Effect of temperature on the bactericidal action of sodium hypochlorite endodontic irrigant. Oral Surg. 50:569, 1980.
9. Martin, H., and Cunningham, W.: An evaluation of postoperative pain incidence following endosonic and conventional root canal therapy. Oral Surg. 54:74, July, 1982.
10. Martin, H., and Cunningham, W.: The effect of endosonic and hand manipulation on the amount of root canal material extruded. Oral Surg. 53:611, June, 1982.

10

Modifications and Special Hints

HAROLD GERSTEIN, B.S., D.D.S.

MODIFICATIONS

After reviewing all the chapters thus far, it must be obvious that the common goal of endodontic therapy is to retain the vitality of the periodontal ligament and eliminate the possibilities for pulpo-periradicular disease. The compromised pulp is sometimes treated to retain vitality in order to maintain the process of root formation. When full endodontic treatment is necessary, a procedure must be used that is most effective for canal debridement and root canal filling.

Although seeing radiopaque material in lateral canals is dramatic, one operator may feel this is most easily accomplished by using a very passive, low pressure technique, whereas another may feel that relatively great pressure is necessary. No one has demonstrated an increased success rate using a technique that emphasizes filling lateral canals.

The following is a technique that the author has used successfully for many years and has found to be easily understood and carried out. It is not intended that these steps be strictly adhered to; rather, utilizing some aspects should be considered.

Filling Technique

A root canal should be filled in a manner that exerts pressure in a vertical and a lateral direction. In order to fill the apical portion of the canal properly, it is necessary to gain optimal access to that area, so the "splugger" (a specially prepared plugger) will exert the desired effect when the canal is filled. This instrument is described later in the chapter.

The process of locating the orifices of canals, preparing the canals to a measured length, and then serially flaring the canals seems to be a backward approach. It is more desirable to "relocate the orifices" further apically before the major canal preparation takes place. In this way, a more direct approach to the apical portion is achieved and the instruments are less influenced by curvature and the cervical dentinal bulge.

If the orifice(s) is(are) located and the canal preparation is carried out, it is obvious that the root canal file must bend around a large arc and be subject

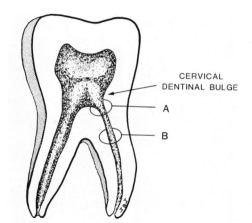

Figure 10–1 Normal cervical dentinal bulge. The objective of preflaring is to relocate the ''orifice'' from area *A* to area *B*.

to the described directional influence (Fig. 10–1). The preparation must take place over a greater curvature. Instead, the operator should locate the canal and effect an initial penetration with small, flexible files (#08, #10, #15 as needed). Then, while the working length film (usually 1 mm short of the radiographic apex) is being processed for verification, the orifice is flared. This is termed ''preflaring'' (Fig. 10–2).

Preflaring

1. Set regular 21 or 25 mm hand root canal reamers so they penetrate approximately 3 to 5 mm into the canal, more if the canal is straight and long enough before reaching a curve. This should be in a relatively straight line (Fig. 10–2*A* and *B*), which is determined by feel and radiographic examination.

2. The reamer tips are blunted by using a diamond nail file or any other suitable grinding instrument (Fig. 10–3). This helps prevent gouging or ledging. As one becomes more adept at this step, blunting the tip becomes judgmental (the author does not blunt).

3. Reamers of appropriate size (#20, #25, #30) are used with a 360 degree turning (reaming) action until the canal wall is firmly felt at the desired depth. It is important to irrigate constantly with sodium hypochlorite and suspend debris and filings for removal. Avoid packing debris into the

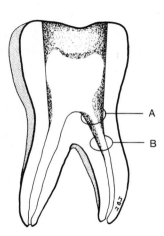

Figure 10–2 After access and preflaring the shaded portion is removed, making area *B* the clinical orifice.

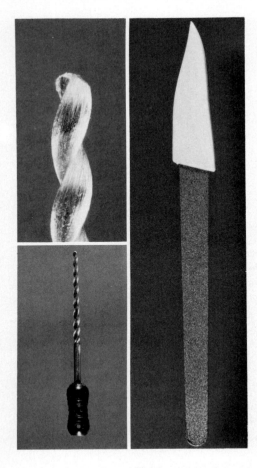

Figure 10–3 *Right,* Diamond nail file. *Lower left,* Reamer with the rounded tip. *Upper left,* Magnified view of the tip of the reamer.

apical third of the canal. Alternate use of Glyoxide* or Perio-Lav† and sodium hypochlorite is advisable. These products contain anhydrous glycerol and urea (carbamide peroxide). Use the aspirator tip over the orifice. The orifice is now transported to mid-root (Fig. 10–2*B*).

4. Mark the working length with stops. Have a definite reference point, as described in Chapter 1.

5. After developing a moderate flare, start the canal preparation at the desired working length, using a strict filing action. If the canal is very tight, create in-between sizes, as described in the following section. Between periods of filing, continue to alternate with the flare preparation. Flare to the desired size — as great as #60 or #70. The preparation then resembles that shown in Figure 10–4.

Many times, the area of greatest resistance is not at the apical portion of the canal but rather at the cervical portion. This is due to reparative dentin deposition as a response to extrinsic factors such as caries, restorations, erosion, and so on. As soon as the orifice is transported apically, the problem becomes negligible, and what was thought to be a very tight canal was in reality a constriction in the cervical canal area or an adverse curvature.

---

*International Pharmaceutical Corp., Kansas City, Mo.
†Spectrumed, Inc., Blue Bell, Pa.

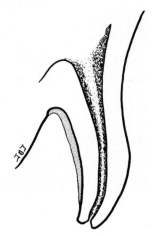

Figure 10–4 Continuous taper from the floor of the chamber of the apex.

The author recognizes the efficacy of using engine-driven instruments such as the Gates-Glidden burs and Peeso reamers but considers hand flaring easier, more predictable, and much safer, since the canal lumen determines the lateral extent of the preparation. The flare is tapered so that the more apical it is, the narrower it becomes and therefore does not endanger the canal wall integrity. During the process of preflaring, pressure can be exerted on one or another of the walls to control the opening. After the canal is filled, there is a ready-made standardized size for future dowel considerations.

The preparation in the apical canal is continued until the desired size is reached. A rule of thumb to employ is that the first file that binds in the apical portion is followed by a file two sizes larger. Use a strict filing action and copious intermittent irrigation. The next procedure is the "single step-back." The stops are set 0.5 mm short of the working length, and the next size instrument is used. The working length is kept patent by returning to the #15 instrument followed in sequence to the last working length instrument. It is important to re-establish patency by returning to the

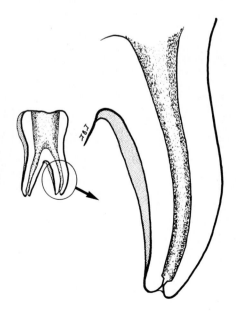

Figure 10–5 Diagrammatic representation of apical step-back. This procedure protects the apical constriction, affords a definite seat for the master cone, and establishes a specific length goal for the master cone.

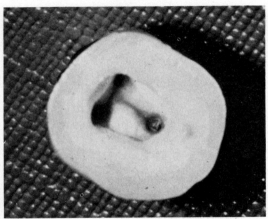

Figure 10–6 Each canal orifice is prepared so each resembles the open end of a funnel.

Figure 10–7 *A,* A #25 file as the final preparation size at the working length (20 mm). This is two sizes larger than the first instrument, which bound. Because of preflaring, the area of binding was not in question. *B,* A #30 file at the single step-back length (19.5 mm), which is 0.5 mm shorter than working length. *C,* Initial working length instrument (#15) in place. There is room for some irrigation, and the debris will be removed. This is followed by use of the #20 and #25 instruments. The next step utilizes the #35 instrument. *D,* The #35 instrument at the single step-back length (19.5 mm), after which Step *C* is repeated.

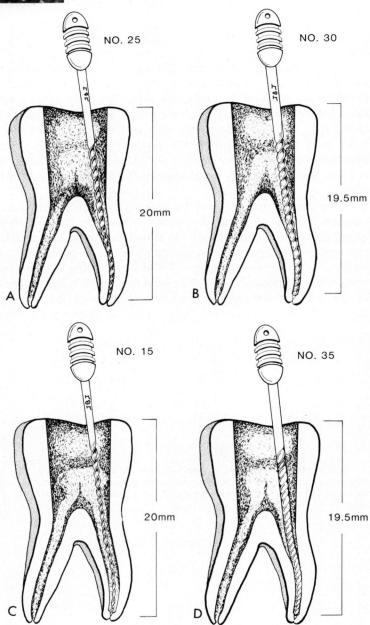

NO. 25

NO. 30

20mm

19.5mm

A

B

NO. 15

NO. 35

20mm

19.5mm

C

D

small sizes because if only the last working length instrument is used, it fills the apical portion so well that it packs debris ahead of it. Another rule of thumb is to increase the preparation by two or three sizes in the step-back position, always returning to the working length #15 instrument and so on. *The step-back position is always 0.5 mm short of the working length.* It is not a sequential step-back. If the canal is very divergent, the walls are planed. Figure 10–5 is a diagram of the theoretical desired result after total preparation.

Note the preparation of the orifices in Figure 10–6. This procedure becomes fast and routine after some practice. Naturally, after reamer preflaring, some operators will follow with the engine-driven orifice openers, which are much safer to use at this time because of the guiding factor of the prepared flare. The preparation technique is illustrated in Figure 10–7. If larger sizes are desired at the step-back length, repeat Step C after each size. The advantages of this preparation technique are:

1. The apical third of the canal is reached by a more direct approach for preparation.

2. A flare is created for "splugger" room. This flare is produced with minimal sacrifice of important dentin, which reduces root strength.

3. There is not a tendency for overpreparation, necessitating the use of larger, stiffer instruments that more easily lead to ledges, perforation, transportation of the apical canal, and weakening of the root. Because of the design of standardized instruments, a relatively flexible instrument at the single step-back length will have the same approximate diameter at mid-root as a stiffer, less yielding, larger file would have at mid-root level.

4. The taper of the canal precludes the possibility of binding at a level coronal to the apical third, which in turn can cause overextension of the master cone during the filling procedure (Fig. 10–8).

5. A more secure apical matrix or stop is created.

6. The length and size of the master gutta percha cone are fixed, so there are no uncertainties as to the desired position.

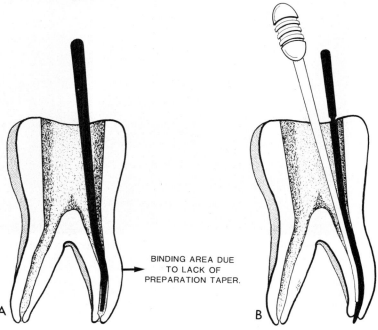

Figure 10–8 *A*, The master cone bound coronal to the apical preparation and was undersized. This problem may be avoided if the apical stop is intact and is well enough developed. *B*, The "splugger" exerts much pressure and if the master cone is grossly undersized and the apical foramen is patent, there is a possibility of overextension.

BINDING AREA DUE
TO LACK OF
PREPARATION TAPER.

A

B

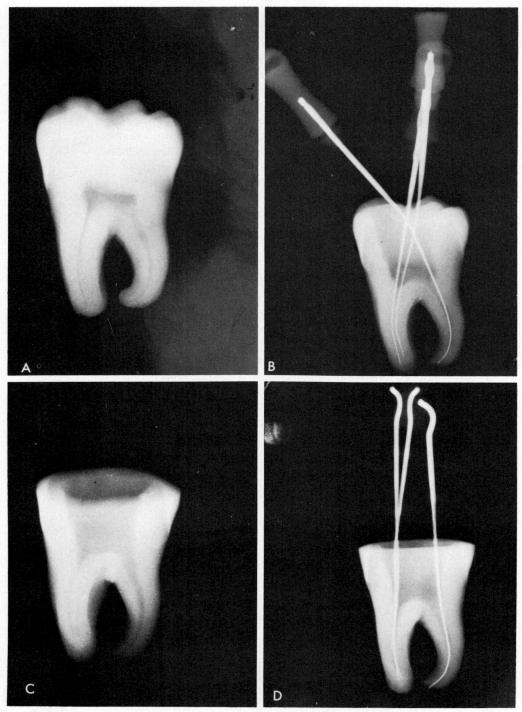

Figure 10–9 *A*, A mandibular molar with representative normal morphologic findings. *B*, Endodontic files used as pathfinders and canal length determinants. Note that the position of the handles is determined by the unprepared orifices and canals. The instruments are in an undesirable working position. *C*, After a preflaring procedure the access to the apical canal is much improved. Note also that the preflare is tapered and does not jeopardize the canal wall integrity. *D*, Instruments in place after preflaring. There is an unobstructed entrance into the apical canal space for better preparation.

7. Length and size are known, which aids in future dowel preparations.

Radiographs of a mandibular molar showing the chamber before and after preflaring are reproduced in Figure 10–9.

Filling the Canal

After the preparation is completed, the clinical and laboratory tests are negative, and the patient is symptom-free (i.e., asymptomatic, dry canal; patent canal; negative bacterial culture), the canal is ready to be filled. The sequence is as follows:

1. Fitting the master cone. The master cone should fit at the specific step-back length (19.5 mm in the example shown). It should be snug and should slightly resist removal (tug-back). The master cone is marked to a reference point by squeezing the cotton pliers to indent the cone. It is advantageous to use a locking pliers, which can be returned in the same direction as it was fitted.

2. Finger pluggers of standardized size are altered so that the tip is slightly pointed. Finger pluggers are used because the taper is approximately the same as that of the root canal instrument and the pluggers match auxiliary gutta percha cones. Also, it is not possible to exert as much torque as with long-handled pluggers or spreaders, which is a cause of root fracture. The pluggers are slightly pointed so that the edges will not bind on the canal wall that curves and there will be an action combining vertical and lateral condensation (Fig. 10–10). The finger "splugger" should fit to within 1 mm of the step-back length (Fig. 10–11). In the illustration a #30 "splugger" is used with #25 auxiliary cones.

3. The canal is thoroughly dried and a coating of the selected sealer is placed on the walls by dipping the last working-length instrument into the sealer and removing it with a counterclockwise motion (Fig. 10–12).

4. The master cone is lightly coated with sealer in the apical third only (Fig. 10–13) and carried to place with a rocking motion (Fig. 10–14). Check the reference point. Too much sealer should be avoided. The sealer is used to soften the gutta percha slightly and takes up minute irregularities in the interface between gutta percha and dentin.

5. The "splugger" is firmly carried to the predetermined length with a slight rocking motion. When there is too much resistance, pause to allow the gutta percha to flow and resume pressure until the proper length is reached. The gutta percha will move into the discrepancy between the working length and the step-back length (Fig. 10–15).

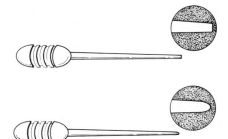

Figure 10–10 *Top,* Finger plugger with a flat end. *Bottom,* Finger plugger with the tip altered by using a sandpaper disc, a finger nail file, a rubber wheel, etc.

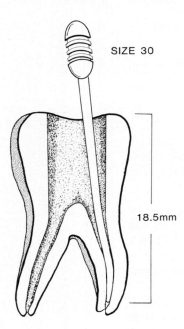

SIZE 30

18.5mm

Figure 10-11 The "splugger" fits approximately 1 mm short of the step-back preparation. Gutta percha does not plasticize enough, with or without heat, to be moved into the full preparation.

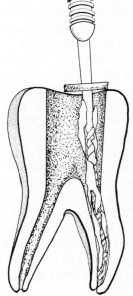

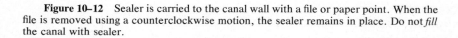

Figure 10-12 Sealer is carried to the canal wall with a file or paper point. When the file is removed using a counterclockwise motion, the sealer remains in place. Do not *fill* the canal with sealer.

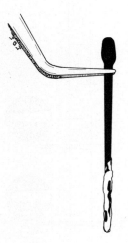

Figure 10-13 Coating the apical portion of the master cone with sealer.

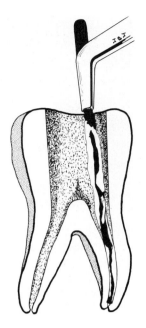

Figure 10–14 Note the relationship of the master cone to the apical walls and the apical stop. The master cone is rocked into position slowly to allow intrusion of excess sealer.

6. Follow with an auxiliary gutta percha cone one size smaller than the "splugger." Some operators like to dip the apical point of the auxiliary cone in a loose mix of sealer to help lubricate and "weld" it to the other cones. This mix is made by taking a dab of the sealer mixture and adding it to pure liquid until the color is the same but the consistency is very loose. The assistant should mix this sealer at the time of the operation.

It is best to add only two or three auxiliary cones at a time and remove the butt ends with a hot instrument before proceeding further. This is to insure that there is no binding in the chamber. Continue adding auxiliary cones until the canal is filled (Fig. 10–16).

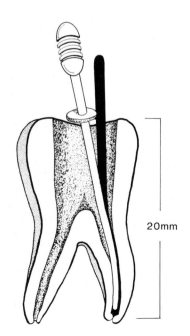

20mm

Figure 10–15 The gutta percha is able to move into the working length patency. Be careful of the amount of pressure applied; wait for the gutta percha to move.

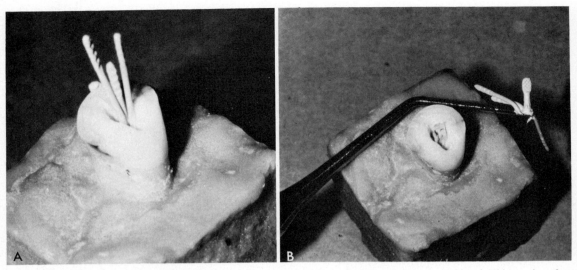

Figure 10-16 *A*, Note that the gutta percha cones bind against one another at the cervical level. This can interfere with the placement of succeeding cones. *B*, By removing the excess cone butts with a heated instrument, the "splugger" can be reintroduced.

7. The chamber is then cleared of gutta percha and sealer, a cotton pellet may be placed over the orifice and a temporary placed, a base and restoration may be placed, or a post preparation made. If no dowel preparation is intended, a strong cement base should cover the gutta percha to protect against gutta percha inadvertently coming in contact with oral fluids. The final restoration should always be placed as soon as possible.

SPECIAL HINTS

As a result of years of clinical practice and teaching, many endodontists have devised "tricks" or "hints" designed to solve certain problems or make them easier to handle. This section is devoted to some random ideas that should be helpful. They are not necessarily originated by the author but are culled from authorities who include such descriptions in their writings and presentations. I particularly recall excellent lectures and papers by Dr. Louis I. Grossman, the contents of which have proved valuable to the profession. Many other lecturers and writers have also indirectly contributed to this chapter. Some ideas are original. I will describe many of these and humbly beg the indulgence of the originators.

Access Opening of the Coronal Structure

The following are helpful hints concerning the process of access opening of the coronal structure:

1. In most cases the initial occlusal outline form should be made without a rubber dam in place, especially if large coronal restorations are present. The original crown and its relationship to the roots are more easily visualized. The root eminences and radiographs are used as references. As soon as the pulp horn or any part of the pulp is reached, the dam should be placed and the area lavaged with NaOCl.

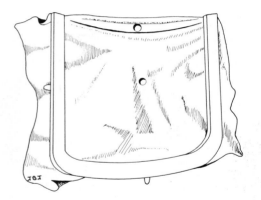

Figure 10–17 A rubber dam with one hole for the tooth and one for orientation. No matter how twisted the dam becomes, it is easy to reorient.

2. The rubber dam should generally have only one hole for the tooth to be treated. A second hole should be placed in the middle of the upper edge of the dam so that the orientation is always known in case the frame has to be removed (e.g., for radiographs) (Fig. 10–17). Generally the hole for the tooth is placed in the center of the dam.

3. Remove any doubtful restorations and all caries in order to preclude leakage.

4. If the tooth cannot carry a clamp because of misalignment, too much crown missing, or other reasons, the dam is placed over the stump, a ligature is tied, and the dam is clamped over another available crown without holes being necessary (Fig. 10–18).

5. At times it may be difficult to place a clamp or a ligature owing to tooth morphology or to the patient's age. The cingulum may be subgingival. With appropriate anesthesia, the clamp may be placed on the attached gingivae. Be careful not to clamp over the sulcus; the clamp must be on attached gingivae in order to preclude loss of gingival tissue (Fig. 10–19).

6. If there is cervical leakage, cement a stainless steel or copper band to circumvent gingival leakage due to a subgingival coronal defect.

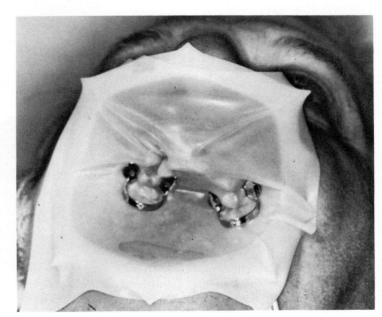

Figure 10–18 Note that the maxillary right lateral is visualized and cannot be clamped. It is ligated and the premolars carry clamps over the dam material. This affords excellent working room.

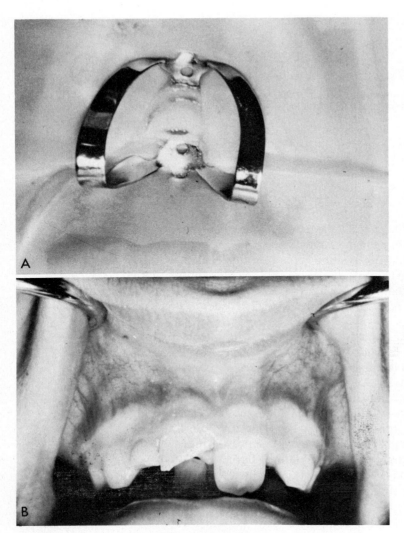

Figure 10–19 *A*, A sterile clamp is placed on the attached gingivae after probing the sulcus to make sure of its depth. *B*, The tissue after 1 week.

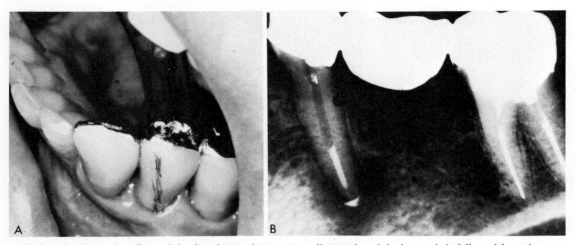

Figure 10–20 *A*, A radiograph is placed over the corresponding teeth and the long axis is followed from the root and marked on the facial aspect. *B*, This radiograph demonstrates the long axis of the root in its relationship to the veneer crown in Figure 10–20*A*.

7. A periodontal pack can be rolled into a ribbon and placed under the clamp to control leakage.

8. Gingival surgery may be necessary to expose sound tooth structure.

9. Use a round diamond stone with much water spray to cut through porcelain. Use a very light pressure.

10. Use a combination taper fissure round bur (700R, 701R, 702R) for access outline and pulpal penetration. Afterward, use this bur in the chamber to remove the roof. The tip of the bur may be made safe by running it against a heatless stone. This procedure is safer and more controllable than peeling the roof off with a round bur (see Chapter 1).

11. If you are not sure of the direction, make a radiograph to reconfirm. Do this before perforating.

12. In cases of crown restorations, it is possible to follow the long axis (in two dimensions) by overlaying a radiograph with indirect light and drawing a line on the crown for proper direction (Fig. 10–20).

13. If necessary, cut the crown down over an elusive orifice (most common for the mesio-buccal orifice of a molar). It is better to sacrifice some coronal structure to insure endodontic success.

14. A Class V cavity preparation may help in locating a canal. Then, with an instrument in the canal, temporary cement is placed into the cavity preparation. While the cement is setting, the file is continuously moved to maintain patency (Fig. 10–21).

15. A transilluminator (fiber-optic) can be useful in locating orifices. It is used on the buccal or lingual surface of the crown and over the root, through bone (Fig. 10–22).

16. Bevel the cavo-surface angle to allow more light to reach the floor and permit easier introduction of instruments (see Chapter 1).

17. Sometimes a stain can be used. Soak a cotton pellet with an iodine solution and place it in the chamber. Remove the excess and wipe the floor with a cotton pellet dipped in alcohol. Many times the stain will remain in the orifice and/or developmental grooves.

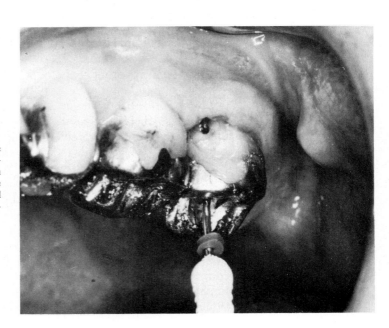

Figure 10–21 A Class V cavity is prepared until the canal is intentionally exposed. The instrument can then be placed through the occlusal access opening and guided into the canal. When temporary cement is then placed, the instrument is moved slightly up and down to maintain patency until the cement hardens.

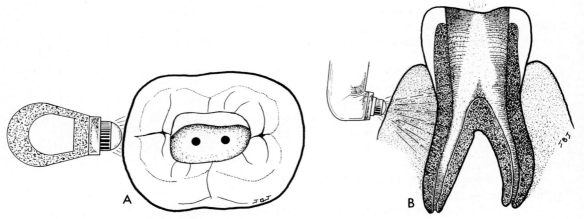

Figure 10–22 *A,* A transilluminator or fiber-optic instrument used through the enamel and dentin illuminates the access opening, and many times the orifice can be seen as a dark dot. *B,* A fiber-optic instrument used through the soft tissue and against the root eminence may, at times, show the orifice lighter than the surrounding floor of the chamber.

18. Use a very sharp endodontic explorer to scratch along developmental grooves and to open tight orifices.

19. Reparative dentin is gray and is darker than the primary and secondary dentin.

Canal Preparation

There are certain helpful concepts that make canal preparation easier. The first section of this chapter described the preflare technique. Some of the following procedures might ease the preparation for a difficult canal:

1. When the orifice is difficult to locate because of sclerotic dentin, do not blindly grind with a bur. Do not use a bur to countersink until you are sure of your orientation. It may be necessary to use a chelating agent containing ethylenediamine tetra-acetic acid (EDTA) as a temporary dressing in the chamber, followed by scraping the floor with sharp endodontic excavators at the next visit.

2. When trying to negotiate a very fine canal with very small instruments (#6, #8, #10), use a vavien motion (slight rock) and exert firm apical pressure. A chelating agent is useless at this stage, since it is effective only when it contacts calcified tissue. In fact, a chelating agent can be self-defeating, owing to its ability to soften calcified tissue at the tip area and cause ledging and false canals. It is desirable to lubricate the file, and a solution of anhydrous glycerin and urea peroxide is the material of choice. This solution lubricates and causes effervescence in the presence of NaOCl, which helps clean out the debris. Be sure that the lubricant is inactivated by using copious irrigation with sodium hypochlorite solution before sealing the access opening, thus eliminating free oxygen.

3. The tip of the root canal instrument should be slightly curved. When it contacts an obstruction, pull back slightly, turn 5 degrees, and try again. Repeat until the instrument bypasses the obstruction.

4. When a tight canal is negotiated, leave the instrument in place until the

instrument length radiograph is made. Fill the chamber with the aforementioned lubricant. Then move the file up and down many times for a very short distance, using an upstroke circumferential motion, until the file is very loose. Do not remove the file until afterward.

5. Always use a small file first, regardless of the canal size. This, plus copious irrigation, helps suspend pulpal debris and dentin filings for aspiration removal. When the initial instrument is a large one that approximates the size of the canal, it will push debris and compact it in the apical canal and possibly inoculate the debris into the periapical tissue.

6. A 15 gauge Luer-Lok needle is effective for aspiration over the orifice. The tip is flattened by removing the bevel, and it is adapted to the suction apparatus. Adapters are available for any suction system and may be purchased from hospital supply companies.

7. When it is difficult to follow a small instrument with the next larger size, the following techniques will help:

   a. Remember to preflare, as previously described.

   b. One can cut the apical 1 to 2 mm of the file, smooth off burs with a diamond nail file, and, in effect, create an in-between–sized instrument. This can be done because in the standardized system the diameter of any instrument increases the same for a given running length (Fig. 10–23).

   c. A compromise to the periapical tissue may be made. A very small instrument may negotiate the canal easily, and if pushed through the apex approximately 3 mm, the effective size within the canal is one step larger (Fig. 10–24). This is to be used only if no other technique is effective, as irritating the periapical connective tissue to such a degree is not good therapy.

8. A chelating agent can be used with #10 or #15 files. It is best to follow this with much irrigation and increase in instrument size to remove the softened dentin.

9. Precurving the root canal instrument helps during the preparation of very curved canals. However, the curve in the instrument should not simulate the shape of the root. Only the tip of the instrument should be curved (Fig. 10–25).

10. One way to minimize cutting in an undesirable area of the canal is to smooth the cutting edge of the instrument with the diamond nail file on the involved side.

11. Remember that the canal tends to shorten as the curves are straightened. Sometimes an interim radiograph is desirable to check the working length.

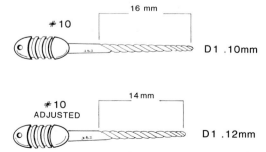

Figure 10–23 A #10 file can be clipped about 1.5 mm from the tip, and this adjusted file is then approximately a #12 instrument.

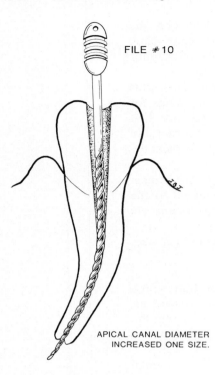

FILE #10

APICAL CANAL DIAMETER
INCREASED ONE SIZE.

Figure 10–24 Note that the diameter of the canal is increased by instrumenting through the apex. The apical constriction must then be artificially reconstructed by the operator.

Figure 10–25 Although file B is shaped like the root, with the curve at point 1, it is obvious that the area between points 1 and 2 is straight. Therefore the instrument will not negotiate this canal any more easily than an entirely straight instrument. The curve should be at the tip, as in file C, regardless of where the curve is in the canal.

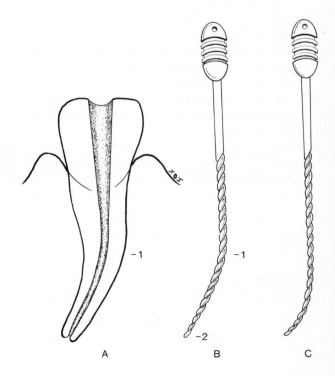

12. Prepare the most difficult canal first in order to determine future action if it is not possible to finish the preparation.
13. If possible, prepare the canal(s) completely at the first visit, regardless of the diagnosis. Early removal of breakdown products and organisms means early favorable body response.

Miscellaneous Procedures

The following are some miscellaneous helpful suggestions:

1. When a vital pulp (usually hyperemic) is extirpated, the bleeding may be hard to control. Formocresol at the tip of a paper point may help stop the bleeding. Epinephrine, 1:100, has also been utilized in the same way. Discretion must be used to avoid chemical burns.

2. When pulp tissue is compressed in the apical tip of the canal, it is sometimes very difficult to remove and may cause severe between-appointment pain. Liquefied phenol, carried to the area by dipping the tip of a file of appropriate size in the solution, tends to coagulate the tissue and break up the ground substance, making it easier to remove. Follow this by heavy dilution with much irrigating solution.

3. If compressed air is used to dry a chamber or remove debris, make sure that the air is blown across the access opening. This will create a vacuum to suck up debris and liquid. Never blow air into an access opening, as it is possible to cause an air embolism as well as inoculate the periradicular tissue with debris, organisms, and so forth.

4. The most useful instrument to create a trench around a silver point or dowel that is to be removed but is too short to lock with a hemostat or Stieglitz forceps is a 701R or 702R series bur with the sides smoothed by a small lathe[1] (Fig. 10–26). The smooth sides must extend slightly around the arc at the tip, so that nothing that touches the object can cut it. Solvent is then placed in the trench, and an attempt is made to work it along the sides and apically. An ultrasonic instrument can be adapted and has been found to be useful in many cases by placing a specially adapted tip in contact with the silver point or dowel. This often breaks the cement bond.[2]

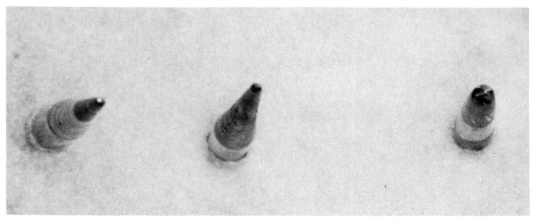

Figure 10–26 Note that the sides of the bur are smooth, as is the arc at the tip. The cutting edges never touch the object to be removed.

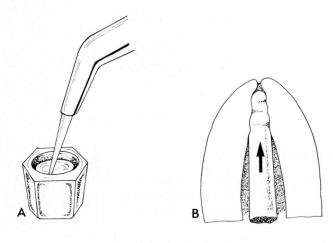

Figure 10-27 The dappen dish (A) holds a small amount of chloroform. The tip of the cone only is dipped momentarily and placed into the canal in a softened state to allow its adaptation to the wall of the canal (B).

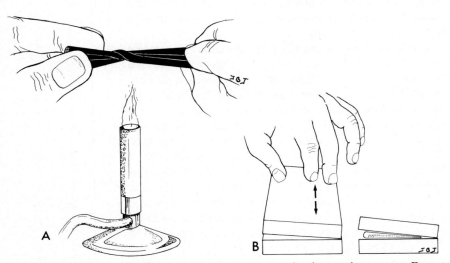

Figure 10-28 A, The three gutta percha cones are twisted over a heat source. Do not place the cones in the flame, as a temperature of 140°F is warm enough. B, The bottom slab is cold. The top slab is gently warmed. The bottom slab is stationary and the top slab is moved foward and backward.

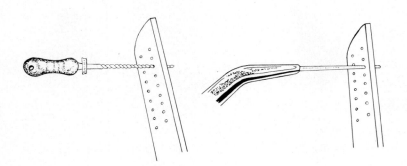

Figure 10-29 A microgauge has American drill gauge numbers, which may be disregarded. Place the file and then the object to be compared in the same hole.

5. In very large, usually immature, canals, it is virtually impossible to prepare the canal properly for the root fill. Do not be led astray by the radiograph. The canals are irregular in cross section. Also a two dimensional radiograph is deceptive as far as apical closure is concerned. A custom gutta percha cone can be made by using an oversized cone that binds 2 to 3 mm short. The canal is lubricated with anesthetic solution, and the tip of the cone is dipped in chloroform and firmly pushed to place, thus creating a pattern of the apical canal (Fig. 10–27). This step may have to be repeated two or three times in order to reach the preparation stop or desired length. Do not dip into chloroform for more than 1 second each time, so as to soften the surface only. Lock the cone in a hemostat or locking endodontic pliers at the desired length, so that it can be returned in the same plane each time it is placed in the canal, including the sealing stage. Another method of customizing a cone is to fill a metal cup (such as a stainless steel crown or aluminum shell) with water and place it in the salt sterilizer so that 1 to 2 mm of the water is above the surface of the salt.[3] When the water is warmed, a gutta percha cone, slightly smaller than desired, is warmed at the tip by placing the tip into the water. This is carried into the canal and, with pressure applied against the apical stop, is soft enough to adapt to the canal wall. An extra-large gutta percha cone can be made by warming three cones laid with two butts in one direction and the third in the other. The cones are twisted and placed on a glass slab. A second glass slab is gently warmed over the flame and used to roll the rough cone until it smooths out. A little practice with tilting the second slab will enable the operator to determine the taper of the final product (Fig. 10–28). The butt end of large gutta percha cones can be used alone for many cases.

6. Many clinicians like to super-dry canals before filling. This can be accomplished by using a solution of 95 % grain alcohol into which several crystals of anhydrous copper sulfate have been dropped. This solution is placed into the canal, and the canal is dried with paper points.

7. Before bleaching a crown of an endodontically treated tooth, the root canal filling should be below the cervical line and a light colored oxyphosphate cement should be placed over the orifice. A cotton pellet is dipped into a chelating agent, and this is carried into the chamber and pressed into the dentinal tubules. After a few minutes, the solution is washed out with NaOCl and hygroscopic alcohol before the bleaching procedure. This opens up the dentinal tubules for better penetration of the bleaching agent. Acid-etched liquid and dilute citric acid have been used for the same purpose.

8. When taking radiographs from two different directions, bend the corner of one film sharply while it is still in the packet. When looking at the two films, one can tell which is which by noting the line created by the bend.

9. When the apex is difficult to see in a film, increase the vertical angle so as to foreshorten the image. Direct the central ray to the tip of the root, even if it means cone cutting the coronal portion.

10. If for any reason, the clinician elects to leave a tooth open for drainage between visits, wiping the cavo-surface with airplane glue or cavity varnish before placing a cotton pellet will help hold the cotton in position.

11. Many times a gutta percha cone may be closely matched to a file or reamer by using a microgauge, which can be purchased in any hardware store. Place the file in a suitable hole so only 1 to 2 mm of the tip comes through. A gutta percha cone is then placed in the same hole and cut so that

the projection is the same. Because of standardization, the sizes will then be similar (Fig. 10–29). This technique can be used with silver cones and endosseous implant stainless rods.

12. When adjoining teeth are to be treated, it is best to treat them at the same time, as periapical contamination from tooth A can cause post-treatment problems in tooth B if the tooth A canal still contains the causative substances. The bone is cancellous and there is danger of apical communication of inflammatory by-products. Use different sets of instruments to avoid cross contamination.

13. The younger the canal, the more coronal the point of apical canal constriction.

14. When there is chronic periapical inflammation with bone resorption, one may safely surmise that some of the apical cementum has been resorbed, even extending into the canal. This affects the area of constriction and, at times, destroys it. Therefore, it is wise to consider a shorter than normal working length for this situation and that described in entry 13.

15. Removing dowels that are firmly cemented can be a frustrating and dangerous procedure. Unless the pressure is exerted in the direction of the long axis, the root can easily be fractured. Also, single rooted teeth have been extracted by a strong pull on the dowel. It is better to use opposing forces, one against the root face and one equal force extracting the dowel, so they counter each other. A crown pulling instrument has been in existence for many years; the author has one dating to the early 1900's (Fig. 10–30).

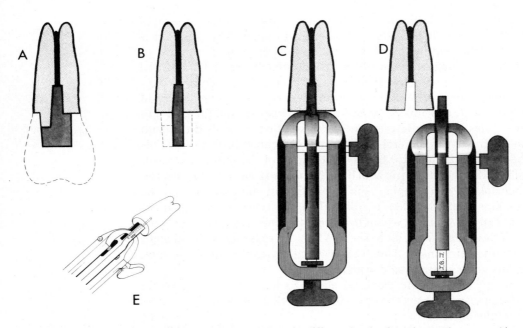

Figure 10–30 *A,* A root with a post and core. Note the different levels of dentin. *B,* The post and its extension after the preparation has been made. In *C,* one set of jaws is tightened against the dowel with the side thumbscrew. In *D* and *E* one can see that turning the top thumbscrew would cause the second set of jaws to remove the dowel with pressure against the root face.

REFERENCES

1. Gerstein, H., and Weine, F. S.: Specially prepared burs to remove silver cones and fractured dowels. J. Endo. 3:408, November 1977.
2. Gaffney, J., Lehman, J., and Miles, M.: Expanded use of the ultrasonic scaler. J. Endo. 7:228, May 1981.
3. Weisman, M.: Warm water technique for sealing large canals. J. Endo. 2:124, May 1976.

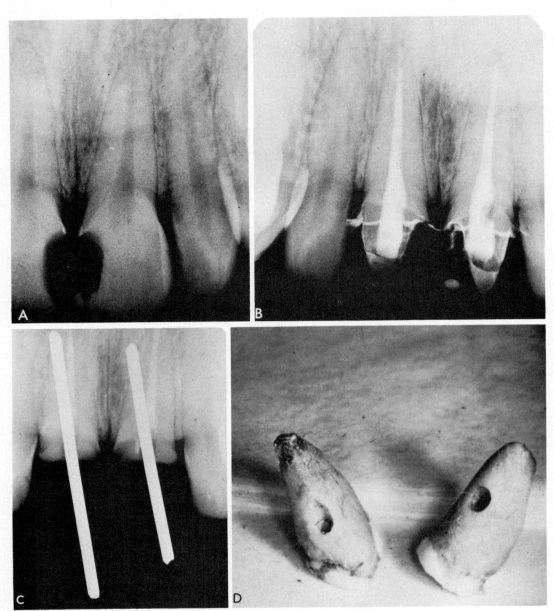

This case tragically illustrates the significance of restorative dentistry in relation to endodontics. A 23-year-old airline stewardess requested conservative replacement of two discolored mesial silicates (A). During cavity preparation, both pulp chambers were iatrogenically exposed, necessitating endodontic therapy. The subsequent preparation for porcelain jacket crowns resulted in excessive tooth loss (B). Dowel space was created with a slow speed bur so that the vertical axis of each post was parallel with the other (C). Massive mid-root perforation resulted in immediate extraction of both teeth (D). This chapter is written in the hope that similar conclusions may be prevented.

11

Restoration Selection Following Endodontic Therapy

GARY N. TAYLOR, D.D.S., M.S.

The proper restoration of any tooth to normal function and morphology following endodontic therapy is a demanding task. The experienced practitioner must thoroughly understand and integrate the clinical disciplines of restorative dentistry, prosthetics, and periodontics. Only then and in concert with an appreciation of fundamental endodontics does it become possible to create a biologically and technically acceptable restoration (Fig. 11–1).

Excellent reviews of the procedures associated with the technical phases of rehabilitation are found extensively in the dental literature in both textbook and periodical form.[1, 2, 3] It is not, therefore, our intent to simply rewrite that which is readily available. We shall, instead, consider the *didactic* and *pragmatic* interrelationship of form and function to best determine, from an endodontic viewpoint, the proper restoration *selection*. Those concepts and procedures pertinent to endodontics, as they apply to reconstruction, will be utilized to temper that decision.

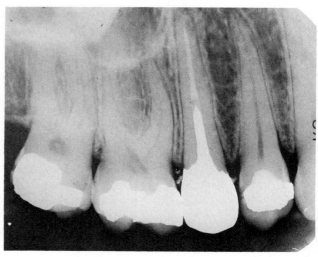

Figure 11–1 Restoration of a maxillary bicuspid immediately following cementation. Acceptable endodontic therapy is complemented by proper radicular reinforcement and coronal protection.

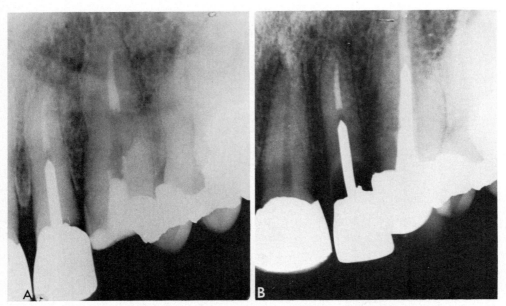

Figure 11–2 *A,* Maxillary lateral incisor recently restored with defective distal margins of core and dowel and crown. *B,* Ten month radiograph following fracture of root and mobility of crown due to recurrent caries.

Unfortunately, the bane of all endodontic practices, or more appropriately of any dentist performing root canal therapy, is the deterioration of a successfully treated tooth into a nonrestorable condition. Many of these situations cannot be prevented, but some most assuredly are iatrogenic. Fractures, for example, are often excused, based on purported brittleness of enormous magnitude, although the true cause of failure was inadequate restoration (Fig. 11–2).

There have been several investigations demonstrating varying degrees of dehydration and desiccation in the dentin of the pulpless tooth. One study reported a decreased water content of up to 9 per cent in the calcified structures.[4] When teeth are properly restored, however, this rarely causes a clinically significant problem. The difficulty experienced during extraction of a pulpless tooth is largely due to the internal loss of coronal and radicular dentin. Thus, the empirical impression is gained of intrinsic weakness and decreased dentin elasticity under the crushing power of the forceps. The correctly reconstructed pulpless tooth should be no more susceptible to masticatory failure than its vital counterpart. This, of course, assumes the prior completion of endodontic therapy (Fig. 11–3).

FRACTURES FOLLOWING ENDODONTIC THERAPY

Different entities contribute to the overt vulnerability of the nonrestored endodontically treated tooth. These include trauma, occlusion, caries, existing restorations, and so forth. Most significant, however, is the loss of circumferential dentin during routine access cavity preparation. Eliminating the transdentinal bridge created by the pulpal roof and direct exposure of the pulp chamber result in the formation of independent lateral walls supported only by cervical dentin. During this interval of treatment, from preparatory appointment to final restoration, the tooth is most subject to fracture. Considering the parameters of functional stress, coronal and root fractures occur in response to, delivery of, and then resistance against applied stress. The anterior and posterior segments differ markedly in their ability to sustain alternate vectors of force.

Anterior Tooth Fractures

Four categories of common fractures occur in anterior teeth following endodontic therapy. The first involves only coronal tooth structure, in which the cervical area is intact or is minimally involved. These pose no particular reconstructive problems since only a horizontal component of tooth structure has been lost near or coronal to gingival and alveolar tissues. The problem is frequently seen in previously crowned maxillary teeth. A palatal access opening sufficiently weakens any existing coronal dentin so that little direct force is necessary to permit cleavage (Fig. 11–4A). This fracture is

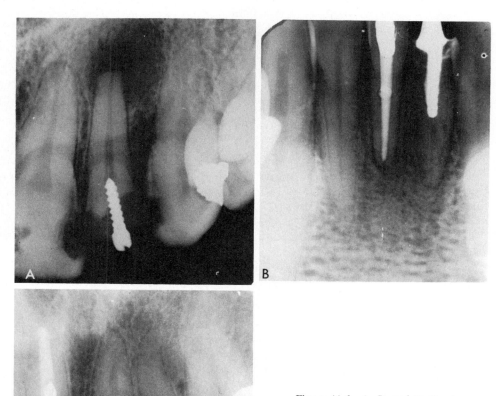

Figure 11–3 *A*, *B*, and *C*, Random examples of dowel utilization for teeth without prior endodontic treatment.

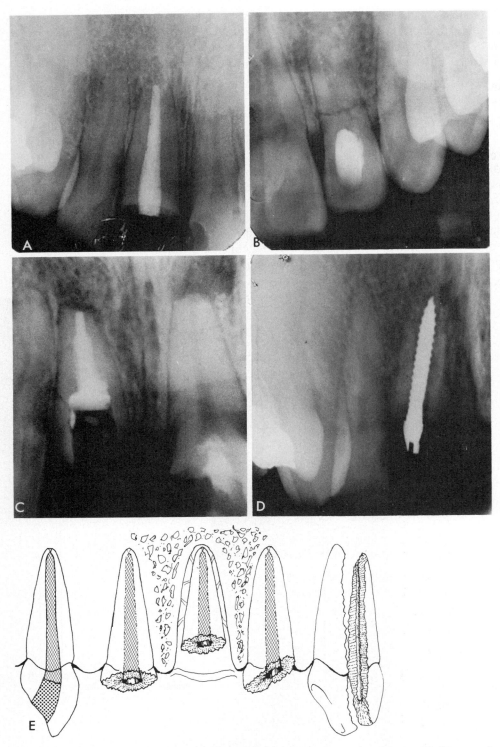

Figure 11–4 Common fractures involving anterior teeth. *A*, Horizontal coronal fracture of maxillary incisor following endodontic therapy. *B*, Horizontal radicular fracture of maxillary incisor 6 months after initiation of calcium hydroxide therapy for open apex. *C*, Horizontal and vertical fractures of maxillary incisor due to short and broad post construction. *D*, Complete vertical fracture of maxillary incisor after placement of oversized screw post. *E*, Illustrative representation of fracture sites.

also encountered in those teeth with proximal surfaces that are cariously or restoratively involved. Fortunately, fracture lines normally pass through sites of least resistance, permitting the radicular structures to remain intact.

The second general fracture type, also limited to a horizontal component, occurs intraosseously in one of the radicular thirds of the root. This results from excessive loss of root structure below the cervical line. Gouging of the root by rotary instruments to prepare the canal for either filling or making post room is usually the cause (Fig. 11–4B). When treatment is warranted, active orthodontic migration to expose clinically restorable margins from the alveolus can be attempted.[5] Limitations are immediate cosmetics, patient age, local periodontal conditions, possible additional root fracture, and practicality.

The third fracture type, having two directional components, occurs horizontally through the body of the crown and then vertically separates the facial and lingual segments of the root (Fig. 11–4C). The term "greenstick" fracture is often applied to this traumatic event. It surprises both patient and dentist, since it occurs in those teeth that are intact save for the access cavity opening. A blow applied across the frontal surface results in a facial horizontal fracture aligned perpendicular to the root canal space. The line then ascends both vertically and apically to involve the palatal surface of the root. The angle created between horizontal and vertical lines is determined by the direction of force, point of contact, size of the root canal space, access cavity, and, most importantly, the inclination of the tooth in the alveolar bone. Successful reconstruction in selected cases is sometimes achieved by periodontal recontouring of soft and hard tissues, when clinically prudent.

A tooth sustaining the fourth fracture type, a single vertical fracture, is absolutely destined for extraction (Fig. 11–4D). Regardless of the minuteness of the crack or stability of the tooth, the segments will eventually separate. The accidental cause is normally a direct vertical force delivered to the incised edge of the tooth. Improper cementation of a dowel by inadequate venting, improper cement consistency, or rapid hydraulic seating pressure may also split roots. Too frequently, screw posts are secured with "just another one-quarter turn," creating a vertical fissure. A chronic inflammatory response ensues adjacent to the defect. The subjective symptoms of ache and tenderness with the objective signs of alveolar destruction, dehiscence, and sinus tract formation become prominent. *No* treatment or restoration should ever be attempted when a complete vertical fracture can be confirmed.

Posterior Tooth Fractures

Shearing type fractures with a single horizontal component are practically nonexistent in posterior teeth. Some authors have suggested that the anatomic constriction found at the cervical line is sufficient to allow this type of fracture.[6] Although theoretically possible, a tremendous horizontal blow would be necessary to cleanly separate the coronal from the radicular dentin. This concept is at the heart of a widespread misconception about dowel placement into the root canal for resistance to fracture without the incorporation of a core as part of the restoration. Conversely, either buccal

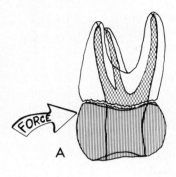

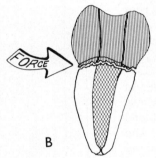

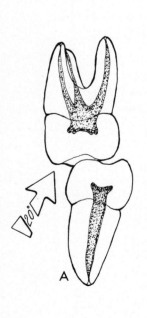

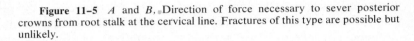

Figure 11–5 *A* and *B*, Direction of force necessary to sever posterior crowns from root stalk at the cervical line. Fractures of this type are possible but unlikely.

or lingual cusps can and do routinely become axially (vertically) displaced from the crown and root stalk. Vertical forces either are dissipated along a least resistant path, normally at the cervical line, or begin in the center of the crown and continue as mid-root involvement. The in toto loss of an entire posterior coronal structure across a single horizontal shearing plane is rare and unlikely (Fig. 11–5).

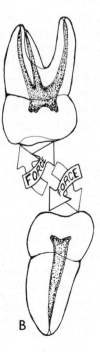

Figure 11–6 Occlusal force vectors. *A*, Positive occlusal relationship of maxillary and mandibular molars. *B*, Normal distribution of force (greatest force in white), showing areas of maximum stress load.

The observation that horizontal fractures predominate in anterior teeth is in direct contrast to the occurrence of vertical fractures in the posterior dentition. Anatomic factors are responsible for a concentration of force through the long axis of posterior teeth to yield either buccal or lingual fracture segments. A normal, yet prominent, 20 degree medial inclination of the mandibular posterior teeth and the accommodating inclination of the maxillary teeth have been implicated.[7] This relationship creates intimate contact between the buccal incline surface of the maxillary palatal cusps and the lingual incline surface of the mandibular buccal cusps (Fig. 11–6). During routine mastication, forces between these surface interfaces are generally not sufficient to produce a fissure within sound enamel that is adequately supported by dentin. However, wedging effects created by the interposition of an unyielding object, such as a popcorn kernel, have the ability to split even a totally intact crown.

The palatal cusps of maxillary molars and the buccal cusps of mandibular molars are described as "supporting" cusps.[8] Their functional relationship to central fossae and/or marginal ridges is normally limited to small circumscribed areas that are sites of immense pressure. Should a tooth in either arch be weakened during endodontic therapy, an opposing intact or restored tooth may be of sufficient unyielding force to independently produce fracture. If the tooth is unopposed or in contact with a denture tooth, the degree of force is reduced and so also the complexity of restoration selection.

Functionally and clinically then, the most common sites for posterior tooth fractures involve the mobile separation of mandibular buccal cusps and maxillary palatal cusps from the remaining secure tooth (Fig. 11–7). The extent of the fracture, whether completely coronal or including some radicular structures, is dependent upon the degree of force, the direction of force, and, most importantly, the amount of remaining dentin. Interestingly enough, those teeth with undermined enamel and virtual loss of all coronal dentin are least likely to result in a nonrestorable fracture. This strongly resembles the analogous phenomenon in the anterior segments. The stress-bearing cusp of a weakened tooth will shear at the site of least resistance resulting from caries or restoration, which is usually at a supraosseous level (Fig. 11–8). Certainly, every restorative dentist has seen the failure of a newly restored tooth in which only unsupported enamel remained for retention of the filling material.

Those posterior teeth, however, with sound dentin supporting the remaining enamel structures are significantly more susceptible to complete vertical fracture, since no particularly weakened areas exist for dissipation of the axially induced force (Fig. 11–7D). Vertical fractures are hopeless situations, creating a "Humpty Dumpty" effect since "all the king's horses and all the king's men cannot put the tooth back together again." The dentist who argues that a conventional amalgam restoration in the coronal access of an endodontically treated posterior tooth is sufficient performs a great disservice to the patient in an attempt to "conserve" tooth structure. The long-term restorative success of all endodontically treated teeth is determined by a primary and a secondary cardinal principle: *First,* the remaining tooth structure must *support* the restoration; *second,* the restoration must *protect* the remaining tooth structure. Only when the "horse is finally put before the cart" and this order of importance understood, can there be a reasonable chance for successful restoration.

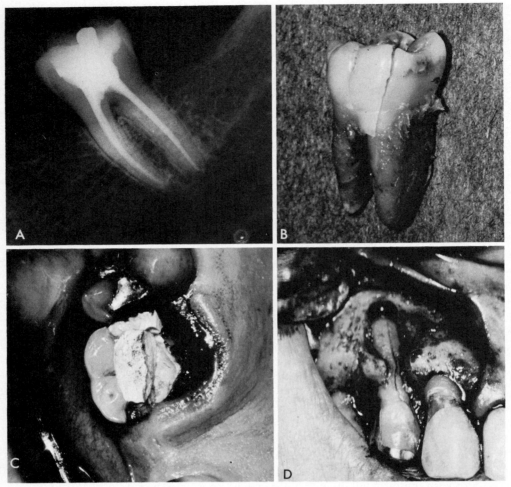

Figure 11–7 Common fractures involving posterior teeth. *A*, Vertical fracture of a mandibular molar that was intact except through its access cavity. *B*, Failure to reduce occlusal contact necessitated extraction within days of completion of endodontic therapy. *C*, Vertical fracture of a maxillary molar. *D*, Vertical fracture of a maxillary premolar.

Figure 11–8 Cariously weakened cusps of maxillary and mandibular molars at common fracture sites.

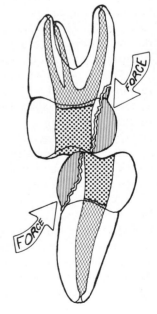

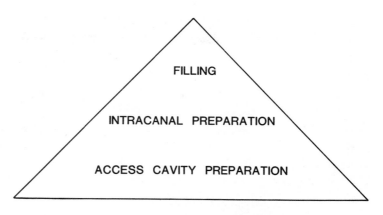

Figure 11–9 The endodontic triad. Each phase of treatment has objective goals. Although the final filling, which occupies the pinnacle of the pyramid, is most important, it can never be accomplished without the broad base of successful access cavity or intracanal preparation.

ENDODONTIC PROCEDURES PERTINENT TO RESTORATION

Not only are the individual disciplines of dentistry important in our reconstructive consideration, but so too are the phases of endodontic therapy. In the most fundamental division, three distinct categories of endodontic treatment are significant: access cavity preparation, intracanal preparation, and intracanal filling procedures.[9] Each should be considered in relation to the final restoration (Fig. 11–9). In other words, the relation of the restoration should never be an afterthought to endodontic therapy but rather a definite goal in the treatment plan, subject to modification and revision when necessary. The endodontic discipline should complement, rather than complicate or defeat, the restorative disciplines.

Access Cavity Preparation

Most authors and clinicians agree that entry to each canal orifice must be direct and unobstructed. Other aspects of the cavity preparation, however, will greatly influence the final restoration. If during this early phase of treatment *all caries and undermined enamel are eliminated,* a tooth originally planned to receive a conservative protective cusp overlay may now require a complete coronal build-up and cast crown. No technique, restorative or endodontic, should involve the wanton destruction of tooth structure. However, conservation at the expense of proper endodontic therapy is poor clinical judgment, especially since most of those structures so meticulously preserved will be eliminated during restoration procedures. Predictably, when a tooth with insufficient structural support sustains normal occlusal forces, fracture of the unprotected enamel results, with subsequent tooth or restoration failure.

Another essential aspect of the access cavity should be to *relieve all occlusal contacts* in posterior teeth or *incisal prematurities* in anterior teeth. In the posterior tooth, this is most effectively accomplished by a uniform reduction 1 mm below each marginal ridge. Such a reduction not only provides better visibility for treatment, but also creates a reproducible flat reference point for instrumentation procedures. Clearly, the greatest clinical advantage is the positive reduction of fracture potential by providing occlusal clearance (Fig. 11–10). Unless a greatly overcontoured temporary filling is placed, the tooth will be free of any occlusal contact and is now

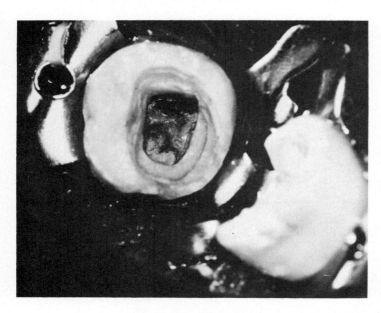

Figure 11–10 Correct access cavity preparation of mandibular molar following caries excavation and occlusal reduction to a level at least 1.0 mm below the normal marginal ridge height.

permanently committed to receive the minimum restoration that includes full cuspal protection.

Intracanal Preparation

All current conventional methods of intracanal debridement and enlargement are based upon form and morphology. Generally, most roots are pyramidal in shape, tapering apically from a broader cervical base. This form provides the rationale for the tapered (stepback) preparation, which modifies the diameter of the existing canal without radical alteration in direction or configuration. In those situations in which a post or dowel is indicated, the most appropriate form is one resembling the gross morphology of the root. Lateral perforation of the root canal into the periodontal ligament space occasionally occurs during overzealous flaring of the root canal or with minimal enlargement when deep proximal concavities are present in ovoid roots.[10] It should *never* occur as a result of post preparation. Therefore, thorough knowledge of root morphology is essential in this phase of treatment.

The logical implication of reproducing external anatomy as part of the post space design dictates that a tapered form be utilized. It may also be advantageous to prepare the post space during the intracanal preparation stage as an endodontic consideration rather than as a latent feature of the dowel technique (Fig. 11–11). Should a problem arise as the result of dowel space preparation, it is better that this complication occurs before endodontic therapy is completed, rather than in the more advanced stages of treatment. Since the tooth is properly isolated and the appropriate hand instruments are readily available, canal enlargement for post room is rapid and the increased diameter of the root canal provides greater access to the apical one third of the canal system. It is interesting to note that the first mention of using root canal instruments for creating post room was not until 1963.[11] The filling procedure is also simplified by the enlarged size of the canal orifice, which allows easier delivery of the filling material. Subsequent

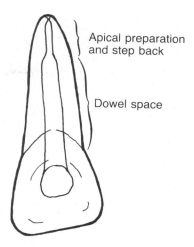

Apical preparation
and step back

Dowel space

Figure 11–11 Dowel preparation included as part of the intracanal preparation. Increased diameter of the root canal allows better access to the apical preparation and facilitates gutta percha removal after endodontic filling.

removal of the filling material (especially gutta percha) for post space is greatly enhanced by a previously prepared canal. Post room of known dimension, both width and length, is then easily cleaned and re-prepared.

Intracanal Filling Procedures

The filling procedure has the least effect on the restorative technique or its selection, assuming it has been accomplished correctly. It is sufficient to say that the filling material must satisfy certain requirements.[12] By this time the dentist must be aware of the intended restoration to be placed and the potential that exists for future restorations. If a core and dowel are required but are deferred owing to the patient's age, questionable treatment plan, economics, and so forth, a full canal length silver point filling would be inappropriate, since eventual re-treatment of the root canal must be performed to create the dowel room (Fig. 11–12). Techniques involving gutta

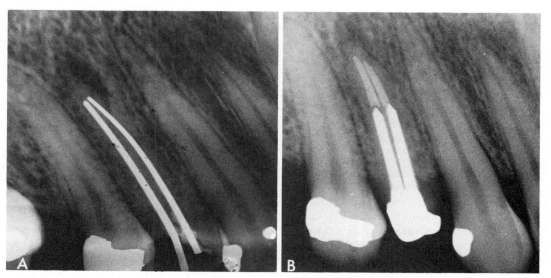

Figure 11–12 Tooth with extensive loss of coronal structure was treated using silver points *(A)*. Re-treatment with gutta percha was necessary to create adequate retention for core and dowel *(B)*.

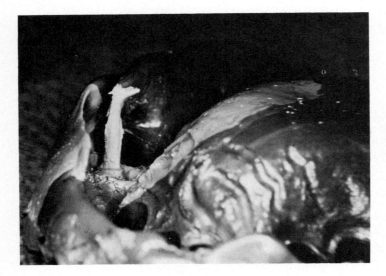

Figure 11–13 Rubber base impression of a maxillary central incisor for a core and dowel, showing canal irregularities and large accessory canal. Exit toward the palatal surface of the root rendered it undetectable radiographically.

percha, on the other hand, must provide for complete filling of the root canal before dowel space is made. Failure to adequately obturate the canal, based on the premise that it will be removed anyway, sometimes prohibits the filling of canal irregularities and large lateral or accessory canals that have the potential for failure (Fig. 11–13). Regardless of the filling material, it must have the potential of partial removal without disruption of the apical seal.

RESTORATION SELECTION

Practically every type of filling material available to dentistry is and has been used for the restoration of the endodontically treated tooth. From the "thumb" amalgam to the most perfect gold casting, it is ironic that the rate of *clinical* success appears so high. The judgment of our treatment's being successful *in spite of what we do* rather than *because of what we do* is a daily rationalization of the techniques practiced. Most of us become myopic in our approach to restorative decisions, for example, the unnecessary placement of posts or full coronal coverage without consideration of the alternatives and variables that are usually present. Exercising the options available requires a parallel but separate consideration of two factors. The first considers the propriety of the restorative material itself, whereas the second is concerned with the site and local conditions under which the material is to be used.

Material Selection

Self-hardening materials such as silicates, composites, and amalgams have varying degrees of hardness, permeability, solubility, and longevity. None are expected to last indefinitely but all should provide normal service following proper placement. A single inherent problem common to all these materials is insufficient strength to withstand occlusal stress. Self-hardening materials derive their clinical success by the design of the cavity preparation and remaining coronal tooth structure. For the endodontically treated tooth, they accomplish only the filling of spaces created by access cavity preparation, unless they are retained by a cemented post or dentinally retained pins. This will remain true until a material is found that will physically unite and bond permanently to tooth structure.

Coronally Retained Restorations

Nonetheless, there are appropriate circumstances for the use of these materials. When strength is not a primary objective to be satisfied, the composite material is esthetically acceptable. It may be placed in any anterior tooth in which there is no break in the integrity of circumferential enamel and in which a normal or non-load–bearing occlusion exists (Fig. 11–14). This material is unacceptable in modified class II malocclusions that produce strong incisal end-to-end relationships or in normal occlusions in which heavy incisal guidance may result in coronal or radicular fracture. An equally unacceptable condition exists when the tooth occupies a prominent frontal position, as in class III skeletal relationships, and in patients who are prone to facial injury, such as adolescent athletes engaged in contact sports. When utilized, a base of relatively high compressive strength cement should be placed adjacent to the canal filling material that has been removed below the cervical line. Zinc phosphate cement or zinc oxide and eugenol (ZOE) are especially appropriate for this purpose.

Various forms of ZOE are now available with fillers and hardeners that yield added strength while maintaining excellent sealing ability. In our filling of the root canal, we attempt to develop a complete hermetic seal of the root canal system but probably do not achieve this goal. A large percentage of endodontic failures are directly attributable to faulty restorations, which allow oral contamination of the root canal system that eventually involves the periapical tissues. This can be seen when re-treating some teeth filled with silver points. Assuming that a less than perfect endodontic filling exists, communication with the oral cavity via a faulty restoration may lead to ultimate failure. Thus, any measure to prolong canal filling intactness must be utilized. The placement of a material known to allow marginal leakage directly adjacent to the endodontic filling jeopardizes the long-term prognosis of the tooth, and for this reason a cement base is recommended (Fig. 11–15).

An access cavity must frequently be made through an existing cast restoration that already provides full cuspal or coronal protection. When the supporting structures are sound and caries-free, a minimal but endodontically adequate access cavity may be filled to restore the occlusal or lingual opening. When active caries exists, the restoration must be replaced, since pulp removal will not arrest bacterial progression and may lead to radicular and alveolar carious involvement. The same precautions for protecting the root canal filling from the oral cavity must be kept in mind in this instance. Amalgam should be placed when gold occlusal surfaces are present, whereas composite materials satisfy cosmetic requirements adjacent to porcelain surfaces (Fig. 11–16).

Tooth-supported complete prostheses (overdentures) are excellent restorations that allow for the preservation of existing alveolar bone. The retained teeth are treated endodontically and then restored in accordance

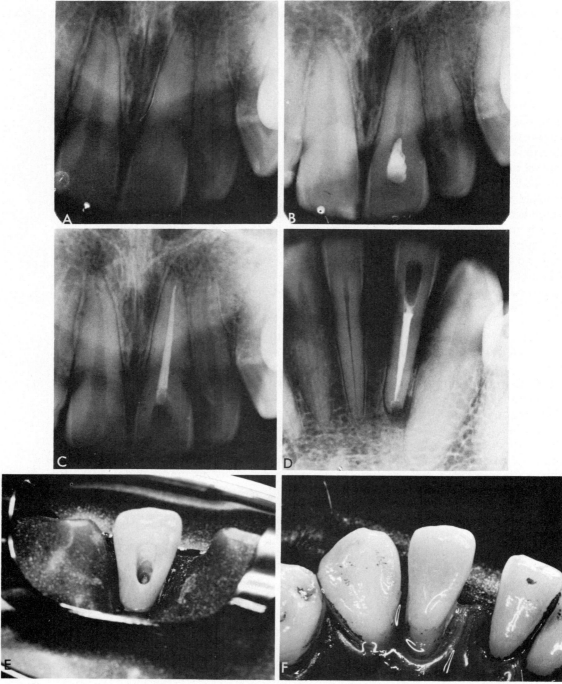

Figure 11–14 In certain instances, the simple filling of an access cavity without radicular reinforcement is possible. *A*, Maxillary incisor with calcification of the root canal system prior to treatment. Noninterfering occlusion exists. *B*, After first appointment, with temporary filling in place. *C*, Endodontic therapy completed and composite restoration. *D*, Mandibular incisor following endodontic therapy. Periodontal involvement and questionable prognosis are indications for conservative restoration. *E*, Access cavity before filling. *F*, Composite material in place.

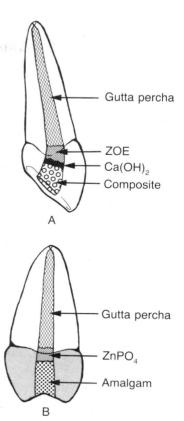

Figure 11–15 *A,* When the root canal is not to be used in the restoration, the endodontic filling must be protected from oral contamination. If strength is not a significant factor, ZOE provides the best coronal seal. It must, however, be covered by calcium hydroxide so that polymerization of the composite is not retarded by the eugenol. *B,* In the posterior dentition, filling of the access cavity through an existing crown is sometimes acceptable. It should always be supported by a cement base of $ZnPO_4$ for strength.

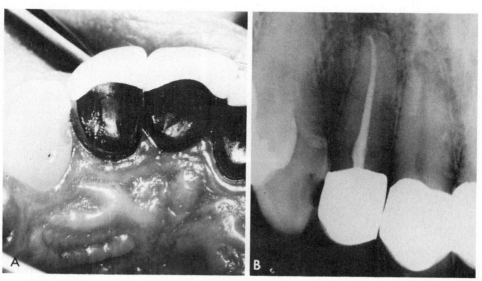

Figure 11–16 *A,* Minimal access cavity of a maxillary incisor with porcelain fused to metal crown that has been filled with amalgam. *B,* Access was adequate to permit endodontic therapy but did not significantly reduce existing coronal dentin.

with the overdenture design. When first introduced, telescoping crowns were thought to achieve the test retention. Unfortunately, many of these teeth developed rapid recurrent caries, necessitating extraction. Since that time, there has been a constant reduction in the amount of coronal tooth structure incorporated into the retentive design of the denture. Most clinicians now recommend simple doming of the radicular stump and filling with amalgam. This has proved to be faster, less costly, and more easily maintained by the patient. When the orally exposed tooth structure has been highly polished and treated with fluoride, it becomes increasingly resistant to caries (Fig. 11–17).

The common practice of placing only a post, whether cast or prefabricated, into the root canal of any tooth for radicular stabilization is unwarranted. This technique has been recommended for decades and reported specifically as a means of reinforcing a sound endodontically treated tooth.[13] Until recently, there have been no studies to substantiate or refute this empirical impression. One in vitro experiment comparing post reinforced anterior teeth with nonreinforced teeth showed no statistically significant resistance to failure loads in the nonreinforced control group.[14] Another showed that virgin pulpless anterior teeth with natural crowns demonstrated greater strength than teeth with pin-retained amalgam cores or cast-gold dowel-cores.[15] A post or dowel as an uncoupled entity merely occupies the canal space and does not protect the tooth from fracturing. An example of this procedure would be a post cemented into the distal canal of a mandibular molar, cut flush with the orifice, and then an amalgam or gold onlay restoration placed. No possible resistance to vertical or horizontal fracture could be realized from this procedure. The tooth most frequently involved is the maxillary incisor, which, when coronally intact, receives a poor fitting dowel through the access cavity (Fig. 11–18). This may not only

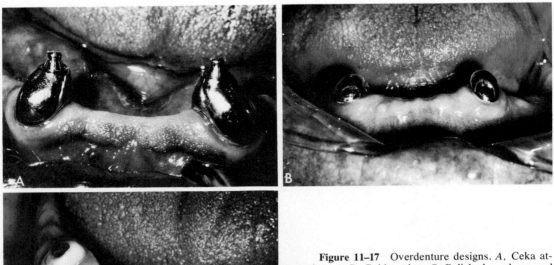

Figure 11–17 Overdenture designs. A, Ceka attachment. B, Gold coping. C, Polished amalgam and tooth structure. (Courtesy of Dr. Robert Mroz, Veterans Administration Hospital, Hines, Illinois.)

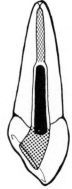

Figure 11–18 The concept of cementing a post into roots to achieve some type of radicular resistance to fracture is unfounded and never recommended.

result in a more serious fracture than if the tooth were traumatized without a post, but may possibly negate future restoration if the post cannot be removed. The principal function of any core and dowel system is to provide intraradicular retention for the core while integrating extracoronal protection into the restorative design. The presence of a post that is occupying space along the vertical axis of the tooth seems to be totally insignificant.

Coronal Reinforced Restorations

Pins, both dentin-retained and cemented, enjoy tremendous popularity in clinical use. The soaring cost of precious metals and laboratory fees has forced some federal, capitated, and private practices to rely on the self-hardening materials as the primary restoration in an increasing number of cases. Other routine indications, such as teeth with a questionable endodontic or periodontic prognosis, patients unable to tolerate multiple visit procedures, high caries index, and anatomic conditions not conducive to dowel placement, have been cited as circumstances not receptive to cast restorative techniques.[16] Referring to our original premise that the "remaining tooth structure must support the restoration," pin-retained amalgams can provide excellent restorative capability in certain select situations.

The most significant criterion for this restoration selection, in addition to adequate dentin support of the remaining enamel structure, is the ability to achieve intercuspal splinting and cuspal protection. These materials may act as a secure interim filling during endodontic treatment, as an essential foundation for complete coverage, or as the final restoration itself. Three general types of pins are available: self-threading,[17] friction-lock,[18] and cemented.[19] The first two are extensively used because of simplicity of placement and immediate retention by threading or wedging into dentin. They are available in multiple sizes, variable lengths, self-shearing designs, and color-coded systems coordinating twist drill to pin size. The third type depends exclusively on cement and pin channel depth for retention.

Historically, cemented pin amalgams gained recognition as a restorative alternative in 1958, and the frictionally retained and threaded types were advocated by 1966.[20] A subsequent study reported that the least retentive pin was the cemented type. However, several reports insist on the use of cemented pins because of the formation of minute fracture lines and crazing of the dentin following threading or friction loading.[21] The latest report to date, utilizing the scanning electron microscope (SEM), showed that dentin-

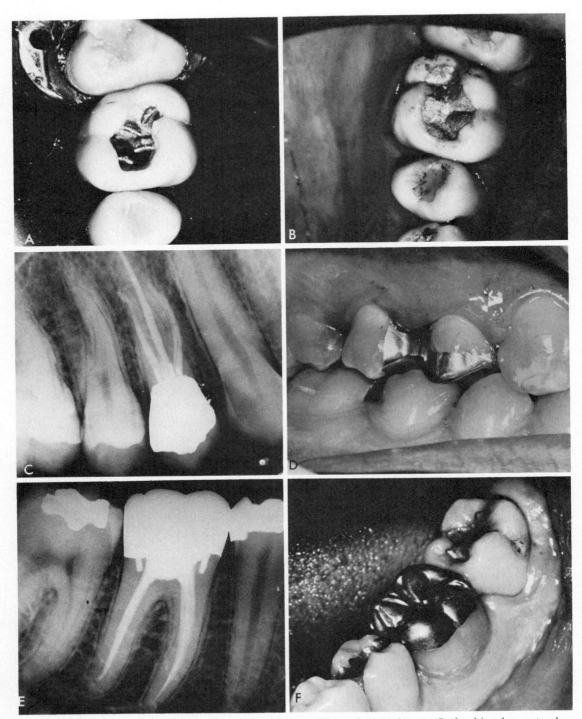

Figure 11–19 Progressive degree of tooth replacement utilizing pin retention. *A*, Occlusal involvement only, with cemented pins positioned for intercuspal splinting of a maxillary molar. *B*, Occlusal restoration after carving. *C*, Radiograph taken before restoration of second premolar. Note vertical axis of the pins in the first premolar. *D*, Cuspal coverage with proper restoration of coronal contours. *E*, Radiograph showing pin placement and proximal contouring. *F*, Mandibular molar with full cuspal coverage. (Restorations courtesy of Dr. S. M. Plies, Suisan, California.)

al damage occurs not during normal channel preparation but rather at the time of forced pin placement. No damage occurred at any phase of the procedure when cemented pins were utilized.[22] These conclusions, combined with a reported 100 per cent incidence of dentinal crazing for self-threading pins in dried, endodontically treated teeth,[23] present a strong case for the use of the cemented pin technique.

Each of the pin types has certain preparation requirements in common. When cusp reduction is necessary, 3 mm is usually sacrificed to provide an adequate bulk of amalgam. Depending on the position of the pin, it may maintain vertical orientation or be bent horizontally toward the midline to achieve a cuspal "splinting" or "tying together" effect of the core material (Fig. 11–19). The vertically intact pins extend occlusally to be incorporated into at least half the length of the reduced cusp. There are no exact guidelines for the number of pins to be used, but one author suggests that the "rule of thumb" be one pin per involved cusp and two per missing marginal ridge. This may be excessive, depending upon the size and shape of the tooth, so that the number and location of pin holes must be dictated primarily by empirical judgment.

Some practitioners mistake the clinical difference between pin-retained and pin-reinforced restorations.[24] The presence of a pin within a self-hardening restorative material such as amalgam not only fails to increase its compressive strength but does not reinforce the alloy. In fact, a significant decrease in tensile strength has been demonstrated in amalgams in which pins were present. Therefore, the cemented pin would seem to be the restorative choice for two reasons. First, it is least destructive to dentin, and second, it provides *retention* for the amalgam while reinforcing (splinting) existing *coronal* structures when the pins are bent medially.

Another requirement is the depth of the pin channel. Serious advocates of pin-retained restorations suggest a recommended depth of 2 to 5 mm in sound dentin, although this is variable, depending upon the type of pin used. This seems to be within the accommodation of average tooth morphology, assuming average competence of the clinician. The danger of lateral and infrabony perforation is a constant problem inherent to the pin technique, which may precipitate the loss of the tooth (Fig. 11–20). If this happens, the

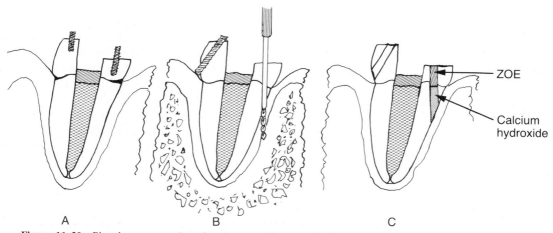

Figure 11–20 Pin placement and perforations. *A,* Correct pin placement. *B,* Supraosseous and infraosseous perforations. *C,* Treatment of the infraosseous perforation.

channel is allowed to hemorrhage spontaneously until normal stasis occurs. The site of perforation in relation to bone should be established either clinically by extracoronal probing or radiographically by the use of bite-wing films. At no time should the channel be re-entered. When the perforation site is above alveolar bone, it must be included within the margins of the restoration. Irrigation of the site with a readily available saline solution will be necessary to cleanse the channel. Local anesthetic solution is particularly good for this problem, since it is sterile, can be gently deposited through the syringe needle into the channel, may have some limited hemostatic action, and is not likely to produce additional tissue injury. With bleeding controlled, the channel can be gently dried using a sterile endodontic paper point and then filled with a paste consisting of calcium hydroxide. The above procedures must always be performed with a rubber dam in place.

It is certainly not within the context of this chapter to discuss the biologic events resulting from the use of calcium hydroxide (see Chapter 7). However, it is important to note that the most appropriate time for treatment is immediately following perforation. The osteoid potential related to this material is probably based upon its alkalinity, which is conducive to the formation of alkaline phosphatase, the deposition of available calcium ions from the circulatory system, and the activation of undifferentiated mesenchymal cells from the periodontal ligament and surrounding connective tissues to form either bone or cementum-like material. The procedure is simple and successful if the perforation is not excessive. The technique for placement of calcium hydroxide after bleeding ceases is as follows: A small portion of calcium hydroxide powder (available from pharmaceutical and dental supply companies) is mixed with several drops of any local anesthetic solution to form a thick compact paste. It is transferred and delivered into the channel by a retro-filling amalgam carrier, which forms a thin dense pellet. A small blunt-ended plugger, such as those advocated for heated gutta percha filling techniques, is then used to gently move the pellet down the channel to the exit site. A normal mix of ZOE should cover the defect within the pulp chamber to seal the channel orifice from the operative field. The restorative procedure can then be continued. Premixed calcium hydroxide paste, available in a syringe with disposable needles, may be applied with equal effectiveness. It is important to inform the patient of the perforation and potential complications.

Perforations can be successfully avoided and pin-channels correctly positioned by paralleling the twist drill with the adjacent root surface so that a medial orientation is maintained. One author, commenting on pin placement within dentin, suggested that the recommended thickness surrounding the pin be three times the pin hole diameter.[25] A general and more widely held conviction is that the pin hole be approximately 1 mm from the dentino-enamel junction.[26] New or sharp-ended twist drills have repeatedly been shown to reduce dentin cracks during the channel preparation.

Each of the pin types has advantages and disadvantages. Two serious disadvantages of the self-threading pins exist in relation to this restoration procedure. As just mentioned, crazing and cracking can be produced by screwing the pin into sound dentin. This may or may not produce a clinically significant problem, but should be noted. Second, bending of these pins, if necessary, is almost impossible without splitting the tooth. For this latter reason, the cemented pin is advocated as the superior technique, since it allows greater versatility in pin design. Normally, a 0.025 inch diameter pin is seated into a properly positioned 0.027 inch diameter pin channel. The pin can then be removed, bent, and adjusted for length before cementation in order to provide the maximum retentive and splint-efficient position possible. Zinc phosphate cement is safely used at this time, since the tooth is pulpless. Delivery via lentula spiral either by hand or by slow speed contra-angle handpiece is most effective in achieving uniform cement distribution within the channel.

The preparation is ready to receive the filling after a 1 to 2 mm base of zinc phosphate cement is placed over the pulpal floor to ensure a reasonably level and secure base for the amalgam. Condensation is modified only by the use of small condensers to negotiate between pins and ensure uniform packing. The final restoration is then carved and checked for proper occlusion. It should also be noted that this technique provides an effective core, to be followed by a cast restoration. Reinforcement can be achieved by peripheral pin placement in addition to a prefabricated dowel extending from the canal into the body of the amalgam or composite core material. Regardless of the modifications or the type of final restoration selected, active interrelationship of remaining tooth structure, retentive core, and final restoration must be produced. Passive filling of the void created during endodontic therapy is inadequate.

Within the group of coronally retained restorations are cast materials that provide cuspal protection by the development of reverse bevels. These are most appropriate for the posterior dentition and include occlusal onlays, inlay/overlay restorations involving multiple surfaces, and modifications of the three-quarter–type crown. As required with all restoration selection, they are dependent upon firm support extending from a dentinal base. Any attempt to include a weak or unsupported cusp will ultimately end in fracture and failure caused by recurrent caries or, more likely, by the physical loss of bulk tooth structure away from the restoration.

The principal feature of overlay restoration is the bibevel occlusal preparation. In schematic form, every portion of the remaining coronal structure is beveled from its median dentin surface to course occlusally over a rounded corner, then reverses gingivally and ends on peripheral enamel. A line drawn from the apex of the bevel to its enamel termination forms a 1 to 2 mm surface that is continuous horizontally along all coronal margins (Fig. 11–21). There are several distinct benefits to justify the time and effort necessary to construct these restorations. Obviously the general contour and morphology of the crown are preserved, since the original crown form is more or less intact. A large percentage of the margins are supragingival, which makes for easier finishing by the dentist and more accessible hygiene for the patient. The increase of tissue acceptance when compared with full coronal coverage is also apparent. This restoration, however, should be considered only for the patient with good oral hygiene.

Modifications involving the different aspects of this restoration are left to the discretion of the clinician, but certain preparation designs are frequently overlooked. For example, both proximal surfaces of posterior teeth are routinely included in the restoration despite the lack of enamel defects or existing caries. Since the endodontically treated tooth is already weakened by the access cavity, a sound proximal surface should always be preserved when possible. The marginal ridge must, however, be protected

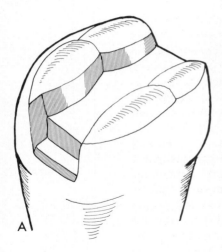

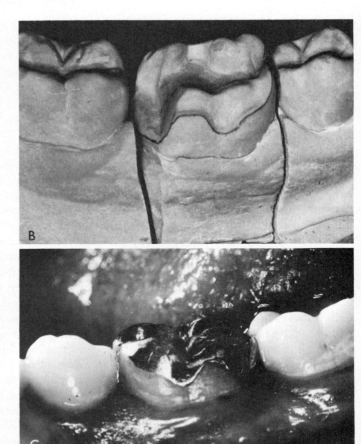

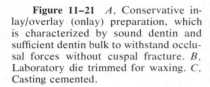

Figure 11–21 *A*, Conservative inlay/overlay (onlay) preparation, which is characterized by sound dentin and sufficient dentin bulk to withstand occlusal forces without cuspal fracture. *B*, Laboratory die trimmed for waxing. *C*, Casting cemented.

and therefore prepared to receive an adequate thickness of gold by troughing the ridge crest with a small round bur. This creates marginal bevels that extend toward, but not into, the contact area (Fig. 11–22).

Unfortunately, not many teeth requiring endodontic therapy have sufficient remaining structure to support this restoration type. When doubt exists as to the long-term success of the restoration, the full coronal restoration should be selected. It has been and will continue to be the restoration of choice following endodontic therapy.

Radicular Reinforced Restorations

The decision to include a post as part of the restorative process has been largely empirical in nature. No exact definition as to percentage of tooth loss or anticipated stress necessary to dictate dowel inclusion has been verified experimentally or clinically. It has been suggested that 25 per cent or more loss of the coronal tooth structure may require some form of artificial dentin augmentation.[27] The prudent choice is to use available root canal space when any doubt exists as to the ability of the final restoration to survive normal occlusion. It is rarely necessary to involve more than a single root of any tooth to provide adequate strength and retention for the restoration.

As previously discussed, the most appropriate time to create post room within the physical confines of the root canal is during intracranial preparation prior to filling. Regardless of the type of filling material or technique, the dowel space is cleared with greater ease if it is already prepared within the canal. This is most apparent when removing gutta percha with a heated instrument, since both size and depth are already known and the instrument can be trial inserted prior to any filling procedure.

Intraradicular Space Preparation for Dowel (Post) Room

The use of any portion of the tooth aside from the root canal to provide restorative retention or strength is poor clinical judgment. The root canals occupy the most median portion of the root and are surrounded by the

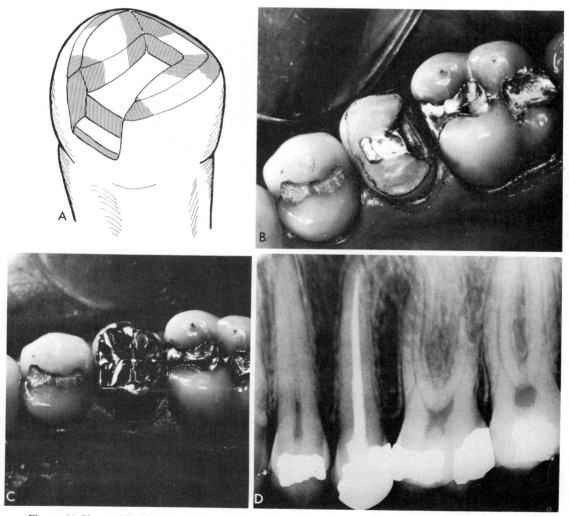

Figure 11–22 *A*, Modified premolar overlay preparation to conserve an intact proximal wall. *B*, Clinical preparation. *C*, Occlusal appearance of cemented casting. *D*, Final radiograph. (Courtesy of Dr. Anthony DeBello, Ocean Springs, Mississippi.)

greatest dentin width available. Even in multi-canal roots there is virtually no chance of failure if a few simple clinical principles are adhered to:

1. Most important is the knowledge of the morphology of the treated root, i.e., approximate width, developmental grooves, number and classification of canal systems, and so forth.

2. Routine utilization of roots that are straight and therefore more likely to accommodate dowel preparation without complication is necessary.

3. Any root has sufficient width to support at least a 0.80 mm (No. 80) dowel but should not exceed a 1.40 mm (No. 140) dowel.

4. At the fabrication stage incorporate the four dimensions of dowel restoration (see below).

Dimensions of Dowel Restoration

There are four dimensions of the canal preparation for a dowel and subsequently of the dowel itself, which correspond to the realities of normal root morphology and applied functional stress. Each dimension may create the opportunity for failure if done improperly. Therefore, it is important for the dentist to be aware of each of these requirements so that modification of one may be compensated by another. It is with particular amazement that we see on a daily basis an incredible array of poorly constructed post systems that have provided years of service. Our belief is, however, that the *ideal* restoration is easily attainable by adhering to a few simple guidelines based on anatomic form. The four dimensions are length, diameter or width, taper, and direction (Fig. 11–23).

Length. The minimum length of the dowel has been suggested as a ratio equaling 1 to 1 or preferably 1 to 1.5 the length of the restored clinical crown (Fig. 11–24). This dimension is variable, depending upon the length of available root, occlusion considerations, and alveolar bone support.[28] Current research indicates that displacement resistance to tensile force applied to a cemented post remains static between 7 and 9 mm but increases 24 to 30 per cent when lengthened to 11 mm.[29] This length is consistent with some crown and root lengths and can be clinically achieved when measured from the most coronal aspect of the cervical line. However, most authorities suggest that a minimum of 5 mm of filling material be left in the apical root canal to ensure the integrity of the endodontic filling. This condition must be met before post length is determined. In certain instances of anatomically, pathologically, surgically, or orthodontically shortened roots, this may be carefully reduced to 3 mm.

Diameter. The diameter or width of the dowel must duplicate in

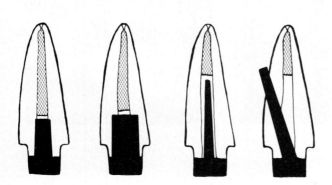

Figure 11–23 The complications relating to the four dimensions of canal preparation to receive a core and dowel: length, width, taper, and direction.

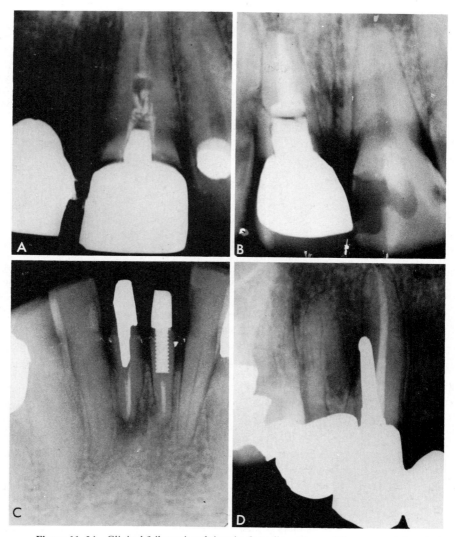

Figure 11–24 Clinical failures involving the four dimensions of the core and dowel. *A*, Length: insufficient retention. *B*, Width: weakened tooth structure. *C*, Taper: morphologic intolerance (lateral perforation). *D*, Direction: vertical axis deflection (axial perforation).

miniature the gross morphology of the root. Several roots are capable of accepting practically any available standardized dowel size. The largest is approximately a No. 140 root canal instrument equaling 1.40 mm at its tip (D_1) and 1.70 mm at the end of its 16.0 mm shaft end (D_2). Such roots are found in maxillary central incisors and palatal roots of maxillary molars. Roots of lesser bulk are weakened when enlarged significantly beyond the normal size of the canal seen during adolescence and are subject to failure dependent upon the tensile, compressive, and shearing forces involved. One study suggested that no statistical difference exists between the retentive ability of a No. 60 or No. 70 dowel diameter.[30] This should not be surprising, since the difference in size is less than a 15 per cent increase. However, a similar study comparing the retentive resistance of No. 80 and No. 120 dowel diameters indicated a 24 per cent increase in retention.[28] As a general

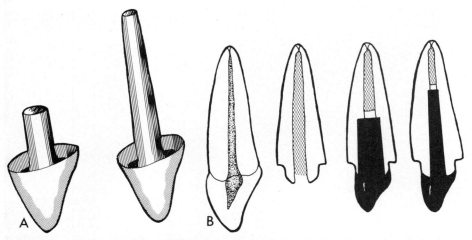

Figure 11–25 *A,* Diagrammatic illustration of two dowels with the same square surface area contact. The long and wide dowel provides neither the strength nor the retention of its correct counterpart. In fact, weakening of the tooth and increased susceptibility to fracture often occur owing to this poor design. *B,* The retentive factor is increased as a function of width or diameter. The longer, tapered post is more anatomically correct.

rule, a root canal should not be enlarged beyond 1.4 mm, since larger diameters tend to gut and weaken the root. At the minimum extreme, the dowel should not be less than 0.8 mm, since there must be sufficient inherent strength within the metal to withstand sustained forces (Fig. 11–25).

Taper. This is the dimension that generates the most heated debate between the restorative dentist and the endodontist. As noted in the opening paragraphs, the improper restoration of a pulpless tooth is frequently worse than no restoration at all. Over the years, endodontists have progressed from making no dowel space for the generalist to routinely providing it in an attempt to reduce the irreparable damage from rotary instruments used within the canal for removing filling material. Some specialists have even included the actual fabrication of the core and dowel as part of the endodontic service for the patient in order to avoid future root weakening restorative procedures.

The classic endodontic texts suggest the routine use of tapered posts. This is correctly justified by two morphologic realities that transcend the pure physics and mechanics of structural design. First, *all* roots are more or less tapered. Any dowel preparation that invades the root canal space and is of a parallel design may significantly weaken the lateral walls and predispose them to horizontal fracture. This is, of course, not absolutely true for all teeth since some roots approach roundness in cross-section and easily accommodate a moderate parallel post. Others, however, are ovoid, having a wide facial-lingual dimension but a narrow mesio-distal dimension (Table 11–1).[9]

Second, and most hazardous, is the presence of proximal developmental grooves or concavities (see Fig. 11–24). Mandibular incisors are notoriously hourglass-shaped when viewed in cross-section. The use of a parallel post in a root with this gross morphology is anatomically unsafe, since lateral perforation commonly occurs and extraction is the only possible remedy (see Fig. 11–33). A review of the literature shows that most endodontists prefer the tapered preparation, since it rarely creates perforation or fracture problems.[31] Prosthodontists, on the other hand, have presented an undeniable body of evidence that the resistance of a post to displace-

TABLE 11–1 Suggested Dowel Size*

Teeth	Indicated Size	Optimal Dowel Size
Maxillary teeth		
Central incisor	90 to 140	110
Lateral	70 to 100	90
Canine	80 to 120	100
First premolar		
Buccal root	70 to 120	90
Lingual root	70 to 110	90
Second premolar	70 to 110	90
First molar		
Palatal root	80 to 120	100
Mesio-buccal root	70 to 100	90
Disto-buccal root	70 to 100	80
Mandibular teeth		
Central	70 to 80	70†
Lateral	70 to 80	70†
Canine	80 to 120	100
First premolar	70 to 100	90
Second premolar	70 to 120	90
First molar		
Distal root	70 to 100	90
Mesio-buccal root	70 to 100	90
Mesio-lingual root	70 to 100	80

*From Tilk, M. A., Lommel, T. J., and Gerstein, H.: J. Endo. 5:81, 1979.
†Endopost.

ment or failure from lack of strength is best provided by the parallel design.[30] All these studies appear sound in their experimental design and statistical analysis.

Under the heading of taper we must include two other major dowel designs. These dowels are of the parallel form and are either threaded or serrated (cylindrical). Common sense impressions were statistically verified in studies in which the tapped threaded post provided greater retention than the serrated post. The former failed because of dentin fracture, whereas the latter failed at the cement margin nearest the dentin wall. These in vitro studies, unfortunately, have not addressed the in vivo consequences of their conclusions. How can data concerned with straight constant vector forces not encountered in the normal occlusion be of benefit in the application of our restorative procedures? It is our firm belief that the well-designed and properly constructed tapered post will sustain any functional stress and is the endodontic restoration of choice. The judgment of the clinician as to the efficacy of the parallel post must be relied upon after considering root shape.

Direction. Errors, modifications, and cumulative problems encountered in the previous dimensions of dowel construction do not equal the devastating effect of failure to maintain proper vertical axis when making post room (see Fig. 11–24). The irreversible damage caused by a lateral perforation is unjustifiable, since almost all such perforations are the result of the use of rotary instruments in the root canal. Many clinicians believe that removal of gutta percha by following shreds of the material is 100 per cent successful. Innumerable extracted teeth are mute testimony to this dubious claim. Peeso reamers, Gates-Glidden burs, Para-post drills, and so on, all have the potential of being deflected by any root canal filling. This is especially true of gutta percha, since it, too, becomes hard and brittle with time. A rotary instrument, if it must be used, should be within the canal only after initial canal clearance by hand instruments. This lessens the possibility of perforation and bur separation. A perforation rate greater than zero cannot and should not be a part of any reconstructive procedure.

The primary dowel requirement is to provide retention and strength to the overall restoration. Retention is a function of square surface area contact, both amount and intimacy. Resistance to fracture is also dependent upon contact, but the dowel must also have the approximate form of the gross morphology of the root. Weakening of the root occurs when inadequate length is compensated by increased width (see Fig. 11–25).

Technique for Dowel Space Preparation

Although new endodontic filling materials have been recently introduced and others are certain to be formulated, gutta percha in its various methods of application (lateral condensation, warm, thermoplastic, chloropercha, vertical condensation, and so forth) dominates as the material of choice. Partial removal from the canal without disruption of the periapical filling is of critical importance. The time of removal may or may not be significant, but since most sealers used with gutta percha have a defined setting period, it would seem that a failure of the sealer interfaces (sealer to gutta percha and sealer to dentin) would be least likely to occur prior to final set. For this reason, whenever possible, we suggest that dowel space be prepared at the canal obliteration appointment. Gutta percha removal done subsequently must be approached more cautiously, since the probability of seal damage increases after setting. If any doubt exists as to the integrity of the apical segment, it should always be replaced, since dowel placement effectively eliminates the possibility of conservative re-treatment.

The length of the entire remaining tooth is determined by previous treatment records or is estimated radiographically (Fig. 11–26). This reinforces the proposal that post room be physically created within the canal prior to filling and recorded in the treatment record. Freshly placed gutta percha is extremely heat sensitive and yields to a soft mass when in contact with a heated instrument. It becomes pliable at 25 to 30°C, becomes a soft mass at 60°C, and melts at 100°C. Several brands and designs of straight plugger type instruments are suitable for this procedure. With a silicone stop placed a minimum of 5 mm short of the apical filling, the instrument tip is heated cherry red in a flame and immediately transferred to the root canal orifice. An apical push forward 2 to 3 mm and then immediate removal allow a clean separation of the coronal one third of gutta percha from the main core. The softened gutta percha generally adheres to the plugger. If the plugger is pushed into the gutta percha mass and allowed to cool in place for more than a few seconds, removal of the entire filling may result. The plugger is now wiped clean, reheated, and another segment of filling removed. This is repeated until the desired length has been achieved. Any attempt to remove too much gutta percha at one time may result in the complete removal of the canal filling. This occurs very infrequently and usually indicates inadequate gutta percha condensation. The root canal space can now be safely enlarged with hand instruments (or rotary instruments in competent hands) to receive the selected post.

Gutta percha has a shelf life of approximately 18 months at room temperature before it exhibits brittleness (aging) and breaks under force.

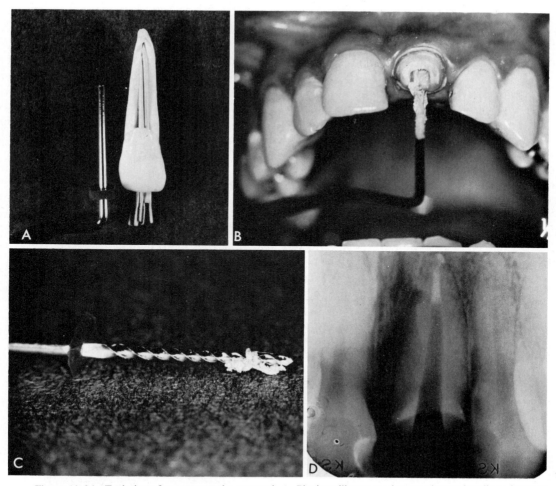

Figure 11–26 Technique for gutta percha removal. *A*, Placing silicone marker on plugger handle to leave at least 5.0 mm of apical filling. *B*, Removal of gutta percha by heated instrument. *C*, Stray gutta percha from canal irregularities removed by file. *D*, Properly prepared canal to receive core and dowel.

This aging also occurs in the root canal, and with additional time the material becomes less susceptible to applied heat. It is now thought that aging is actually a transformation of gutta percha to a more highly crystalline form.[32] Removal, as mentioned previously, must be performed cautiously. The recommended technique at this later time involves the use of hydrocarbons such as chloroform. This liquid can be slowly deposited by means of a disposable syringe into the pulp chamber until flooding occurs. A small reamer or file that does not easily bend (No. 20 or 25) is then started into the gutta percha for 1 or 2 mm as a probe. It should then be withdrawn, wiped clean, and inserted back into the gutta percha mass. The dissolving effect of the chloroform will soften the material so that it can be easily removed to the desired length. If any doubt exists concerning the remaining apical filling, the entire mass should be removed immediately and the root canal retreated.

It is assumed without further mention that all the above procedures are done with the rubber dam in place. There is *no* defense, technical or legal, after a patient swallows or aspirates any material, whether solid or liquid.

Temporary Restorations

Temporary restorations pose peculiar problems during endodontic therapy. Although required to satisfy either a cosmetic need in the anterior segment or a protective function in the posterior dentition, at no time must the interappointment seal be jeopardized prior to root canal filling. Posteriorly, rapid gross occlusal reduction renders the tooth less likely to fracture by eliminating functional contacts with little esthetic compromise. Generalized instructions to the patient to avoid the side involved and slight diet adjustment are usually sufficient to maintain the temporary restoration intact.

The anterior teeth provide a special complication because of our youth and beauty conscious society. Even the suggestion of leaving the office *without* an anterior crown is unacceptable to most patients. The key factor is the maintenance of the coronal seal. In routine lingual access cavities, no problem exists. However, when an existing crown is displaced or fractured (i.e., P.J.C.), it can be replaced by one of the polycarbonate forms if the access seal is first placed independently of crown cementation and sufficient coronal structure remains for retention. This will guard against seal breakage if the crown is lost again.

When little coronal structure is present, either no crown should be placed or a treatment partial denture (i.e., flipper) should be fabricated to cover the gingivally flattened crown (Fig. 11–27). Using the root canal for retaining a dowel- or pin-constructed temporary crown often leads to contamination and is never recommended, even at the strongest insistence of the patient. Gross microorganismal contamination of the root canal from

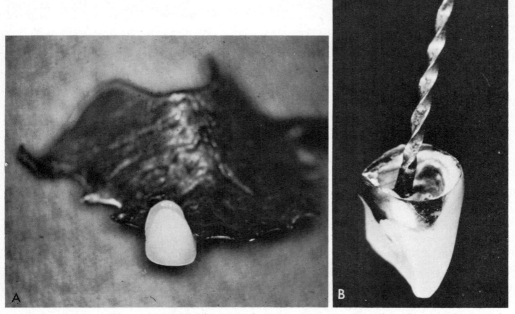

Figure 11–27 *A*, The recommended inter-appointment temporary restoration of an anterior tooth is the use of a treatment partial denture. At no time should the canal be utilized for crown retention until the apical foramen has been sealed. *B*, The use of a file to retain a pre-existing veneer crown after root filling.

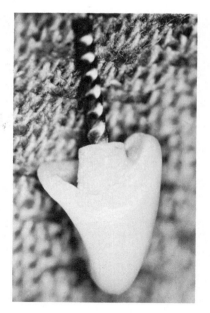

Figure 11–28 Recommended temporary crown fabricated after root canal therapy has been completed.

the oral cavity can lead to acute exacerbation, periapical infection, or ultimate failure of the endodontic therapy. This principle can never be compromised.

Once the root canal is filled, an excellent temporary crown may be made after post room is present. The largest file used in the canal to dowel length is cut so that 4 to 5 mm of the shaft extends from the canal orifice. Incisal clearance must be checked. After the separated file is removed from the canal, a polycarbonate temporary crown is selected for size and contoured both incisally and gingivally to replace all missing tooth structure for cosmetic purposes. With the file segment replaced in the canal, the crown is replaced to check for internal clearance of the file. When this is achieved, a regular mix of self-curing acrylic is spatulated into the crown and placed over the tooth and protruding file. The soft acrylic will fill the canal orifice and make an impression of the remaining coronal tooth structure. It is allowed to set, with removal tested several times before final curing so that undetected undercuts do not prevent removal. After trimming and polishing, the post crown is cemented with a mix of calcium hydroxide cement (Dycal, Hydrex) so that removal will be uncomplicated (Fig. 11–28).

Dowel Techniques

Four broad classifications of dowel types are presently utilized: base metal screw posts, cylindrical parallel posts, semiprecious metal pre-cast posts, and the custom precious metal cast posts.

The (self-threading) screw posts are broad threaded and tapered and resemble a sheet metal screw (Fig. 11–29). They are available in various sizes and lengths and rely principally on physical scoring of the dentin for retention, but may be assisted by cements. Two serious problems exist with this system. First, there is no correlation with the standardization of endodontic instruments. Thus the selection of the post is largely by trial and

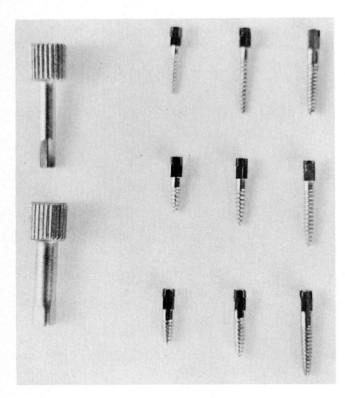

Figure 11–29 Screw posts and handles necessary for insertion.

error, which unfortunately results in inadequate adaptation to the canal space (Fig. 11–30). Second, the tendency to turn the post more than the suggested one quarter to one half rotation after dentin has been engaged is too great a temptation for many clinicians. Depending upon the amount of circumferential surface contact between post and dentin, splitting of the root can easily occur (Fig. 11–31).

The most common predictable fracture occurs when the post is screwed directly into gutta percha. Tremendous hydraulic-like pressure is created within the canal, since the material is laterally displaced by penetration of the post. Since gutta percha is not compressible, a well-filled root will

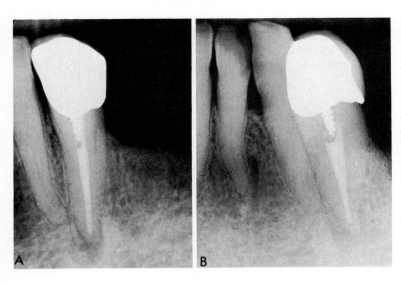

Figure 11–30 Screw post placed within root canal appears to fit canal well in straight-on radiograph *(A)*; whereas angle radiograph *(B)* shows poor adaptation of post to canal.

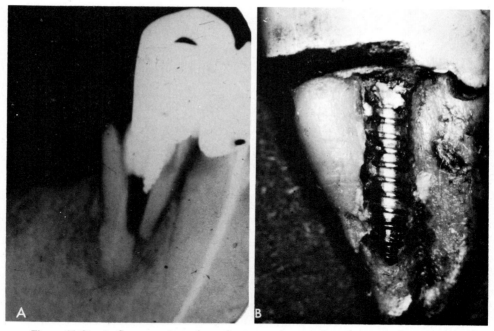

Figure 11–31 *A*, Screw post causing a fracture and separation of root. *B*, Screw post exiting through distal surface of a mandibular molar root.

succumb to fracture regardless of the thickness of the root or the lack of dehydration.

Cylindrical parallel posts are now widely used (Fig. 11–32). The canal space is created by a long shank drill that is slightly larger than the post. Again, it is important to reiterate our conviction that a rotary instrument

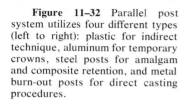

Figure 11–32 Parallel post system utilizes four different types (left to right): plastic for indirect technique, aluminum for temporary crowns, steel posts for amalgam and composite retention, and metal burn-out posts for direct casting procedures.

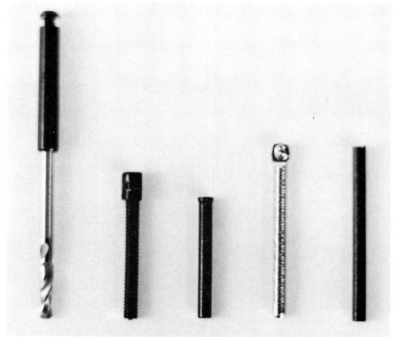

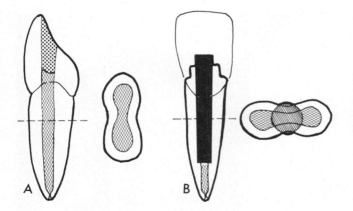

Figure 11–33 Morphologic intolerance of radicular structures to receive a post. *A*, Typical hour-glass root configuration common to ovoid roots (horizontal section). *B*, Placement of nontapered post. Radiographically, this post would appear to be within the lateral perimeters of the root (see Fig. 11–24*C*).

should *not* be used to remove gutta percha because of the risk of perforation. If the canal is cleared to the necessary length before using the drill, the possibility of lateral deflection is significantly reduced. The dowel is principally retained by cement. The fundamental clinical problem inherent in its use is placement into roots not morphologically capable of accommodating this shape. Lateral perforation is common in roots with moderate to deep proximal developmental grooves (Fig. 11–33) after post preparation with a rotary instrument (Fig. 11–34).

Both the screw post and parallel post are used to retain coronal self-hardening materials such as amalgam and composite via their coronal extension out of the canal orifice. The irregular coronal ends aid in retention, as do the serrations or threads along the shaft of these posts. A composite of both these posts is the Kueur type. This parallel threaded and dentinally tapped post is screwed into the dentin of the root canal. Its coronal end is large and replaces much of the lost tooth structure, but realistically its use is appropriate only for single rooted anterior teeth.

If we wish to achieve our structural goal of coronal protection and radicular stabilization, neither of the above systems is adequate. Although they do provide sufficient retention of the core material, they do not impart any coronal-radicular protection from the relationship of core to dowel or resist-

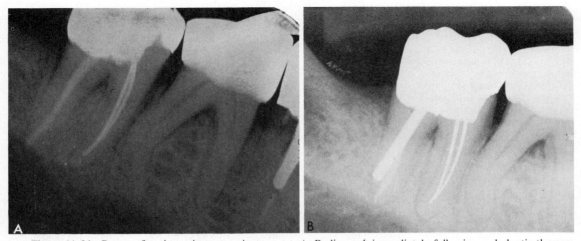

Figure 11–34 Post perforation using rotary instrument. *A*, Radiograph immediately following endodontic therapy. *B*, Post preparation and gutta percha removal by rotary drill, resulting in perforation.

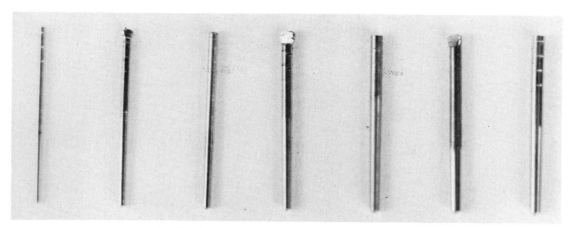

Figure 11–35 Standardized pre-cast posts of regular and high fusing metals.

ance to shearing forces, if these are present. All coronal protection must be developed by the subsequent placement of a crown with margins extending onto radicular dentin. The primary difference between screw and cylindrical posts, when compared with pre-cast and custom posts, is that the former require extensive canal modification to accommodate the post, whereas the latter rely on the post's fitting the existing canal — a very significant factor having great morphologic and clinical ramifications.

Semiprecious pre-cast posts are standardized metrically from sizes 0.70 mm (No. 70) to 1.40 mm (No. 140) having the D_1 to D_2 dimensions of root canal instruments. They are designed principally for a cast-to-dowel technique, which is compatible with gold. Two metal types, first introduced in 1964,[28] are available: *regular* for use with regular casting golds and *high fusing* (high-platinum gold) for use in porcelain fused to metal restorations (Fig. 11–35). These posts are reported to have two to four times the tensile strength of a cast post. A significant advantage of their use is the rigid aspect of the dowel to the root canal space during core fabrication for accurate alignment and easy insertion.

The last dowel type is the custom precious metal cast post. These provide the most accurate relationship of dowel surface to canal walls in the majority of teeth. Standardized color-coded dowels made of plastic were developed by Kahn and Gerstein so that the post-core restoration could be cast in a single metal.[33] Available in sizes No. 80 to 140, the dowels can be used in either direct or indirect methods (Fig. 11–36).

The direct method, using either wax, acrylic resin, or a combination of both, faithfully reproduces the internal anatomy of the root canal. This technique requires removal of all undercuts within the canal. Since the posts are plastic, resin bonds directly by monomer contact, whereas small wedges cut into the posts are necessary to retain wax. Application of either material by an add-on technique reproduces the irregularity of the canal.

The core itself may be built-up in the identical build-up process or by a new technique developed by Kahn utilizing a "core-form,"[34] which consists of thin, transparent polyeythylene in general shapes and sizes of the core. The core is filled with wax or resin, placed over the dowel until set, and then removed and trimmed (Fig. 11–37). When the core is completed by either method, the plastic post acts as the sprue so that only the casting procedure can be responsible for a noninsertable restoration (Fig. 11–38).

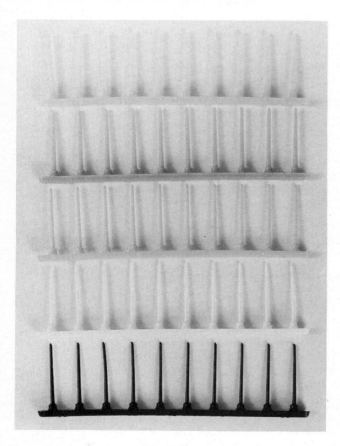

Figure 11-36 Plastic tapered posts available in standardized sizes and colors from 80 to 140 instrument numbers.

The core must be of a specific design and not merely a mass of solid substance replacing coronal structures (Fig. 11–39). It should provide extracoronal protection by a coping-like design that surrounds and overlies the remaining dentin (Fig. 11–40). In this way, the core and dowel become an integral part of the tooth and root canal system. Weine suggests groove placement in round canals to prevent rotation and to aid in proper insertion as a keyway. A square-sided well, 1 to 2 mm deep, directly over the canal orifice may also be used as a lock. Regardless of the root (internal core) preparation design, it must allow for easy placement. Failure to adequately seat the casting results in poor internal approximation of the dowel and

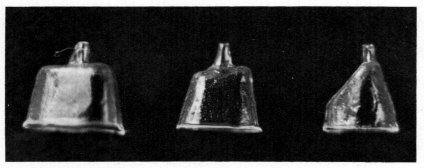

Figure 11-37 "Core form" kit with necessary polyethylene core sizes to simplify construction of the core and dowel using the direct technique.

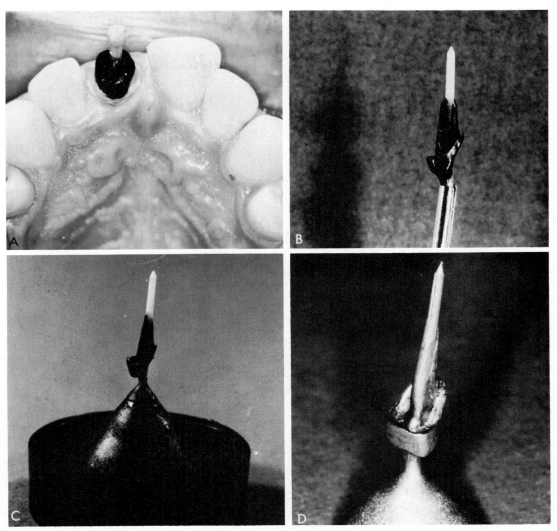

Figure 11–38   Direct core and dowel fabrication. *A*, Direct pattern made of either inlay wax or acrylic resin. *B*, Completed direct pattern reproduces root canal asymmetry. *C*, Plastic post acts as sprue pin. *D*, Completed casting.

subsequent failure due to excessive cement thickness, easy displacement of the post, and increased likelihood of root fractures from fulcrum movement within the canal (Fig. 11–41).

The indirect method is best performed using a dense impression material such as rubber base. The post must be painted with adhesive for retention in the impression. Before inserting the post, some material should be injected into the orifice and then the post forced through it down the canal. This causes flow and displacement into irregularities and complete canal preparation reproduction. After removal, the usual method of die preparation is modified only to accommodate the dowel length. The finished core and dowel can then be cemented in place after casting and trial insertion. Venting, thickness of cement, insertion pressure, and speed are all details of clinical experience and judgment.

Our belief that this system is clearly superior to contemporary techniques is based upon our knowledge of the roots and canal systems present

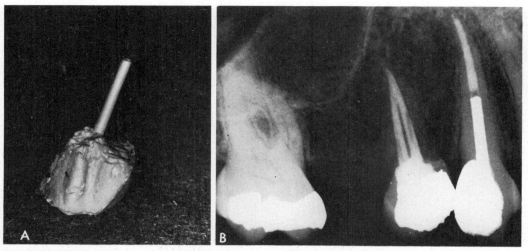

Figure 11–39 *A*, Core and dowel integrated as a final restoration. *B*, Casting provides no protection for remaining coronal structures and increases the possibility of radicular fracture.

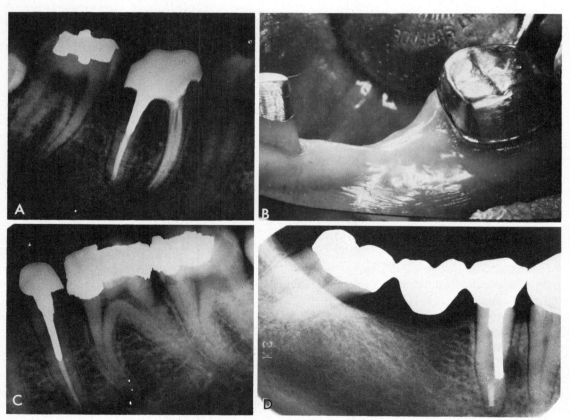

Figure 11–40 Core requirements. *A*, Radiograph of mandibular molar after receiving a core and dowel. Note positive seat provided by the pulpal floor and bevel effect created by casting. *B*, Mandibular molar and premolar with core and dowels. Sufficient dentin remained to support simple core for premolar. Inadequate coronal dentin necessitated coping-type core to completely surround the radicular structures. *C*, A groove or well acts as both a key way to aid insertion and a positive seat to insure complete placement of the casting. *D*, Improper seating of adequate dowel resulted in fulcrum movement and fracture of the root.

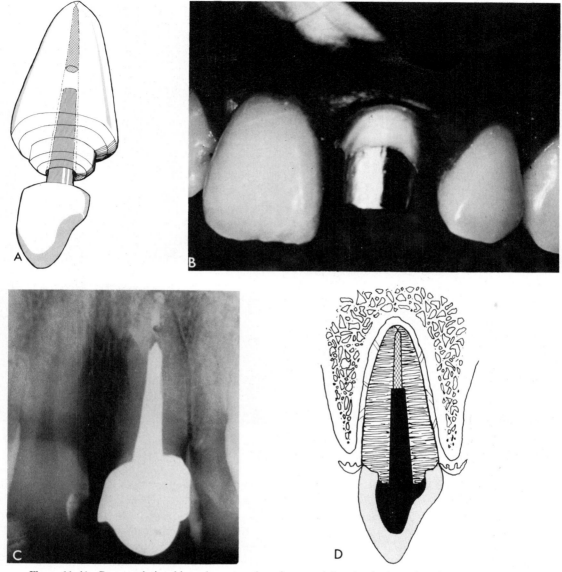

Figure 11–41 Proper relationship and construction of core and dowel to both tooth and cast crown. Post system provides intracanal retention and extracoronal protection, while cast crown unites all components into an integral unit. *A*, Proper construction for cast core and dowel. *B*, Coronal preparation. *C*, Radiograph of final restoration. *D*, Diagrammatic illustration of individual reconstructive components.

in most teeth. We do not argue that better experimental retention or tensile strength is created by other systems, but that these systems are also more conducive to complications. Although more time consuming than the others, this procedure can be virtually 100 per cent successful. We believe this not to be overstated, since no chance for perforation exists and the intimate relationship of the dowel to the true configuration of the root canal provides excellent retention and strength.

Finally, the properly designed core and dowel consists of a dowel that satisfies the requirements of length, width, taper, and direction to provide intraradicular retention for the core that imparts extracoronal protection.

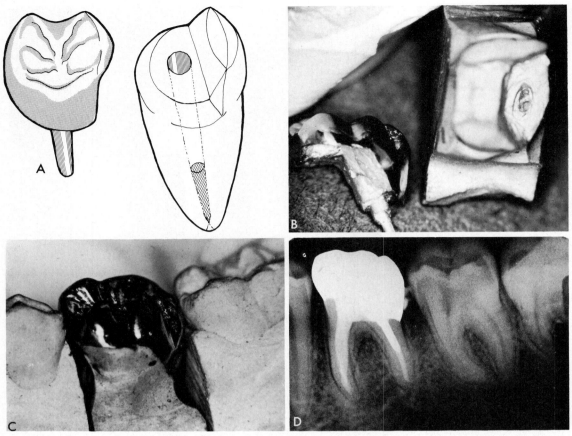

Figure 11–42 Single unit internal-external casting modified: *A,* Three-quarter type crown with retention assisted by the post. *B,* Casting and die separated. *C,* Casting and die. *D,* Radiograph of cemented restoration.

The placement of a crown is a final reinforcement that unites the tooth with the core and dowel as a single integral unit (see Fig. 11–41).

Some textbooks suggest the construction of a Richmond-type crown. This consists of a single gold casting in which the core and dowel and crown are one unit. Although technically and clinically possible (Fig. 11–42), the fabrication deformities associated with expansion and contraction of the materials make internal and external adaptation very difficult. This restoration is not recommended for routine use.

Many restorations and techniques have been omitted in this chapter. Some do not merit our consideration, whereas others require an exemplary level of clinical sophistication. Regardless of the restoration selected for the endodontically treated tooth, it must provide for the functional integrity of the remaining coronal and radicular structures. In the final analysis, the clinical success of the pulpless tooth is often significantly more dependent upon the quality of its restoration than the quality of the root canal therapy performed.

Acknowledgments

To Mary, my daughters, and Pete, who gave up another summer and accept that we will "do it next quarter." Special thanks to James Cockerill, photographer and assistant, for his dedication and time to this project.

REFERENCES

1. Ingle, J. I., and Beveridge, E. E.: Endodontics, 2nd ed. Philadelphia, Lea & Febiger, 1976, pp. 773–796.
2. Weine, F. S.: Endodontic Therapy, 2nd ed. St. Louis, The C. V. Mosby Company, 1976, pp. 444–475.
3. Cohen, S., and Burns, R. C.: Pathways of the Pulp. St. Louis, The C. V. Mosby Company, 1976, pp. 537–575.
4. Helfer, A. R., Melnick, S., and Schilder, H.: Determination of the moisture content of vital and pulpless teeth. Oral Surg. 34:661, October 1972.
5. Simon, J. H., Kelly, W. H., Gordon, G. G., and Erickson, G. W.: Extrusion of endodontically treated teeth. JADA 29:17, July 1978.
6. Cohen, S., and Burn, R. C.: Pathways of the Pulp. St. Louis, The C. V. Mosby Company, 1976, p. 539.
7. Pokorny, D. K.: Current procedures in fixed prosthodontics. Dent. Clin. North Am. 15:693, July 1971.
8. Kraus, B. S., Jordan, R. E., and Abrams, L.: Dental Anatomy and Occlusion. Baltimore, Williams & Wilkins, 1969, pp. 234–235.
9. Tilk, M. A., Lommel, T. J., and Gerstein, H.: A study of mandibular and maxillary root widths to determine dowel size. J. Endo. 5:79, March, 1979.
10. Weine, F. S.: Endodontic Therapy, 2nd ed. St. Louis, The C. V. Mosby Company, 1976, pp. 152–262.
11. Gerstein, H., and Evanson, L.: Precision posts or dowels. Ill. Dent. J. 32:70, February 1963.
12. Grossman, L. I.: Endodontic Practice, 7th ed. Philadelphia, Lea & Febiger, 1970, pp. 331–332.
13. Waliszewski, K. J., and Sabala, G. L.: Combined endodontic and restorative treatment considerations. J. Prosthet. Dent. 40:155, August 1978.
14. Guzy, G. E., and Nichols, J. I.: In vitro comparison of intact endodontically treated teeth with and without endo-post reinforcement. J. Prosthet. Dent. 42:43, July 1979.
15. Lovdahl, P. E., and Nicholls, J. I.: Pin-retained cores vs. cast-gold dowel-cores. J. Prosthet. Dent. 38:507, November 1977.
16. Brown, D. R., Barkmeir, W. W., and Anderson, R. W.: Restoration of endodontically treated posterior teeth with amalgam. J. Prosthet. Dent. 41:40, January 1979.
17. Going, R. E.: Pin-retained amalgam. JADA 73:619, September 1966.
18. Goldstein, P. M.: Retention pins are friction-locked without use of cement. JADA 73:1103, November 1966.
19. Markley, M. R.: Pin reinforcement and retention of amalgam foundations and restorations. JADA 56:675, May 1958.
20. Moffa, J. P., Razzano, M. R., and Doyle, M. G.: Pins — a comparison of their retentive properties. JADA 78:529, March 1969.
21. Boyde, A., and Lester, K. S.: Scanning electron microscopy of self-threading pins in dentine. Oper. Dent. 4:56, Spring 1979.
22. Collard, E. W., Caputo, A. A., and Standlee, J. P.: Rationale for pin-retained amalgam restorations. Dent. Clin. North. Am. 14:43, 1970.
23. Chan, K. C., Svare, C. W., Williams, R. H., and Khowassah, M. A.: Comparison of the retentive property and dentinal crazing ability of retention pins and machinist's taps. J. Dent. Res. 53:1425, 1974.
24. Markley, M. R.: Pin retained and reinforced restorations and foundations. Dent. Clin. North Am. 11:229, 1967.
25. Gourley, J.: Favorable location for pins in molars. Oper. Dent. 5:2, Winter 1980.
26. Courtade, G. L.: Pin pointers. III. Self-threading pins. J. Prosthet. Dent. 20:335, October 1968.
27. Johnson, J. K., Schwartz, N. L., and Blackwell, R. T.: Evaluation and restoration of endodontically treated posterior teeth. JADA 93:597, September 1976.
28. Gerstein, H., and Burnell, S. C.: Prefabricated precision dowels. JADA 68:787, June 1964.
29. Johnson, J. K., and Sakumura, J. S.: Dowel form and tensile strength. J. Prosthet. Dent. 40:645, December 1978.
30. Standlee, J. P., Caputo, A. A., and Hanson, E. C.: Retention of endodontic dowels: Effects of cement, dowel length, diameter and design. J. Prosthet. Dent. 40:152, April 1978.
31. Gutmann, J. L.: Preparation of endodontically treated teeth to receive a post-core restoration. J. Prosthet. Dent. 38:413, October 1977.
32. Sorin, S. M., Oliet, S., and Pearlstein, F.: Rejuvenation of aged (brittle) endodontic gutta-percha cones. J. Endo. 5:233, August 1979.
33. Weine, F. S., Kahn, H., Wax, A. H., and Taylor, G. N.: The use of standardized tapered plastic pins in post and core fabrications. J. Prosthet. Dent. 29:542, May 1973.
34. Kahn, H., Fishman, I., and Malone, W. F.: A simplified method for constructing a core following endodontic treatment. J. Prosthet. Dent. 37:32, January 1977.

INDEX

Numbers in *italics* indicate illustrations; those followed by (t) indicate tables.